The Story of Nursing in Briti[sh] Mental Hospitals

From their beginnings as the asylum attendants of the nineteenth century, mental health nurses have come a long way. This is the first comprehensive history of mental health nursing in Britain in over twenty years, and during this period the landscape has transformed as the large institutions have been replaced by services in the community. McCrae and Nolan examine how the role of mental health nursing has evolved in a social and professional context, brought to life by an abundance of anecdotal accounts.

The nine chronologically ordered chapters follow the development from untrained attendants in the pauper lunatic asylums to the professionally qualified nurses of the twentieth century, and, finally, consider the rundown and closure of the mental hospitals from nurses' perspectives. Throughout, the argument is made that while the training, organisation and environment of mental health nursing has changed, the aim has remained essentially the same: to nurture a therapeutic relationship with people in distress.

McCrae and Nolan look forward as well as back, and highlight significant messages for the future of mental health care. For mental health nursing to be meaningfully directed, we must first understand the place from which this field has developed. This scholarly but accessible book is aimed at anyone with an interest in mental health or social history, and will also act as a useful resource for policy-makers, managers and mental health workers.

Niall McCrae is a lecturer in mental health nursing at Florence Nightingale Faculty of Nursing & Midwifery, King's College London. As well as the history of mental health care, his research interests include the therapeutic role of the nurse, and evaluation of training and treatment innovations in psychiatric services. His previous book, *The Moon and Madness*, examining the legendary notion of lunar influence on behaviour, featured on the BBC radio series, *All in the Mind*.

Peter Nolan has worked for over fifty years in various capacities within mental health services, both in the UK and abroad. The focus of much of his research has been on how service users make sense of mental health services and the degree of understanding they bring to what is being provided. Though now retired, he continues to write about how and whether people with mental health problems benefit from interventions, how nurses interpret what they do and the likely changes that services will undergo in the future. He has a long-term interest in the evolution of psychiatric ideas and practices and the various factors that influence them. This book, he believes, is important in enabling the voices of the predecessors of mental health nurses to be heard, voices that for too long have been silent.

Routledge Key Themes in Health and Society

The Story of Nursing in British Mental Hospitals

Echoes from the corridors

Niall McCrae and Peter Nolan

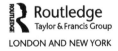
Routledge
Taylor & Francis Group

LONDON AND NEW YORK

First published 2016
by Routledge
2 Park Square, Milton Park, Abingdon, Oxon OX14 4RN

and by Routledge
711 Third Avenue, New York, NY 10017

First issued in paperback 2017

Routledge is an imprint of the Taylor & Francis Group, an informa business

British Library Cataloguing-in-Publication Data
A catalogue record for this book is available from the British Library

Library of Congress Cataloging-in-Publication Data
McCrae, Niall, author.
    The story of nursing in British mental hospitals : echoes from the
    corridors / Niall McCrae and Peter Nolan.
        p. ; cm. – (Routledge key themes in health and society)
    Includes bibliographical references and index.
    I. Nolan, Peter, 1942– , author. II. Title. III. Series: Routledge key
    themes in health and society.
    [DNLM: 1. Psychiatric Nursing – history – Great Britain.
    2. Deinstitutionalization – history – Great Britain. 3. History, 19th
    Century – Great Britain. 4. History, 20th Century – Great Britain.
    5. Hospitals, Psychiatric – history – Great Britain. WY 11 FA1]
    RC450.G7
    362.2'10941-dc23   2015034994

ISBN 13: 978-1-138-55682-9 (pbk)
ISBN 13: 978-0-415-73895-8 (hbk)

Typeset in Baskerville
by HWA Text and Data Management, London

'Niall McCrae and Peter Nolan have considerable expertise in the history of mental health services. The "readability" of their book is one of its most pleasing features and the authors have the skill of making the complex simple and fascinating. This book, while of interest to mental health nurses, should be required reading for all members of the multi-professional mental healthcare team. Entering the mental health professions today without knowing their histories would be like starting a journey without a map. This book is one of the best maps of the historical terrain that I have come across.'
– **Hugh McKenna**, *Professor, Pro-Vice Chancellor (Research and Innovation)*
University of Ulster, UK

'At last, due credit to nurses who devoted their careers to the vulnerable in an impoverished yet caring environment: good work was done.'
– **Jo Brand**, *comedian and former psychiatric nurse*

'A thought provoking and comprehensive history of mental health nursing based on a rich variety of sources, this is a detailed, far ranging and accessible overview. McCrae and Nolan have produced what should become the seminal work on the history of British mental health nursing.'
– **Claire Chatterton**, *Chair, RCN History of Nursing Society, UK*

Contents

Illustrations

Figures

Plates

Tables

Preface

History has, among its many purposes, that of exploring and explaining how the past has shaped the present. Closely aligned to this is assisting us to resolve the mystery of who we are.[1] In taking an active interest in our background, we come to appreciate that while we don't live in the past, the past lives in us.[2] A major benefit of history is in enabling us to understand our reality, and its limitations and possibilities. To become more aware of the dimensions of that reality is especially important when seeking to understand the lives of those who are marginalised, by social class, gender, culture or ethnicity, or anyone on the lowest rungs of a hierarchy. Those who ignore what the past has to teach us have a very restricted vision.

Although the discipline of history can be described in many ways, it should not be confused with nostalgia, rose-tinted reminiscence or mourning for the dead. It can, however, reveal the resourcefulness of the human spirit and inspire, and perhaps warn, the living. Studying history helps us to lament what should be lamented, to honour what should be honoured and to celebrate what should be celebrated.[3] 'Doing history' requires open minds and hearts and a refusal to allow others to predetermine the findings. Historians tend to be cautious in accepting the interpretations of other historians, regardless of the evidence they cite and what they claim to know. It is an endless quest for 'truth', a quest that can never fully be realised.[4] As well as being a continuous dialogue between the present and the past,[5] it is also our best means of challenging our taken-for-granted concepts of institutions and practices and of the assumptions that underpin them.[6]

Conscientious historians, committed to guarding the integrity of their discipline, strive to abide by methodological conventions. Careful selection of sources, objectivity of analysis and the formulation of valid conclusions are required to ensure a rigorous enquiry. Philosopher RG Collingwood saw history not as a luxurious indulgence to fill hours of leisure, but a means by which reason is maintained and the human mind acquires knowledge of itself.[7] For Collingwood, the study of history shows us not only what has been achieved in the past, but also the diverse potential of human beings. Understanding the motives that drove people to behave in certain ways expands our collective memory and enables us to appreciate how the political, economic and social values of the past have shaped the world that we inhabit today.[8] History is a job never done, because interpretations of the past are constantly being reconsidered in the light of new evidence and the formulation of new questions. As no authoritative truth exists for the past, revisionism is necessary and meaningful. Otherwise we would lose that sense of a human civilisation that is constantly evolving and never fixed.

While traditional approaches to history have tended to focus on the great and the good, revisionist historians have a much broader gaze; uppermost in their minds is their responsibility to ensure that some stories are not lost or deemed too unimportant to record.[9] Psychiatry has been criticised for over-emphasising certain aspects of its past while ignoring others, endorsing the observation that 'there is a history that remembers and a history that forgets'.[10] History of 'ordinary people' seeks an understanding of the lives of those who have been denied authorship and are consequently in danger of being forgotten, thus redressing that most final and brutal of life's inequalities: whether or not you are remembered in the pile of historical debris left to modernity.[11] Contrasting with traditional top-down approaches, history from below is largely the history of the disadvantaged. EP Thompson[12] posited four fundaments of social history:

1   History must be our collective conscience
2   It tells the stories of as many people and as many ways of being in the world, as it can reasonably do
3   It presents the complexity and context of human experiences in the past to the readership of the present
4   It is the engine of our collective social maturity

Until recently, the history of mental health services was largely presented as the history of psychiatry, written by psychiatrist-historians who depicted their predecessors as working inside a unified system of thought and practice that represented a benign progression towards the alleviation of human suffering. It was, in essence, a history from the perspective of doctors and in attempting to own the past, they were laying down their claim to the future. These medical authors were articulate, had access to a substantial corpus of primary data and found it relatively easy to publish their material. They had a vested interest in conveying a favourable image of institutions and of the influence that they exercised inside them. They monopolised credit for 'advances' in the care and treatment of the mentally ill, giving the impression that all progress was essentially *medical* progress. In taking this position, they did disservice to those who were closely involved in the day-to-day lives of patients, consigning their stories to a footnote in the history of psychiatry.[13]

Like researchers in other disciplines, historians are obliged to be scrupulously honest about their sources, transparent in their analyses and logical in the conclusions they draw from their data. Readers should be wary of any tendencies to resort to myth-mongering or peddling fantasised versions of the past.[14] Those who set out to paint a positive picture of psychiatric care and treatment were either deluding themselves or hoped to delude their readers, as many mental hospitals throughout the world were terrifying institutions in which people were subjected to extreme and unproven treatments, and where their rights and dignity were disregarded.[15] Berrios and Porter[16] concluded that the majority of the early histories of psychiatry were no more than poorly collated collections of opinions and conjecture, betraying an ignorance of historical method. As Healy[17] explains, conscious or unconscious distortions of the past have exaggerated the knowledge and skills of asylum doctors, inflated the effectiveness of treatments and ignored the contributions of other members of staff, consequently overlooking the inadequacies and abuse within the system. Cannadine[18] condemns the 'lazy approach to history' that accepts unquestioningly the conclusions of others and is satisfied with simplistic explanations. Change grabs our attention, but stability is ignored because it is taken for granted at the time, and it appears less interesting than the story of seminal events and innovations. However, the astute historian accepts nothing as read.[19] Indeed, such events and innovations may have had limited impact on the everyday reality of institutional life, and only years later are they honoured as historical milestones or turning points.

In recent decades there has been tremendous development in the history of psychiatry and mental health care, inspired by the likes of social historian Roy Porter. Launched in 1990, the *History of Psychiatry* journal is a rich resource of critical accounts of the evolution of psychiatric theory and practice, with a plethora of fresh insights Meanwhile, other mental health professions have been examining their past. This embryonic activity has not evolved in synchronicity due to disparities in availability of educational and research opportunities, accessibility of archival resources and whether the discipline has an interested readership. Early studies of the nursing in mental hospitals demonstrate the problems of naïve enquiry. In his book *The Waiting Room to Hell*, Cubbin[20] described conditions in Shelton Hospital (the former Shropshire asylum) in the 1950s, while admitting that his desire to tell the story outweighed his ability to do so. Such humility is admirable, and should be more widely acknowledged in the annals of psychiatry and its associated disciplines.

Since the closure of mental hospitals at the turn of the century, numerous books have been written on these defunct institutions. Many are flimsy in their sources and writing, but there are also some exemplars of scholarly but accessible accounts. Diana Gittins,[21] for example, applied sociological critique in her book on Severalls Hospital in Essex; while deservedly highlighting the exploits of medical superintendent Russell Barton, she also brought patients, nurses and other underlings to the fore. Nonetheless, despite their vital role, nurses remain marginalised not only in the history of mental health care, but also in the present multidisciplinary system. Boschma[22] attributes this to a lack of role clarity and a lack of robust history to underpin nurses' professional status. Disciplines with clearly demarcated boundaries are able to confine themselves to rewarding areas of work, leaving everything else to nurses, whose role in mental health care is consequently amorphous. Boschma suggests that if nurses felt more secure in their role, they could work as equal partners with other professions in improving mental health services, ensuring that theory and practice are informed by nursing experience. Professional confidence is necessary to challenge mediocrity and to shape new ways of working, and to nurture a professional culture that allows

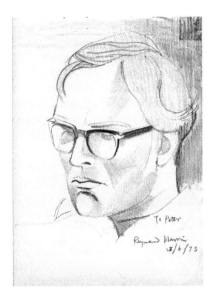

Figure 0.1 A portrait of Peter Nolan, drawn by a West Park patient in 1973

change to occur. Playing their part in expanding the therapeutic imagination is important in a climate in which nurses' humanistic values are trumped by financial targets and bureaucracy.[23]

Perhaps neglect of its history has contributed to the decline of mental health nursing in recent years.[24] Knowledge of professional background confers an understanding of how we got where we are, and where we may be heading, but nurses have tended to be dependent on others who purport to know more about it then we do ourselves. Mental health nurses are insufficiently assertive in drawing attention to the factors that are threatening their existence, such as poor recruitment, inadequate training, high levels of attrition among both students and qualified staff, and underfunding. Warelow and Edward[25] argue that current training and education of mental health nurses is culpably deficient in failing to transmit an identity with the history of the profession. Hence, they argue, historians of nursing have an important responsibility:

> To account for the endurance of traditions, understand the complex interplay between continuity and change and explain the origins, evolution and decline of institutions and ideas.[26]

Researching and writing this book has been a labour love for both authors. From our own professional practice, we appreciate how much valuable information and insight is lost when nurses with vast experience leave the profession, retire or die. We want to help nurses to examine their past and learn from it; to tell the stories of those who spent whole careers caring for people shunned by society. In the course of our research we have interviewed many ex-nurses whose perspectives were never previously sought or valued, in a process of triangulation with documentary records and published literature. Undoubtedly there are many stories still waiting to be told and our wish is that these should be heard before they disappear into the ether. However, we have guarded against selective portrayal, following the principle of EP Thompson that if history is comforting, it is not doing its job.

This book has four main objectives: to contribute to the growth of historical enquiry into mental health care in general and mental health nursing in particular; to examine the many and varied influences that have shaped the evolution of mental health care; to reveal hitherto unexplored material; and, finally, to assure mental health nurses of their rightful place in history.

Peter Nolan and Niall McCrae

July 2015

Notes

1   Carr EH (1990): *What is History?*
2   Phillips UB (1968): *The Slave Economy of the Old South.*
3   Schama S (2009): *A History of Britain (volume 1): At the Edge of the World.*
4   Popper K (1976): *Unended Quest: An Intellectual Autobiography.*
5   Carr EH (1990).
6   6 Porter R (1992, ed.): *Myths of the English.* London:
7   Harris EE (1957): Collingwood's theory of history. *Philosophical Quarterly.*
8   Thompson P (1978): *The Voice of the Past: Oral History.*
9   Rowbotham S (1992): *Women in Movement: Feminism and Social Action.*
10 Marx OM (1970): What is the history of psychiatry? *American Journal of Orthopsychiatry.*
11 Hitchcock T, Sharpe P (1997, ed.): *Chronicling Poverty: The Voices and Strategies of the English Poor 1640–1840.*
12 Thompson EP (2002): *The Making of the English Working Class.*
13 Walk A (1961): The history of mental nursing. *Journal of Mental Science.*
14 Porter R (1992, ed.).
15 Willmuth LR (1979): Medical views of depression in the elderly: historical notes. *Journal of the American Geriatrics Society.*
16 Berrios G, Porter R (1995, ed.): *A History of Clinical Psychiatry: The Origins of Psychiatric Disorders.*
17 Healy D (2001): The dilemmas posed by new and fashionable treatments. *Archives of Psychiatric Treatment.*
18 Cannadine D (2013): *The Undivided Past: History Beyond our Differences.*
19 Berrios GE (1995): Research into the history of psychiatry. In *Research Methods in Psychiatry: a Beginner's Guide* (eds C Freeman, P Tyrer).
20 Cubbin JK (2006): *The Waiting Room to Hell.*
21 Gittins D (1998): *Madness in its Place: Narratives of Severalls Hospital, 1913–1997.*
22 Boschma G (2012): Community mental health nursing in Alberta, Canada: an oral history. *Nursing History Review.*
23 Holmes C (2006): The slow death of psychiatric nursing: what next? *Journal of Psychiatric and Mental Health Nursing.*
24 Crowther A, Ragusa A (2011): Realities of mental health nursing practice in rural Australia. *Issues in Mental Health Nursing.*
25 Warelow P, Edward K (2007): Evidence-based mental health nursing in Australia: our history and our future. *International Journal of Mental Health Nursing.*
26 Leishman J (2004): Back to the future: making a case for including history of mental nursing in nurse education programmes. *International Journal of Psychiatric Nursing Research.*

Acknowledgements

The following nurses discussed their experiences in mental hospitals with the authors:

The female side

Angela Ainsworth (St Luke's)
Annie Altschul (Royal Edinburgh)
Joyce Archer (All Saints)
Kay Baggins (Gartloch, Napsbury)
Yvonne Beaumont (Parkside, Lancaster Moor)
Ruth Benbow (Claybury)
Brenda Billings (Graylingwell)
Jo Brand (The Maudsley)
Patricia Burdett (Coney Hill)
Imelda Bures (Netherne)
Alison Bussey (Hill End)
Val Canty (Fairmile)
Louise Clark (Parkside)
Fiona Couper (Tooting Bec)
Bridget Dickson-Wild (Netherne)
Mary Everett (Cane Hill, Netherne)
Sharon Frood (Carlton Hayes)
Morah Geall (Hellingly)
Velvendar Godfrey (Runwell)
Beryl Hepworth (St Bernard's)
Janet Herd (Warlingham Park)
Mary Hicks (St Lawrence's)
Louise Hide (Fulbourn)
Irene Jones (St Bernard's)
Jayne Love (St Augustine's, Fair Mile)
Judy Lunny (Graylingwell)
Fiona Nolan (Banstead, Horton)
Ann O'Donnell (Netherne)

Carmel Piris (Netherne)
Olive Slattery (Gartnavel, Highcroft, All Saints)
Mary Slevin (All Saints)
Sophie Slevin (All Saints)
Felicity Stockwell (Holloway Sanatorium, Whittingham)
Judith Watson (Goodmayes, Warneford)
Brenda Wild (Graylingwell)

The male side

Philip Barton-Wright (High Royds, Scalebor Park)
Neil Brimblecombe (Hill End)
Paddy Carr (Parkside)
Tom Chan (Park Prewett, Brookwood)
Eric Chitty (Moorhaven)
Alistair Clark (Ravenscraig)
Bryn Davis (The Retreat, Holloway Sanatorium)
Carlos Forni (Bexley)
John Greene (Moorhaven)
Kevin Halpin (Oakwood)
Dermot Hennessy (Banstead, Netherne)
Allan Hicks (St Lawrence's, Goodmayes)
Tom Hopkinson (Rubery Hill)
Barone Hopper (Graylingwell)
John Kelly (Hartwood)
Jack Lyttle (Gartloch)
Andrew McCrae (Denbigh, Hill End)
Tim Mosses (Bexley)
Jim Newlands (Hartwood)
Ronnie Newman (Roundway)
Ian Norman (Long Grove)
Mike O'Connor (Park Prewett)
John Pay (Graylingwell)
Tony Quinn (Tooting Bec)
Teerenlall Ramgopal (St George's Stafford)
Peter Robinson (Cane Hill)
Mark Rudman (Whitecroft)
Charlie Russell (Hartwood, Cane Hill)
Iain Tulley (Hartwood, Exminster)
Jim Vaughan (Barrow)
Peter Walsh (Woodilee, Banstead, Horton)
Tom Walsh (West Park)
Herman Wheeler (Rubery Hill)

Other informants

Julia Brooking (professor of nursing, University of Birmingham)
Maureen Gomez (laundry manager, Netherne)
Mary Gutierrez (nursing assistant, Netherne)
Tom Harrison (psychiatrist, Hollymoor)
Jean McFarlane (professor of nursing, University of Manchester)
Alan Packham (estates foreman, Horton)
Bill Reavley (psychologist, Graylingwell)
Peter Scarrett (social worker, Netherne)
George Townsend (electrician, Horton)
Tony Tramalgini (nursing assistant, Netherne)
William Trethowan (professor of psychiatry, University of Birmingham)
Bob Wycherly (psychologist, Middlewood)

1 The pauper palace and its servants

In the beginning, there was care in the community. *Homo sapiens* has always been a social animal, whose bonds stretch beyond blood relations to tribe or townsfolk. Throughout the Middle Ages feudal communities looked after their own. The Church preached compassion for the mad as for the sick, and the 'village idiot', a medieval caricature of the odd or mentally impaired person, received parish alms. The term 'lunatic', derived from the legendary belief in mental derangement provoked by full moon, applied to people with temporary or permanent loss of mental faculties. Some lunatics wandered from town to town – their liberty to roam only curtailed if they became troublesome, when they might be punished at the stocks, whipping post or ducking pool.

Since the fifth century monasteries had been established in Britain. The monastic life demanded unquestioning obedience, self-restraint, humility and commitment to improving one's spiritual life through service to the community, asceticism and celibacy. As in secular enslavement, monks' heads were shaved to confirm their capitulation to God's will. In a frugal existence, devotees sought to overcome the desires of the flesh by fasting, manual work, prayer and study. They laboured in the fields, the mill, kitchen and gardens; skilled 'brothers' were deployed as smiths, leatherworkers, masons or carpenters, and a scribe produced the chronicle of the monastery.[1] By around the twelfth century Benedictine monasteries began to reach out to people with sickness or disability in the community. Peripatetic monks visited sufferers of mental disorder in their homes and gave practical and spiritual guidance to their family and friends. Anyone who did not recover was invited to submit to the ordered life of the monastery until able to return home.[2]

Despite such caring provision, some people of wayward mind and spirit were seen as a danger to society, drawing not sympathy but severe penalty. In the religious turmoil of the late Middle Ages, insanity and evil were often conflated. The omnipotent Catholic Church responded to deviance and dissent with the *Malleus Maleficarum* (*Hammer of the Witches*), a missive credited to two celibate Dominican theologians, Heinrich Kramer and Jacob Sprenger. The *Malleus* asserted the dangers of witchcraft, and guided magistrates on interrogation and torture.[3] Witches were known as libidinous women who copulate with incubi, casting spells in cahoots with the Devil to spread evil throughout the land. While some men were also persecuted, the misogynistic *Malleus* asserted that women, due to their vanity, proneness to lying, weak intellect and lust, were most prone to diabolical possession. Between 1580 and 1650 there were 200,000 prosecutions in Europe; the guilty were burnt at the stake, thereby destroying both body and spirit.[4] The sixteenth and seventeenth centuries were dangerous times for anyone behaving oddly.

As society recoiled from witchcraft hysteria, theological interpretations of madness began to be eclipsed by the advance of medicine. Dominating Western medicine was the ancient Greek system of four humours: blood, yellow bile, black bile and phlegm. These humours governed behaviour: mania was due to bile boiling in the brain, while excessive black bile caused melancholia; imbalances were treated by purging, blood-letting and sudden plunging in hot or cold water. A more humane treatment of madness was promoted by maverick Swiss physician Paracelsus in the sixteenth century. Having observed healing practice in Tibet, Constantinople, Arabia, Egypt and the Holy Land, Paracelsus rejected harsh physical methods and medicinal concoctions as guesswork, emphasising instead the moral virtue of the lunatic's carer or physician.[5] Eventually humoural medicine was undermined by revelations in anatomy and physiology, and discovery of the nervous system relocated the seat of insanity from visceral organs to the brain.[6] However, this was not readily followed by advances in treatment: Thomas Willis, reputedly the first neurologist, saw torture as the most reliable means of imposing order on unruly minds. Insanity, according to medical opinion, needed robust treatment:

> I do advertise every man the whiche is madde or lunatyke or frantyke or demonyacke, to be kepte in safegarde in some close house or chamber where there is lytell light; and that we have a keeper the whiche the madde do fear.[7]

From alms to the madhouse

The only institution specifically for care of lunatics was the Bethlem Hospital in London. Built in 1247 as a priory dedicated to St Mary of Bethlehem, this establishment moved in 1676 from its monastic buildings to a larger site beyond the city wall at Moorfields, with accommodation for 120 lunatics. Public viewing was offered for a small fee, and 'Bedlam' (a truncated name that became synonymous with madness) was as popular as the zoological gardens; inmates were encouraged by their keepers to growl like wild beasts for their audience. The governors extracted donations from affluent visitors, in whom pity might be aroused; this was a major source of profit until the notorious parade was abolished in 1770.[8] Although the hospital was run by a religious organisation, the mostly male staff was not averse to brutality. Treatments included bleeding, blistering and beating, but as insanity eluded cure, Bethlem rested on the assumption that the best that could be done for the insane was to restrain them.

A corrective to Bedlam was Robert Burton's *The Anatomy of Melancholy*, published in 1621.[9] An Oxford don and celibate priest, Burton was afflicted with physical and mental maladies throughout his life. He saw melancholy as an imbalance of body, mind and spirit, which could be corrected by the restorative powers of blood-letting, exercise, good diet and country air. It was the responsibility of the medical profession to help people whose affliction alienated them from their fellow beings. Sufferers needed a calm and restful environment, supported by kindly, tolerant people. For Burton, lasting recovery depended not on the quantity of medicinal concoctions but on the quality of human relationships.

Since 1634 the Bethlem keepers had been subordinated to a salaried physician. Nepotism was evident in a 125-year medical dynasty beginning with the appointment of James Monro in 1728.[10] The Monros refused to take medical students and were intolerant of anyone who doubted their methods. Despite its worsening reputation, Bethlem had a lengthy waiting list. James was succeeded in 1751 by his son, John, in the same year that a rival institution opened across the road. Appointed as physician in charge of St Luke's Hospital for Lunatics was William Battie. Son of a vicar, Battie's commitment to improving conditions for the mentally ill was inspired by the Enlightenment philosophy of Hobbes, Rousseau, Voltaire and Locke. Hobbes' *Leviathan*, published in 1651, presented the ideal of a social contract whereby the State would control greed and protect the weak from brutishness and misery. Battie's *Treatise on Madness*, published in 1758, criticised the coercive and barbaric treatment and cramped cells at Bethlem Hospital. Monro was infuriated by this slur from a commercial rival.

While differentiating lunatics from other itinerant outcasts, the Vagrancy Act 1744 could only enforce their removal to a house of correction, but in the eighteenth century various institutions for the insane emerged. Some of the general hospitals that opened in larger cities, funded by public subscription schemes, included an annexe for lunatics (as at Guy's in London). The Manchester Lunatic Hospital of 1766 was administratively attached to the general infirmary, an arrangement followed in Liverpool in 1792. Meanwhile private madhouses proliferated. Typically owned by clergymen or doctors, these establishments catered for private lunatics or recipients of Poor Law assistance. Unsurprisingly, the latter class got the worst deal; head-shaven inmates were perpetually shackled to the walls of dank and dingy cells. Concern at abuses led to appointment of a parliamentary committee to enquire into care of lunatics; the resulting Madhouse Act of 1774 required a licence for owners, and in the London environs madhouses were to be inspected by a body of five commissioners from the College of Physicians. As the only sanction was that details of irregularities were displayed at the madhouse entrance, proprietors remained a law unto themselves. It was the rough treatment meted to King George III during his episodes of madness that brought the plight of the insane to public attention.

Philanthropists' stone

Exempt from the Madhouse Act was the care of pauper lunatics. In 1806 High Sheriff of Gloucestershire and prison reformer Sir George Onesiphorus Paul, after visiting several madhouses, highlighted the dreadful plight of the insane poor to the Secretary of State for the Home Department. This led to the appointment of a Select Committee, chaired by Charles Williams-Wynn and comprising several members of the Clapham Sect, an influential society for humanitarian reform.[11] At this time the number of identified lunatics was small: only 2,248 in England and Wales (2.26 per 10,000 population), of whom 1,765 were in workhouses and 140 in gaols. In its report in 1808 the Parliamentary Committee presented a catalogue of cruel and degrading treatment, demonstrating urgent need to protect lunatics – particularly paupers, who had no choice in where they were sent. A law was subsequently passed for the provision of county pauper lunatic asylums.

To understand these developments, we must consider the political and social context of Britain at the beginning of the nineteenth century. Parliamentarians at this time were aristocrats, and parochial authority rested with the landed gentry: the few governed the many. Men (rarely women) of high social standing were selected as magistrates by the county's Lord Lieutenant for formal appointment by the Home Secretary (a system that continued until local government legislation in 1888). Any transfer of power to the State was likely to be opposed as a threat to local autonomy. The County Asylums Act of 1808 was a tentative step, merely giving English and Welsh county justices the option to build an asylum at ratepayers' expense.

The 1808 Act recommended that asylums be built on an airy, south-facing site with good water supply. They would be located on the outskirts of a market town, thus within reach of medical assistance. The reformers were inspired by a model establishment in York founded in 1792 by William Tuke, a tea merchant and philanthropist. The Tuke family were Quakers, a minor religious group whose basic tenets were peace and simplicity. The ethos of The Retreat was moral management, based on the notion that even the most frenzied lunatic could return to lucidity if treated well. Each of the thirty residents was allocated a personal attendant, and troubled minds were diverted by fulfilling occupation, prayer and recreation. The spacious grounds were aesthetically pleasing, with gardens offering views over the surrounding countryside, and domesticated rabbits and fowl in the airing courts. The Retreat was not only a haven but also a therapeutic environment, and its recovery rate impressed the humanitarian reformers.

As presented in Samuel Tuke's *Description of The Retreat*,[12] published in 1813, the principles and practice of moral management required little medical input; visiting physicians merely treated bodily illnesses (not until forty-two years after its opening was a medical superintendent appointed). By contrast, patients in other lunatic hospitals and asylums were subjected to regular purgatives and cold baths, phlebotomy of the arteries of the head and neck, and contraptions such as the gyratory chair. The Tukes saw such interventions as distasteful. As eloquently discussed by Michel Foucault in *Madness and Civilisation*,[13] it was incidental to the development of the medical profession that a system of institutional care was founded for the insane. In the guise of 'alienists', doctors appointed to manage the new county asylums had more appeal in social stature than in clinical expertise. However, the asylum movement sowed the seeds of a medical monopoly of madness, in which the scope of practice expanded from individual treatment to an overall therapeutic regime.

Alongside the Tukes the greatest pioneer in the institutional care of lunatics was physician Philippe Pinel, who in 1792 was appointed head physician at the Bicêtre, a large hospital for the insane in Paris. This was a time of turmoil in France, as Robespierre pursued his *Grande Terreur* against the aristocracy and 30,000 died at the *guillotine*. An erudite humanist, Pinel took no part in the political upheaval, but he implemented the revolutionary doctrine of *liberté* at the Bicêtre, where he was shocked by the brutal treatment of lunatics. Freeing inmates from fetters, blood-letting and ducking, Pinel practised *le traitement moral*, emphasising individualised care and meaningful occupation. Like the Tukes, he believed that care of inmates depended on the character of attendants. Jean-Baptiste Pussin and his wife Marguerite were employed as head attendants, with whom Pinel visited each patient daily to review progress, carefully recording their observations. The Tukes and Pinel independently devised similarly enlightened therapeutic approaches, but the latter attracted doctors with its emphasis on 'treatment', unlike the non-medical language of The Retreat.

Public asylums did not suddenly appear on the horizon after the permissive 1808 Act. The first, in Nottingham, began to receive patients in 1810; it was built on a site of five acres, with a lawn in front and two airing courts behind (additional land was later purchased for growing crops). Unlike The Retreat, the architecture of the first generation of public asylums prioritised confinement over comfort, with custodial manifestations throughout. Walls were of great thickness, in locally quarried stone, as in the imposing bastion of the Kent Asylum at Barming Heath. Of some influence was the 'Panopticon' model for institutions devised in the late eighteenth century by philosopher-jurist Jeremy Bentham. This circular structure had cells or wards radiating from the centre like spokes of a cartwheel, thereby maximising surveillance and reducing the need for physical restraint. Although applied at the Glasgow Asylum of 1814 and in amended form in the Cornwall and Devon asylums, Bentham's model was generally deemed too oppressive for county asylums, being favoured instead for the prison-building programme.[14]

The typical linear structure comprised a series of wards each side of a central administration block, where the office and residence of the medical superintendent were situated. Contrasting with the grand facade, the corridors to the male and female sides led to a Spartan interior of bare walls, asphalt floors and minimal furnishing. Each ward consisted of a wide gallery and adjacent sleeping quarters, where patients slept in wooden boxes with straw bedding. Heating was by open fires, quite inadequate for large dormitories in winter, while oil lamps effected modest illumination. Narrow iron casement windows afforded little daylight and fresh air, resulting in persistent stale odours. Yet the asylum was an improvement on the hovels to which many patients were accustomed.

From the outset of the public asylum system, power of admission was invested neither in physicians nor Poor Law officers. Parish overseers were legally bound to report a lunatic, who would be examined by a justice of the peace and, if certifiable, sent to the asylum. A visiting committee was appointed by county magistrates to oversee the management of the institution. The official visitors were distinguished gentlemen, and some ladies, of philanthropic bent; they held monthly meetings at the asylum, scrutinising the accounts and offering patients an audience for any grievance.[15]

Meanwhile, dreadful conditions persisted in private madhouses and lunatic hospitals. Magistrate Godfrey Higgins found that a patient he had sent to York Asylum, a charitable establishment founded in 1777, had been repeatedly flogged. The asylum governors denied any wrongdoing, but Higgins pursued the matter and an investigation began in November 1813. On 26 December there was a serious fire at the asylum, when most of the staff members were absent: two male attendants were taking Christmas leave and the doctor was attending a private patient thirty miles away. Four patients perished in the blaze. Higgins subscribed to become a governor of the asylum and in this capacity he was able to see the conditions for himself. Squalid cells housed several incontinent lunatics, with walls daubed in excrement, the stench causing Higgins to vomit. A single airing court was provided for each sex, where the meek melancholic mingled with the agitated maniac. Male and female patients were inadequately segregated with the result that ten women were impregnated (in one case a child was fathered by an attendant named Backhouse, who was required to pay maintenance to a poorhouse).[16]

These atrocious conditions led to appointment of a Select Committee in 1815 to enquire into regulation of the care of lunatics. The investigators were not easily fooled, and at York they found handcuffs and chains concealed under filthy straw. Bethlem Hospital was indicted by the notorious case of William Norris. An educated man, Norris had allegedly tried to kill attendants; for twelve years he had been continually chained so that he could barely stand, with an iron ring around his neck. John Haslam, apothecary to Bethlem, was asked by an investigator about the treatment of inmates:[17]

> *Would you treat a private individual patient in the same way as has been described in respect of Bethlem?*
> No, certainly not.
> *What is the difference of management?*
> In Bethlem, the restraint is by chains, there is no such thing as chains in my house.
> *What are your objections to chains and fetters as a mode of restraint?*
> They are fit only for pauper lunatics; if a gentleman was put in irons, he would not like it.

Social class division was pronounced in treatment of the insane, with a hierarchy of care from the comfortable private asylums, where moneyed patients were waited upon by servants, to the windowless dens for paupers, staffed by illiterate 'keepers'. Bethlem was far from perfect, but Haslam drew a distinction between the staff at such charitable institutions and the private madhouse:

> With respect to the persons, called keepers, who are placed over the insane, public hospitals have generally very much advantage. They are better paid, which makes them anxious to preserve their situations by attention and good

behaviour: and thus they acquire some experience of diseases. But it is very different in the private receptacles for maniacs. They there procure them at a cheap rate: they are taken from the plough, the loom, or the stable; and sometimes this tribe consists of decayed smugglers, broken excise-men, or discharged sheriff's officers. If anything could add to the calamity of mental derangement, it would be the mode which is generally adopted for its cure. Although an office of some importance and great responsibility, it is held as a degrading and odious employment, and seldom accepted but by idle and disorderly persons.[18]

Keepers maintained order and attended to basic needs, but these poorly paid workers received little guidance from proprietors, who were mostly ignorant of therapeutic endeavour. Indeed, perpetual incarceration was profitable. Despite damning evidence of mistreatment of pauper lunatics, a proposed inspection regime was rejected four times by the House of Lords between 1814 and 1819. Local magistrates did not see statutory control as the solution. However, the shameful revelations caused growing unease in the ruling class and in 1827 another enquiry was conducted, which led to two Acts of Parliament. There was no public asylum serving the London conurbation, where paupers went to one of many private madhouses or to Bethlem or St Lukes. Some licensed houses were large: Hoxton House, Peckham House, Camberwell House, Grove Hall in Bow, and the Red House and White House in Bethnal Green held between 200 and 400 inmates. The Select Committee led by Dorset magistrate Robert Gordon told the House of Commons of miserable conditions in madhouses containing Middlesex paupers, particularly at Doctor Warburton's madhouse in Bethnal Green. Violent inmates were kept in a 'crib room', each chained to a box of straw where they were left for entire weekends without attention, until Monday morning when they were taken into the yard and doused by pails of cold water to wash them of excrement.

The Madhouse Act of 1828 tightened regulation of private madhouses and charitable lunatic hospitals. In the London area, the ineffectual College of Physicians inspectors were replaced by the Metropolitan Commissioners in Lunacy, a new inspectorate appointed by the Secretary of State, despite opposition from the College and madhouse-owning doctors as an infringement on medical practice. Five of the fifteen commissioners were to be medically qualified, and the legal profession secured representation in an amendment in 1832, requiring at least two barristers. The Metropolitan Commissioners could revoke a licence and discharge anyone improperly detained. Commissioner Lord Ashley, who had seconded the legislation, became chairman in 1834. A tireless campaigner for the care of lunatics, Ashley[19] was spurred to social activism by an unhappy upbringing relieved only by the housekeeper, whose affectionate care taught him that compassion conquers all. His day would come.

While the new public asylums were exempt from inspection, the County Asylums Act 1828 imposed new requirements, including a resident medical officer, whose order was necessary for any use of restraint. Annual reports of admissions, deaths and discharges were to be sent to the Home Office. Alongside statutory obligations, a code of practice was prepared by parliamentary reformers as a blueprint for moral treatment. However, merely nine of the fifty-two counties of England and Wales had opened asylums: Nottingham, Bedford, Norfolk, Lancaster, Stafford, West Riding of Yorkshire, Cornwall, Lincoln and Gloucester. The average capacity was 116, well within the maximum of 300 recommended by the 1808 Act. The largest was the West Riding Asylum at Wakefield; having opened in 1818 with 150 beds, its capacity had expanded to 250. Elsewhere, county justices eschewed such a costly venture, arguing that their number of pauper lunatics was negligible. Parish guardians were required to keep record of all lunatics receiving indoor or outdoor relief. By this time 9,000 pauper lunatics were registered in England and Wales – a substantial increase on 1807. For them, the foundations had been laid for a proper system of care.

Forward and back

The men and women drawn to work in the county asylums were a mixed bunch. Ideally recruits were of good physique, practical ability, basic literacy – and deference. Previous experience could not be expected, although some may have worked in private asylums or workhouses. The asylums lured domestic servants, whose pay was considerably lower. Young women were initially posted as kitchen maids or laundresses, before promotion to a caring role. As well as employees of the gentry, previous occupations of male staff included farmhands, artisans, soldiers and sailors. Male wards were thus staffed by stout labourers who could be relied upon to keep order, and men with skills such as carpentry or tailoring who could practise their former trade in the service of the institution.

As in the madhouses, the term 'keeper' was initially used in county asylums, until this was replaced by the more humanitarian 'attendant'. Some matrons referred to their care staff as 'nurses'. The three job titles were used interchangeably by WC Ellis,[20] resident medical officer at Hanwell Asylum, in his treatise on the treatment of lunacy. A convenient arrangement was for the institution to be run by a husband and wife partnership, as at Hanwell, where Ellis was in overall charge but the matron effectively managed the female wing; she was consequently paid more than the head attendant on the male side.

As described in LD Smith's[21] study of attendants in the early years at Stafford Asylum, incentives were introduced for continual service. Keepers in the principal gallery and in the basement storey both received £25, and on the two upper galleries £20 each. In 1825 annual increments began for staff on the lower rate: an additional £1 per year, until they reached parity with those on £25. Volunteers for a weekly night shift gained an extra £5, but this was seen as an unnecessary expense by the Stafford visiting committee and in the 1840s night duty was included in the employment contract for new recruits. Attendants on the night rota were not excused from the normal shift starting at 6 a.m.

At the Surrey Asylum, which opened in 1841, male attendants received from £25 to £31, and female counterparts from £12 to £16.[22] Such differential was the norm at a time when a man's wages supposedly covered his family upkeep.

However, only the most senior male attendants were allowed to marry and to live with their wives and children in the asylum. Otherwise, marriage was deemed incompatible with the requirements of the job; attendants lived in rooms off the patients' dormitories, and could be summoned to duty at any time during the night. The marriage bar was a major factor in the attrition of younger female staff, but spinsters or widows tended to stay. Attendants enticed their relatives to asylum service, thus beginning the intergenerational continuity and informal power bases that became prominent features of life in the mental institution.

Attendants were expected to keep the patients occupied, both for therapeutic benefit and for the self-sufficiency of the asylum. Wards were emptied in the daytime as female patients went to work in the laundry, kitchen or sewing room, and the men in the workshops or outdoors. The derogatory term 'funny farm' originated in the scene of supervised gangs of patients toiling in the fields. Asylum land was fruitful, with sufficient acreage and livestock for ample crops, meat and dairy produce. Alongside the farm account, asylum reports listed the clothing, bedding and tools produced over the year. Some patients remained on the wards, cleaning and polishing the dormitories and galleries. Ellis described Hanwell as a veritable house of industry:[23]

> There are two keepers to each ward, one of whom is a mechanic. Before breakfast, both are employed in the getting up, waking and shaving the patients. After breakfast the mechanic leaves the ward in charge of the other, and he selects from his own ward, and from the other male wards, such patients as are able to work with him at his trade. The keeper who is left in the ward, attends to the patients, takes care that the beds are made, the rooms and the gallery thoroughly cleaned, and employs the patients in picking coir, twine-spinning, or any other in-door employment … Each female ward has two nurses: at nine o'clock the junior nurse, whenever the weather permits, collects those patients in her ward who are to be employed out of doors, and assists and watches over them whilst in the cultivation of the ground. The necessary ward duties, mending the clothes for the male and female patients, the making the whole of the house linen, and assisting in sewing the men's clothes, the superintending the twine-spinning, basket-making, pottle-making and other works, afford sufficient occupation to the nurse who is left in charge.

Many inmates were unable to work, such as the acutely disturbed and the senile infirm. In reality, managing large groups of insane patients, some with proclivity for violence, suicide or escape, was difficult without recourse to physical methods of control. Moral management may have worked at The Retreat, but the large pauper asylum was not so amenable. The dangerousness of lunatics was demonstrated by a dreadful incident in the annals of the Kent County Asylum:[24]

> John Nicols Thom, a Cornishman, was admitted to the Asylum with delusions that he was Sir William Courtenay, King of Jerusalem, Knight of Malta, etc. His wife, having some influence, obtained an order for his release,

notwithstanding the protests of the Medical Officer, with the result that he organised a riot among the poor ignorant hop-pickers in the neighbourhood of Canterbury; obtained arms for them and fought the King's troops in the Blean Woods, where Lieutenant Bennett and 16 soldiers were killed, and Thom and a number of his followers also lost their lives.

Violent inmates were strapped into chairs fixed to the wall, or chained to beds. Among various items of restraint was the straitjacket, which was made of strong material tied from behind, binding hands and arms to the torso. Manacles were used to lock the patient's wrists together. Such restraint was excessively applied by the untrained and unsupervised attendants, and consequently the county asylums were in danger of becoming little different from penal institutions. This was a trend that offended some medical superintendents: they had qualified as doctors, not prison governors. Yet medical treatments were no more beneficial, as WC Ellis explained:

> Very copious evacuations and profuse bleeding from the system are resorted to, and after the animal strength of the patient is exhausted, he becomes quiet, but the mental delusion still remains.[25]

In his book on the treatment of insanity, Ellis presented the following as one of several examples of individualised moral management:

> A female, discharged as incurable from an hospital near London, was, on her admission at Hanwell, one of the most distressing patients among the six hundred. The wringing of her hands, with her constant moaning, almost night and day, rendered her unfit to be amongst the other patients. Liberty and confinement, indulgence and privation were tried without effect; she still persevered in the deplorable noise and wringing of her hands. As she seemed to dislike the open air, she was ordered to be taken out of doors every morning, and kept there the whole day. For a long time no alteration seemed to take place; but the plan was still continued. In about two months her bodily health had greatly improved, and, although she refused to work, her noise was diminished, and she expressed her dislike of the going out of doors. This was a great point gained. She was told, that if she should conduct herself so as not to annoy the other patients, and amuse herself with a little work, she should remain in the house. On the promise of good behaviour, the experiment was tried, and it succeeded. She has, for weeks, daily occupied in sewing. She has little indulgences, the fruits of her labour; and she rarely attempts to wring her hands or to repeat her moaning: when she does, a hint that she be removed from her nurse – to whom she is much attached – and again sent into the garden, is quite sufficient to recall her to order.[26]

Appointed as house surgeon to the Lincoln Asylum in 1835, Robert Gardiner Hill continued the work of visiting physician Doctor Charlesworth, who had considerably reduced instances of restraint. Regarding its use as unjustifiable in any circumstances, Gardiner Hill entirely abolished mechanical restraint by 1838. Against the doubts of the visiting committee, this was a courageous strategy which could not have succeeded without cooperation of the attendants. Staffing was increased and a night watch was posted. Selected for physical strength, attendants were allowed to restrain a violent or disturbed patient manually, but only with use of the hands. Solitary confinement was also permitted, but cold baths and drugs were regarded as mechanical restraint in disguise.

The most celebrated reformer of asylum care was John Conolly, who had abandoned his professorship in medicine at University College London, where his efforts to integrate the mind and its disorders in medical training were frustrated. On succeeding Ellis as resident physician at Hanwell Asylum, Conolly visited Lincoln in 1839 to assess whether non-restraint could be applied at a large pauper lunatic asylum, then housing eight hundred lunatics. Conolly regarded physical coercion as detrimental to recovery, as it made patients morally indifferent. Within seven months he removed all instruments of restraint, including hundreds of leglocks and handcuffs. Conolly had no doubt about the crucial factor in the proper care of lunatics:

> Everything that a judicious committee wishes to be carried into effect – every comfort that the benevolence of the officers would wish to confer – every appliance of daily treatment every curative means, will be either realized or withheld, according to the character of the attendants. They are the instruments by which every great and good intention is brought into hourly practice. It is not necessary to say more, to prove how important it is that they should be well chosen, well governed, well taken care of, well supported in their duty, and well paid.[27]

Within a year of his appointment as medical superintendent at Lancaster Asylum in 1840, Samuel Gaskell abolished manual restraint and removed the iron bars and gates. Gaskell emphasised classification of patients by behaviour, separating the quiet and compliant from the dirty and turbulent, so that moral reinforcement replaced physical coercion. The non-restraint doctrine became a new focus for reformers, although arguably this overshadowed the positive goals of moral treatment. Draconian devices could be withdrawn, but attendants could abuse their power in other ways. Occasionally attendants were sacked for mishandling of patients, although sometimes they were excused by circumstances. The Hanwell regulations stated that 'any keeper striking or ill-treating a patient will, for the first offence, be fine five shillings, and be dismissed for the second'.[28]

Improving the quality of attendants was the key to proper care of the insane, asserted prominent Scottish alienist WAF Browne in his book *What Asylums Were, Are, and Ought to Be*. Browne, having once taken advice that he must fix the attendants before proceeding to cure the patients, was not impressed by the general standard of such workers:

Keepers are the unemployed of other professions. If they possess physical strength, and a tolerable reputation, it is enough: and the latter quality is frequently dispensed with. They enter upon their duties altogether ignorant of what insanity is, fully impressed with the idea that the creatures committee to their charge are no longer men, that they are incapable of reasoning or feeling, and that in order to rule or manage, it is necessary to terrify and coerce them.[29]

Browne wrote this treatise while at the Royal Montrose Asylum. Having opened in 1781, this was the oldest of the chartered asylums in Scotland. Others granted royal charter had opened at Aberdeen (1800), Edinburgh (1813), Glasgow (1814), Dundee (1820) and Perth (1826). These privately owned establishments received two classes of patient: private and rate-aided. While paying 'boarders' benefited from superior accommodation, the principles of moral treatment were earnestly applied throughout. A Bill for provision of district lunatic asylums in 1818 was vehemently opposed as a needless imposition when institutional provision already existed. The latest of the chartered asylums opened at Dumfries in 1839, where the wealthy benefactor enticed Browne to take charge of the Crichton Institution for the insane poor, which stood adjacent to the asylum for private patients. Under Browne's direction, a hundred lunatics benefited from an exemplar of humane care.

In 1842 the foundation stone was laid for the new Glasgow Royal Asylum, which moved to larger premises at Gartnavel. Inscribed in stone above the entrance was the legend: 'Employing no mechanical restraint in the treatment of patients'. Five hundred patients were accommodated, with the affluent class in the west wing, and paupers and lower-rate boarders in separate wards to the east. There was limited space for exercise, or for expansion. In a rapidly growing city, the number of insane was growing, and many were confined at unregulated private premises. Despite progressive ideals, Scottish lunacy provision was slow to respond to the social turmoil wreaked by the Industrial Revolution.

The sweeping drive

As Parliamentary reformers continued to press for a national, regulated system for lunacy, an Act of 1842 empowered the Metropolitan Commissioners to visit asylums and madhouses throughout England and Wales. Written by Lord Ashley, the detailed report in 1844 described much variation in care and conditions. The benefits of inspection were confirmed by dramatic improvements at Warburton's madhouse: in 1828 up to two hundred inmates were held in leg-locks and chains at night, whereas in 1844 only five of the 582 patients were so restrained. Overall, despite some deficiencies in design, county asylums were found superior to other institutions housing the insane. Yet half of English counties lacked an asylum, and there was none in Wales. The population of England had doubled from 7.4 million in 1790 to 14.8 million by 1840, and susceptibility to insanity appeared disproportionately high among the labouring class. The number of registered lunatics was six times greater than in 1807, although this was partially explained by better recording.

Table 1.1 County asylums, 1844

County	Location	Year of opening
Nottinghamshire	Nottingham	1811
Bedfordshire	Bedford	1812
Norfolk	Thorpe, near Norwich	1814
Lancashire	Lancaster	1816
Staffordshire	Stafford	1818
West Riding, Yorkshire	Wakefield	1818
Cornwall	Bodmin	1820
Lincolnshire (for private patients only)	Lincoln	1820
Gloucestershire	Gloucester	1823
Suffolk	Woodbridge	1829
Cheshire	Chester	1829
Middlesex	Hanwell	1831
Dorset	Forston, near Dorchester	1832
Kent	Barming Heath	1833
Leicestershire	Leicester	1837
Surrey	Wandsworth	1841

The asylum movement was driven by two contrasting socio-political motives, leading to the same destination. The unsavoury conditions for the teeming masses in mill towns offended the sensibilities of radical idealists such as Lord Ashley, who channelled their Christian faith into social reform. Alongside this evangelical zeal was the philosophy of utilitarianism, as expressed by Jeremy Bentham's tenet of the greatest good for the greatest number. In a burgeoning capitalist economy that required a large supply of labour, a rationally organised system for the non-productive elements of society supported the progress of society. With philanthropy on one hand, and the utilitarian goal of order on the other, a consensus formed for a centrally controlled institutional response to lunacy.

By 1844 only a quarter of the 16,000 lunatics and idiots chargeable to parishes in England and Wales were accommodated in county asylums. Nine thousand were in workhouses, where they cost parishes about 2 shillings per week, compared to 9 shillings at an asylum. Benthamite ideology spurred the Poor Law Amendment Act of 1834, which imposed the principle of less eligibility: no able-bodied recipient should live better than the lowest-paid worker. Handouts were perceived as encouraging idleness and thereby perpetuating pauperism. The shift from outdoor to indoor relief required substantial expansion of the workhouse system. Although explicitly designed to discourage destitution, union workhouses shared by neighbouring parishes rapidly grew as depositories for all kinds of society's rejects, but they were not designed for care of the insane. Workhouse masters found insane inmates disruptive to productivity and discipline, and in the larger institutions a separate lunatic ward was provided, typically in the worst part of the buildings. The Metropolitan Commissioners visited five such establishments during their tour and were not impressed.

Overall the Metropolitan Commissioners' report demonstrated inadequacies in the care of the insane, reinforcing the case for statutory provision for pauper lunatics and a national inspectorate. Consequently, lunacy legislation was consolidated by two statutes passed by Robert Peel's government. Building of county asylums was mandated by the Lunatic Asylums Act of 1845, while the Lunatics Act of the same year introduced a national body of Commissioners in Lunacy to inspect every public asylum, licensed madhouse and hospital for the insane in England and Wales. At last, the reformers had triumphed.

The Lunacy Commissioners included five lawyers, three medical commissioners and five laymen. As chairman, Lord Ashley doubted whether the medical and legal professions could be relied upon to protect the welfare of pauper lunatics, and he continued to argue that lay people could understand insanity as well as a doctor. In his experience medical inspectors often tolerated or defended substandard conditions. Indeed, the reforms pursued by Ashley had been consistently opposed by a profession with pecuniary interests in the madhouse business. While having no statutory authority over asylum management, the Lunacy Commissioners wielded power through their rigorous inspection and reports that could name and shame a medical superintendent and his employing authority. Their recommendations led to a proliferation of rules governing all activity in the asylum; for example, each use of mechanical restraint was to be documented and justified by a doctor. The Lunacy Commissioners tended to focus on occupation and material comfort, and often enquired into attendance at religious services. They persisted with their notion that the insane could recover, given the right environment and care.

An important role of the Lunacy Commission was to oversee the construction of county asylums. There was much to learn, as serious defects had arisen with ventilation, water supply and drainage. At the recently built Surrey Asylum, patients were endangered by the flawed central heating system:

> Iron pipes had been laid to carry steam throughout the wards but they proved too thin, and explosions throughout the wards were frequent, as the pipes burst and the patients were injured. Within a few years, almost the entire system had to be removed and new fireplaces installed.[30]

Frugality was regarded by the Lunacy Commissioners as a false economy that demoralised patients. Richard Eager described the austere Devon Asylum, which opened in 1845:

> The original building was in the form of a semicircular corridor with galleries 150 feet long radiating from the convexity like the spokes of a cartwheel. The walls were rough brick, painted with whitewash, and the floors black

asphalt. The furniture consisted of heavy tables screwed down to the floor and wooden forms built into the walls so that they could not be moved. There were no chairs and the beds were made of wood with wooden 'stretchers' on which to lie. Mattresses were stuffed with coir, no upholsterer being appointed before 1893.[31]

Unlike official visitors to county asylums, patients did not enter the front porch and wood-panelled reception hall, but were swiftly processed at a side entrance to the male or female side. For the class of patient in county asylums, according to WC Ellis, solidity trumped comfort.

> In asylums designed for paupers only, it is unnecessary to have any plaster on the walls: lime-wash on the bricks is all that is required…in a large building the saving of money is considerable. The doors, both of the galleries and the rooms, should be made substantially strong; none of them panelled. Doors of this description are burst open by a madman without the slightest difficulty.[32]

The average size of the twenty-four county asylums in 1850 had crept up to 297, and demand was rising. A spate of asylum building resulted from the Act, but justices of some counties continued to drag their heels. There were difficulties in purchasing a site that fulfilled the requirements of the Lunacy Commissioners, and landowners were wary of the impact of a lunatic asylum on their estate. Gardner described the prevarication of the authorities in Sussex, who had prioritised the building of a gaol at Lewes. The last county in England to plan its asylum, Sussex eventually erected an impressive structure at Haywards Heath in 1859.[33]

Lord Ashley had specifically criticised the absence of lunacy provision in Wales. The registered insane were widely dispersed in the undeveloped counties of the Principality; most lived in private dwellings supported by parish relief, but unmanageable lunatics, of whom many spoke only their native language, were sent to asylums in England. When the first asylum in Wales opened in 1848, the founders made the first rule that all officers must be conversant in Welsh. While official records were written in English, Denbigh Asylum was a preserve of Welsh culture in Anglicised surroundings.[34] As at Denbigh, smaller counties combined to fulfil their obligations: Brecon, Radnor and Monmouth established the United Counties Asylum at Abergavenny in 1852, with a capacity of 250. Meanwhile urban authorities in England began to build their own institutions, beginning with the Birmingham Borough Asylum at Winson Green in 1850.

The mid-nineteenth century was the zenith of asylum architecture. County authorities responded to their obligations with decorous expressions of civic pride: this was caring intent cast in stone. Modelled on the pleasure grounds of the gentry, the landscaping would have impressed the visitor, who passed through an ornate gate lodge to a sweeping drive flanked by evenly spaced trees, leading to a stately reception block with columned porch. Unlike the picturesque gardens to the fore, aft were fields for farming and sewage. Vast sites were necessary for the recommended maximum of four patients per acre. The Derbyshire Asylum at Mickleover opened in 1853 on an estate of 79 acres for its 360 patients, a ratio of 0.21 acres per head, compared to 0.07 acres at Hanwell Asylum. Elevated sites were chosen, several miles from the nearest large town, affording fresh air and a pleasant aspect, albeit exposed to the elements. Each ward had access to an airing court, with benches and shelters. The perimeter wall was built on a decline, which reduced its height on the outside, while on the inside a *ha-ha* (a ditch dug on the inside perimeter) prevented escape without spoiling the view.

Architectural embellishment was eschewed by the Lunacy Commissioners, who were more concerned with therapeutic milieu than aesthetic extravagance. Nonetheless, while they could reject indulgent designs, the Lunacy Commissioners approved a degree of tasteful stonework to relieve the monotony of a very large building. Among the masterpieces of craftsmanship were the Warwickshire Asylum at Hatton with its Dutch gables and ornate belfry, the lengthy Byzantine yellow-brick range of the Sussex Asylum, and the neo-Gothic Essex Asylum at Brentwood with its steep gables, turrets and gargoyles. In older asylums large tanks in the roof had sufficed for water supply, but as asylums grew, greater gravitational pressure was necessary. Ready availability of a large volume of water was vital for tackling a fire, which might rapidly envelop buildings of combustible material. Piercing the horizon, the lofty water tower became the indelible image of the Victorian asylum.

Medical masters and their minions

Asylum doctoring was not a prestigious pursuit. Although the medical superintendent was in charge of the day-to-day management of the institution, ultimate power rested with the visiting committee. Barred from employment elsewhere, he needed permission to spend a night away from the asylum. Asylum doctors had no say over who was admitted, and patients could be discharged by the visiting committee as they saw fit, although this was rarely done against medical advice. Supported by only one or two assistant medical officers, the medical superintendent's work was more administrative than clinical. With his residence in the main block, he had little respite from the noise and smell of the wards. At Hanwell, for example, the medical superintendent's garden was between male and female airing courts.

Yet the asylum offered alienists a platform on which to develop their professional expertise and authority. At a meeting in 1841 at Gloucester Asylum, the Association of Medical Officers of Asylums and Hospitals for the Insane was founded, with the aim of promoting asylum doctoring as a specialised discipline, to develop its scientific discourse and to set standards for treatment. In 1853 this association started its professional bulletin *The Asylum Journal*, edited by John Bucknill of Devon Asylum. With its case studies, pathological investigations and philosophical discourse, this monthly publication was renamed *Journal of Mental Science* in 1858. At the inaugural meeting it was agreed that the terms 'lunatic' and 'asylum' should be replaced by 'patient' and 'hospital'. While Lord Ashley was sceptical about doctors running asylums, he was persuaded by the therapeutic optimism of alienists such as Browne, who promised much of the asylum as a place of cure. Unintentionally, Ashley's emphasis on treatment (albeit moral rather than medical) gave impetus to medical claims of jurisdiction.

Tension often arose between medical superintendents and the Commissioners in Lunacy. None of the medical commissioners had asylum experience, until Samuel Gaskell's appointment in 1848. Some medical superintendents saw the Lunacy Commissioners as an ally against their parsimonious lay employers, but others resented the perceived interference and petty criticisms of the inspectors, and broadsides were frequently fired from the pages of the *Asylum Journal*. A recurring controversy was the use of restraint. Most asylum doctors deemed this a necessary contingency for violent or disturbed patients, but the Lunacy Commissioners queried its wide variation in usage.

A case at the Surrey Asylum in Wandsworth showed how treatment could overlap with discipline. A mole-catcher admitted in 1855, Daniel Dolley had a strong physique for his age of sixty-five. On one occasion when he became excitable the medical officer for the male side Charles Snape ordered a shower-bath. As Snape was departing from the scene he was violently struck on the back of his head by Dolley. The shaken doctor demanded that the patient be showered for at least half an hour, followed by a dose of antimony. Shivering after the prolonged onslaught of cold water, Dolley had a seizure and died. His death was attributed to a diseased heart, but after an inconclusive post-mortem examination, medical superintendent Hugh Diamond secretly sent the heart to two London surgeons who found no pathological cause. The heart was returned to the asylum where Diamond burnt the evidence. The Lunacy Commissioners decided to investigate, and on hearing from alienists Charles Hood and John Conolly that such use of the shower-bath was dangerous, they instituted a charge of manslaughter against Snape. The jury found no case to answer and Snape was reinstated, but the debacle showed that the Lunacy Commissioners would not shirk from confronting dubious medical practice, and the case led to a decree that the shower-bath should never be used for more than three minutes.

The medical superintendent could be held to account not only for his own actions but also those of attendants. At the pinnacle of a rigid hierarchy, he hired and fired, while delegating supervision of junior staff to the head attendant and matron. Each supported by a deputy, the head attendant and matron inspected the wards in their respective departments daily, and completed a summary of the number of patients, staffing changes and any untoward incidents. At some asylums, annual reports featured contributions by the matron and head attendant, but this input was dropped in the later nineteenth century when the standard format comprised reviews by the medical superintendent, chaplain, steward and chairman of the visiting committee. For positions of such responsibility, asylum committees sometimes looked beyond their county for candidates experienced in care of the insane. The managers of the North Wales Asylum at Denigh prepared resident medical officer George Turner Jones, matron Nichols and head keeper Robinson by sending them to Gloucester Asylum for instruction by reputable medical superintendent Samuel Hitch.[35]

To the dismay of libertarian doctors such as John Conolly, men and women of desirable character were not readily found. Turnover was high, as many attendants found the work too demanding and the conditions of service too restrictive. Any breach of discipline by attendants was reported by their superior to the medical superintendent, who might summon the miscreant to his office for a reprimand if not summary dismissal. Asylum reports provide copious detail on staff discipline; for example, John Blewer and David Jones, two of the five male attendants initially appointed at Denbigh Asylum, were sacked after being seen climbing over the perimeter wall for an evening in town.[36]

In crowded and understaffed wards without recourse to effective drugs, inevitably there was rough handling by nurses, sometimes causing serious injury to patients. Signs of abuse were sometimes found by medical examination. The head attendant and matron were expected to report bruising or other injury detected while supervising the bathing of patients. Bathing was a potentially violent situation, with numerous shivering and agitated patients standing in line, and harried attendants trying to complete the task as quickly as possible. Occasionally criminal proceedings against attendants were initiated by the Lunacy Commissioners, if they were not satisfied that the medical superintendent had taken appropriate action. As the asylum system expanded, some attendants moved from one institution to another, and the Lunacy Commissioners proposed a national register to prevent the incompetent or troublesome from gaining employment elsewhere.

Some medical superintendents faced insurgency. In 1854 Doctor Grahamsley at Worcester Asylum responded to female attendants' objection to revised staff rules by dismissing them all. He then rejected a pay rise for the matron, who was his sister-in-law. Amidst the unrest, Grahamsley took his life in the retort room of the gasworks, and the matron was subsequently sacked for insubordination. The *Asylum Journal* regretted the 'melancholy end of this promising physician';[37] the same edition of the journal carried an advertisement for Grahamsley's successor. At the Buckinghamshire Asylum, the libertarian approach of medical superintendent John Millar dissatisfied the visiting committee.[38] Millar let the matron take his young daughter around the female wards, believing that this stimulated a maternal instinct in patients. Long before parole was introduced at other asylums, he allowed male patients to visit the Aylesbury Fair. When attendant Henry Brown arrived for night duty intoxicated, he was replaced by Millar and his wages for the shift forfeited, but the chairman of the committee insisted that Brown be dismissed. Struggling to recruit locally, Millar appointed as head attendant Thomas Lissaman, who he knew from a private asylum in London. Lissaman took liberties with the relaxed regime and after several incidents of impropriety the visiting committee demanded Millar's resignation. This provoked action by the Association of Medical Officers of Asylums, with a petition signed by eighty-five members sent to the Lord Lieutenant of the county, but to no avail. This battle against lay control was lost, but the professional body of asylum doctors was beginning to assert itself.

To improve discipline and quality of care, attendants needed guidance for their demanding role. In 1841 Doctor Kirkbride, head physician at the Pennsylvania

Hospital for the Insane and an honorary member of the British asylum doctor's association, produced a manual for attendants; he later recommended that the association introduce a formal qualification.[39] Other pioneers were Alexander Morison at the Surrey Asylum, who began lectures in the 1840s on humane principles of care for the insane, and WAF Browne in Dumfries, who introduced the first training course for attendants in 1854. A silk purse, however, could not be made from a sow's ear. Men and women of suitable disposition were needed, as described by a French alienist in the *Journal of Mental Science*. Berthier, physician at Bourg Asylum, suggested that the job might be best suited to members of religious orders who had cultivated reflection, self-denial and generosity of spirit. He also emphasised obedience: only by following the doctor's orders meticulously would successful outcomes be achieved.

> He needs to apprehend not only the duties of his calling and the instructions given to him, but must realise his true position as one raising him above that of servant, or prison-warder, to that of controller and yet withal, the benefactor and friend of his patients.[40]

So much for the expectations of their masters, but what did attendants seek in return? Here was a stable job with board and lodgings, but the wages hardly compensated for the arduous work, strict discipline and limited time off duty. At the Warwickshire Asylum, for example, attendants worked from 6 a.m. to 8.30 p.m. They had one evening off per week, finishing duty at 6.30 p.m. There were no full days off, but they had two half days in each three-week period, finishing at 2.30 p.m.[41] Arriving late on duty incurred a fine. At night the attendants retired to their rooms with perhaps twenty minutes to read a book before the strictly applied 'lights out' at half-past ten. A good sleep could not be guaranteed due to their proximity to the patients, as in this description at the Lincolnshire Asylum:

> The attendant's bed room is placed between two of the dormitories, from which it is only separated by a swing door with perforated zinc panels, and the under attendant sleeps with the most tranquil patients in the third dormitory.[42]

Wards were staffed at night, the daytime attendants being required to deal with any nocturnal disturbance. Special duty was sometimes ordered to watch a disturbed or suicidal patient overnight. In 1861 medical superintendent Lockhart Robertson reported the benefits of a dedicated night staff introduced at the Sussex Asylum; he described the attendant's role in checking epileptic patients, changing the bedding of the incontinent, and if necessary removing a disruptive patient to a side-room.[43] Each side of the asylum was covered by one attendant, who visited each ward at two-hourly intervals. As urged by the Lunacy Commissioners, hourly visits later became standard. This was a gradual development; Devon Asylum, for example, managed without a night watch until 1878.[44]

Discipline was symbolised by uniform. Attendants on the female side wore dark petticoats with white aprons and cloth caps, the apparel of domestic service that evolved as the uniform of the nurse (by around the 1860s female attendants were ordinarily known as 'nurses'). The men wore a blue serge suit of jacket, waistcoat and trousers, with brass buttons and a number on the jacket sleeve. This smart but custodial garb was completed by a peaked cap bearing the county arms. Both male and female attendants had a bunch of keys and whistle dangling from a belt. Losing this set of keys was the swiftest route to the gate.

Bread and beer

In 1851 the Middlesex justices opened a colossal second asylum. Hanwell had become the largest in the country with over 1,000 patients, and despite Conolly's humanitarianism, an accumulation of chronic cases with no prospect of discharge inevitably detracted from the therapeutic atmosphere. Asylum managers were fighting a losing battle and had no choice but to extend buildings, which consequently bore little resemblance to the homely model of The Retreat. Proposals to double the size of Hanwell were rejected in favour of the new institution, built six miles north of central London. With its majestic Italianate frontage, crowned by an imposing dome with cupolas and campaniles, Colney Hatch was showcased at the Empire Exhibition as the most modern asylum in Europe. Although the grounds were mostly enclosed by a wall ten feet high, a stretch of railings alongside the railway allowed passengers to marvel at the great edifice.

Beside the gate lodge was stabling for the horses of magistrates and visitors. A straight drive led to the main entrance, with lanes left and right leading to the male and female wings and respective medical quarters. The chapel, with capacity for 600, was next to the reception lobby; to the rear was a vast hall with orchestra, waiting room, committee room, a dining room for magistrates, servants' quarters, steward's office, general store and dispensary, kitchen and bakehouse. The boilers for laundry and kitchen were served by a huge steam engine. An artesian well bored to a depth of 330 feet had a daily yield of up to 120,000 gallons of water. Off the corridor leading to the male side were the brewhouse and workshops of the tinman, plumber, upholsterer, printer, tailor, shoemaker, turner and carpenter; the laundry and sewing rooms were towards the female side. The farm had a livestock of twenty-eight cows, one bull, two calves, 152 pigs, forty sheep and seven horses.[45]

With the largest workforce of any asylum, Colney Hatch was staffed on the male side by a head attendant, fourteen senior attendants each in charge of a ward, and twenty-five ordinary attendants; on the female side the matron and deputy matron supervised forty-none attendants. The perambulatory night staff was supplemented by two stationary attendants on each side watching over a dormitory of epileptic and suicidal patients. Male wards were numbered 1 to 14, each holding thirty patients; female wards 15 to 32, with thirty-four patients. Each ward comprised a wide gallery, dining room, washroom, bathroom, scullery, store and two water closets, and rooms for attendants.

The Lunacy Commissioners soon found faults in the Colney Hatch fabric. They insisted that the asphalt ward floors be replaced by wooden boards. As the only corridor was on the ground floor, doctors passed through the gallery of each ward to get to the next, although such throughput may have kept attendants on their toes. In 1857, a less impressive aspect of Colney Hatch was presented in the *Quarterly Review*:

> Its façade, of nearly a third of a mile, is broken at intervals by Italian campaniles and cupolas, and the whole aspect of the exterior leads the visitor to expect an interior of commensurate pretensions. He no sooner crosses the threshold, however, than the scene changes. As he passes along the corridor, which runs from end to end of the building, he is oppressed with the gloom; the little light admitted by the loop-holed windows is absorbed by the inky asphalte paving ... the staircases scarcely equal those of a workhouse; plaster there is none ... whitewash does not conceal the rugged surface of the brickwork. In the wards a similar state of things exists: airy and spacious they are without doubt, but of human interest they possess nothing. Upwards of a quarter of a million has been squandered principally upon the exterior of the building; but not a sixpence can be spared to adorn the walls with picture, bust or even the commonest cottage decoration.[46]

Asylum patients were bathed on admission and weekly thereafter. During water shortages (a frequent problem before connection to the public water main), bathing was often postponed; in hot summers, body odour pervaded the wards. Reminders of the bathing regulations by the Lunacy Commissioners suggest that the practice of using the same water for several patients persisted. Patients' clothes and other belongings were removed on admission, including dentures, spectacles and jewellery. Items were recorded and stored, to be returned to the patient on discharge or to the family on death. Many patients arrived in workhouse clothing, which was returned on admission. Clothes were pooled for each ward, stamped with the ward number.[47] Mangled at the laundry, trousers and petticoats were often baggy or too short, and ill-fitting boots caused sores and a hobbling gait. The Lunacy Commissioners frowned upon regular use of a strong dress or jacket. Made of thick material and buttoned at the back, this was a form of restraint that had reappeared at Hanwell:

> The patients who destroy their dresses are put into strong canvas garments, bound round with leather and fastened with padlocks.[48]

Some individuality was permitted. Men were allowed a beard if they kept it clean, and female patients adorned themselves with their embroidery. Indeed, the *Quarterly Review* writer found the austerity relieved by patients:

> There is no more touching sight at Colney Hatch than to notice the manner in which the female lunatics have endeavoured to diversify the monotonous appearance of their cell-like sleeping rooms with rag dolls, bits of shell, porcelain, or bright cloth in the light of the window-sill. The love or ornament seems to dwell with them when all other mental power is lost.[49]

Moral management was in tune with the Protestant work ethic later described by Prussian sociologist Max Weber, but inmate labour was not only for salvation of lost souls; it was vital for the running of the asylum, and thus required incentives. Some inmates were deployed as ward workers, cleaning the dormitories and making beds, and performing basic care for other patients; for this they were rewarded with extra tobacco or a side-room. For patients, the most important factor in their quality of life was the character of their room-mates. Wards were categorised by conduct, as recommended by medical superintendent Robert Boyd at the Somerset Asylum:[50]

> It would be very desirable to make a subdivision amongst the curable and industrious patients, by separating those who are talkative and otherwise annoying from the quiet and convalescent, without placing them with the idle or mischievous class. The females are at present divided into five classes, of which the curable and industrious form the first class, or those who are chiefly employed at needlework or sedentary occupation, and amongst them are to be found many of the most useful patients but some of whom are excitable and at times very troublesome. The second class includes chiefly working patients who are employed in the laundry, kitchens and out of doors, consisting principally of cases of mania, monomania, and imbeciles, some epileptics, and perhaps a few convalescents. The third class consists of the noisy, violent, and those of disagreeable and destructive habits, including maniacs, some epileptics and idiots. The fourth class includes the chronic and infirm, cases of dementia, melancholia, some epileptics and imbeciles. The fifth class, the sick or infirmary patients.

The architect's plans for Worcester Asylum, which opened in 1852, featured one airing court for 'the violent and dirty', a second for 'the imbecile and epileptic' and a third for 'the tranquil and convalescent' (the latter was nearest the medical superintendent's office).[51] This organisation of living space motivated patients towards productivity and compliance.

While exasperated by cheeseparing authorities, the Lunacy Commissioners persistently sought to improve the lot of the powerless inmates of lunatic asylums. In the better institutions, male wards were furnished with a billiard table, and female wards with a piano. Reading materials were provided, although the Lunacy Commissioners often found nothing more interesting than discarded Latin school books. Patients' relatives were not allowed into wards, their visits restricted to an hour on Sundays and perhaps a midweek session, in the main hall. Patients' letters were scrutinised and destroyed by the medical superintendent if likely to cause trouble. Nonetheless, efforts were made to bring normality to asylum life. In summer there were walking parties and picnics; at Colney Hatch patients enjoyed annual outings to places such as Crystal Palace, the zoo and Epping Forest.[52] Winter gloom was lifted by a weekly dance, to the tunes of the asylum band. This rare opportunity for socialisation of male and female patients was first introduced at a pauper asylum by Samuel Hitch at Gloucester in 1841. The *Quarterly Review* contributor described how strict segregation of sexes was relaxed for the Monday ball at Hanwell:

> Shortly after six o'clock the handsome assembly room, brilliantly lit with gas, becomes the central point of attraction to all inmates, male and female, who are considered well enough to indulge their inclinations for festivity … In a raised orchestra five musicians, three of whom were lunatics, soon struck up a merry polka, and immediately the room was alive with dancers … At nine precisely, although in the midst of a dance, a shrill note is blown, and the entire assembly, like so many Cinderellas, breaks up at once and the company hurry off to their dormitories.[53]

Chapel services were attended by large numbers of patients and attendants. The chaplain had an important role in the asylum, with its emphasis on moral rectitude. As well as conducting services, he visited individual patients, and ensured adequate supply of prayer books in the galleries. In English asylums the chaplain was Anglican, but in counties with a large Irish immigrant population, a Roman Catholic priest also held services. A high proportion of patients were of non-conformist faith. At the Leicester Asylum, for example, alongside many Baptists, Congregationalists, Methodists and members of the Salvation Army were patients declaring themselves as a 'Calvanistic dissenter from the Trinity Chapel', a Russian Jew, a follower of the Latter Day Saints, a spiritualist and a 'free thinker'[54]. Religious enthusiasm was a common factor in asylum admissions, some patients being described in the Leicestershire records as 'ranters'. Many patients had a prominent religious theme in their madness, but ministrations were restricted. At Lancaster the chaplain needed permission from the medical superintendent to administer Holy Communion to any patient.[55] As the status of the chaplain declined, so did his remuneration.

The chaplain also offered spiritual guidance to staff, from supporting the homesick to giving succour to sick attendants, some of whom died in residence at the asylum. For their work, there was perhaps no more appropriate use of the Christian dictum 'All things whatsoever ye would that men should do to you, do you even so to them'.[56] Henry Hawkins, chaplain at Colney Hatch from 1854 to 1900, wrote several tracts for attendants on coping with life in the asylum:

> After your duty has been done on the ward and the time for rest has come, do not let your mind be in the wards still. Even though you may remain in the Asylum during the remainder of the day, do not let your thoughts and your talk be only about Asylum matters. Asylum gossip is poor conversation. Interest yourself in what is going on outside. Form a habit of reading if only a page everyday, some book of history, poetry, biography, wholesome fiction. Self-improvement should never be neglected.[57]

Some asylums had private patients, who were allowed to wear their own clothes in a relatively comfortable block separated from the main buildings. Such patients were a source of income, but in the rigid class structure of Victorian Britain, the county asylum was primarily for paupers. Sometimes a middle-class patient was admitted if no longer able to afford the fees at a private sanatorium. Certification instilled fear in affluent society, as the lunatic asylum was dreaded not least for the genteel person's exposure to the lower orders, as conveyed in Mabel Etchell's account of her transfer from a private asylum:[58]

> 'I am to go to a county asylum, Ada.' She burst into tears. 'Now that's what I call really wicked, amongst such a low set! O Miss, you will never be happy there … Don't you know they are all paupers, and you will have no drawing room, but all herd together in one ward, and anybody goes there, the refuse of the workhouses even! O Miss Mabel! And the food is only fit for pigs.'

The asylum diet was a morbid fascination to Etchell:

> On Saturdays there was a perfect army of meat pies all standing in rows, which, when cooked, were conveyed to the dining rooms in wheelbarrows or handcarts. I cannot say much of the quality of these dishes, for the crust was very heavy and indigestible, and wheat of course quality; but lunatics are supposed to be indifferent to the epicureanism of the table, and perhaps their internal organisation can relish deleterious substances more readily than sane people.

In most asylums the main meal of the day was served in the dining hall around one o'clock, after grace was recited. Cold meat, broth, suet pudding and pies were the staple fare, served with seasonal vegetables and washed down with table beer. Food for epileptic patients was cut into small pieces to prevent choking during seizure. Mealtimes were arduous for attendants in the sick and infirm wards, where many patients were spoon-fed. After the last meal of the day at five o'clock, a humble repast of bread and butter taken on the wards, there was a long wait until breakfast. The Lunacy Commissioners tasted the food on their annual visits, commenting in their reports. Great quantities of milk, eggs, pork and vegetables were produced, but it was insufficient for a rising population. Cheaper food was bought, and this was not always to satisfaction, according to Lunacy Commissioners' reports. Tinned corned beef from the Argentine, unpalatable to some patients, became a staple item in winter.

Working patients also had a light 'lunch' around 11 a.m., comprising bread and cheese with a half pint of ale. Produced on site, beer was supposedly nutritious and a safer beverage when water supply was prone to contamination. Male patients typically received a daily pint in the ordinary diet, plus another pint during breaks in the farm or workshops; women received half or two-thirds of the male ration. Attendants also received a share from the barrel. Buckinghamshire Asylum, for example, issued two pints daily to men, and one pint to female employees.[59] The staff brew was of superior strength and quality to that given to patients. Medical Superintendent Lockhart Robertson at the Sussex Asylum noted: 'The home-brewed beer of the attendants is the best I've ever tasted in an asylum.'[60] Until its removal by Doctor Hood in 1851, a hydraulic tap at the Bethlem Hospital was constantly accessible to attendants, according to Russell 'making the fat and formidable keepers look more satisfied than cheerful'.[61]

Rising tide

By the mid-nineteenth century it became clear that Britain was experiencing an escalation in lunacy. Despite its capacity of 1,250 beds, Colney Hatch was already being expanded in 1857, when it was subdivided into five departments each supervised by a matron or head attendant.[62] In the rapidly industrialised county of Lancashire, despite two additional asylums built at Rainhill and Prestwich, demand continued to outpace supply. By 1865 there were forty county and borough asylums, with a total population of 22,284. The London asylums were largest, with 1,945 inmates at Colney Hatch and 1,609 at Hanwell. Lord Shaftesbury (Ashley having succeeded to earldom on his father's death in 1851) argued that new asylums should not be built for more than 600 patients. In 1857 they were unable to prevent the Surrey magistrates adding 700 places to their asylum at Wandsworth; a site initially deemed sufficient for 500 patients would now hold 1,500. In 1864 three-storey blocks were hurriedly erected at Prestwich Asylum, increasing the capacity to over a thousand.[63] While they disapproved of extension of existing asylums, the Lunacy Commissioners accepted this as the lesser evil to severe overcrowding.

The cause of this 'great confinement'[64] has been much debated. For sociologist Andrew Scull, the asylum system was a conspiracy of capitalism and professional interests. His economic determinism and cynicism towards the medical profession has been criticised, yet his thesis is compelling: the increase in insanity seems inextricably linked to the rise in pauperism, and it created an expanding empire for doctors. Rapid transformation from a pastoral to urban society shattered the social equilibrium, and whereas close-knit communities had traditionally looked after their own kind, economic hardship and social breakdown left families unable to support the sick or disabled. Whenever industries wallowed in the troughs of economic cycles, destitution pervaded the masses. As Scull explained in *Museums of Madness*,[65] responsibility for unproductive members of society switched to an institutional mechanism of social control. The feeble-minded, frail elderly, epileptic and insane were a drain on relatives, and could not avoid the clutches of the Poor Law or the pauper lunatic asylum. The latter became the last resort for those of no use in the workhouse. The proportion of lunatics per 10,000 of population in England and Wales doubled from 12.66 in 1844 to 24.13 in 1870, an increase from 20,893 to 54,713 registered cases.[66] Although the largest asylums were in densely populated areas, the prevalence of lunacy was relatively higher in counties such as Wiltshire, where agricultural unemployment was rife.

An emerging feature of lunacy was the disproportionate increase in female patients. Women were more vulnerable to institutionalisation due to their economic disadvantage, and a condescending attitude of the male establishment towards the 'weaker sex', a notion given credence by the medical profession. In her book *The Female Malady*,[67] Elaine Showalter showed how male doctors imposed cultural ideas about 'proper' feminine behaviour. Governed by their reproductive system, women were regarded as primarily emotional, unlike the male agent of reason. Hysteria was the classic female madness. Once roughly equal by sex, the asylum population became skewed, as women consistently accounted for three-fifths of the total. Accordingly, there was more building on the female side, and the number of nurses overtook that of male attendants.

Although dozens of new asylums had opened since the 1845 Act, the workhouse continued as a staging post for the insane. In 1857 there were 14,393 lunatics in county asylums, and 6,800 in workhouses. To reduce costs, boards of guardians were inclined to avoid admission except for the worst cases, which required an order by a justice of the peace and a medical certificate. By 1865, 104 of the 688 workhouses in England and Wales had lunatic wards, but this arrangement was more for maintaining order than providing care. The oppressive workhouse environment contrasted with the spacious grounds and healthful regime in asylums. Boards of guardians were often criticised for their lack of proper facilities, most notably in a scathing supplement to the Lunacy Commissioners' annual report in 1859.[68] Inmates were forced to work, typically picking oakum, cutting their fingers on the tarred chunks of rope.[69] Lunatics were spared regular punishments such as birching, but physical restraint was common, and in one workhouse the mortuary was used for seclusion. The Lunacy Commissioners decreed that any lunatic restrained in a straitjacket should be removed to an asylum.

Despite its horrors, the workhouse had advantages over the asylum, as shown by Peter Bartlett's[70] research in mid-nineteenth-century Leicestershire. There was more shame in being certified as a lunatic than to be destitute, and a workhouse inmate was free to leave.[71] The Lunacy Commissioners did not oppose accommodation of chronic harmless cases in the workhouse, and sometimes they praised the care. In response to overcrowding, the Lunacy Amendment Act 1862 permitted transfer of such patients from the asylum. In the late nineteenth century Poor Law institutions continued to house about a quarter of the lunatics in England and Wales. However, asylum doctors frequently complained of being sent moribund senile patients, many of whom died within a few days of admission, while potentially curable cases languished in the workhouse. Furthermore, infirm patients sent from workhouses were unfit to work, detracting from the asylum's self-sufficiency.

In popular imagination, the asylum was a fearsome place, holding the wildest madmen at the outer margins of humanity. Such perceptions were occasionally challenged, as in this positive portrayal in the *Quarterly Review*:

> The furious maniac who arrives at Colney Hatch or Hanwell in a cart, or handbarrow, bound with ropes like a frantic animal, the terror of his friends and himself, is no sooner within the building which imagination invests with such terrors, than half his miseries cease. The ropes cut, he stands up once more free from restraint, kind words are spoken to him, he is soothed by a

bath, and, if still violent, the padded room … calms his fury, and sleep, which has so long been a stranger to him, visits him the first night which he spends in the dreaded asylum.[72]

Yet alleviation of acute disturbance did not always lead to recovery. In their report of 1844, the Metropolitan Commissioners had warned that if admission was delayed until lunatics were in an advanced state of insanity, the therapeutic potential of the asylum would decline. Finding that 85 per cent of the 4,356 in county asylums had been resident for more than two years, the report had expressed concern about the accumulation of incurable cases, and pressure was mounting. Ward 19 at Colney Hatch, for example, held ninety patients – three times its initial capacity.[73] As more patients were crammed into wards, the asylum became not a place of sanctuary but an environment hostile to recovery. The cure rate plummeted from around 15 per cent in the 1840s to 8 per cent in the 1860s.

In Scotland, meanwhile, the seven Royal Chartered asylums were rapidly becoming unfit for purpose. Lord Ashley had told the House of Commons in 1845 that Scottish facilities for lunatics were worse than anywhere in Europe or America. A Bill renewed the push for public asylums in 1848, but was rejected as an excessive burden on ratepayers. The catalyst for change was an American campaigner for the insane.[74] In 1855 retired schoolteacher Dorothea Lynde Dix came to Britain to recuperate after President Pierce rejected her proposal for federal aid for lunatics. Staying in Yorkshire with her acquaintance Daniel Hack Tuke, Dix heard that all was not well north of the border, and so she embarked on an *impromptu* tour. Although welcomed at Gartnavel, she had difficulty in gaining access to many private asylums, but saw enough to raise urgent concern with Lord Shaftesbury. A Royal Commission was rapidly established, and this led to the Lunacy (Scotland) Act 1857.

Scotland was divided into districts for lunacy administration, with each required to build an asylum for pauper patients. In 1863 the first district asylum opened at Lochgilphead for the county of Argyll. The first report of the Scottish Lunacy Commissioners[75] noted that the entire Highlands, far north and Hebrides lacked provision apart from a few cells in the basement at Inverness Infirmary and a pauper institution in Elgin. Opening in 1864, Inverness District Asylum had the largest catchment area in Britain. Casting a wide shadow, it took patients from outposts such as Barra or Benbecula, or from remote crofts in northern Sutherland or Caithness, who might never see their families again. For the populous industrial belt, much larger institutions were necessary. In 1875 the Barony Parochial Asylum, the first of several public asylums on the outskirts of Glasgow, opened at Lenzie with 400 beds; soon the second city of the Empire would be ringed by mental institutions. Renowned for its medical schools, Scotland produced many prominent alienists, who were libertarian in their management of asylums. A radical change was the 'open door' system; at Lochgilphead, for example, all wards were unlocked from 9 a.m. to 6 p.m.[76] Parole was widely permitted, and boarding out was introduced, whereby patients were taken into private dwellings for lengthy periods.

Such innovations were scarcely applied in England, where an overwhelmed system was stagnating. As expectations of asylum care lowered, so did staff morale. Working a ninety-hour week, attendants herded inmates to and fro in an unbending routine, with a constant jangle of keys as doors were locked and unlocked. The priority was containment, preventing escape or access to potential weapons or implements for suicide. Cutlery was counted before and after each meal. Patients were counted in and out of the airing court and dining hall, and frisked before returning from workshops. This did not prevent serious incidents, and sometimes a cunning patient slipped away, resulting in a fine for the careless or unfortunate attendant. Suicide was also seen as a failing of duty, but a determined patient could find the means. At the Sussex Asylum, for example, there were hangings from a towel in the bathroom and from a branch in the shrubbery, and fatal ingestion of poisonous berries in one case, and nails and shoelaces in another. Incidents led to tightening of procedures, reinforcing the custodial atmosphere. The patience of the most caring attendants was tested in wards of up to a hundred inmates. Living cheek-by-jowl in packed dormitories, patients squabbled and sometimes fought. Noting the number of black eyes during their inspection visits, the Lunacy Commissioners disapproved of too many refractory patients being placed in the same ward.

In 1863 a popular novel by Charles Reade presented a vivid account of asylum life. *Hard Cash: A Matter of Fact Romance* was not a fully accurate portrayal, drawing on earlier madhouse scandals, but it highlighted how patients had minimal contact with medical officers and were at the mercy of attendants. Responding to criticism that he had exaggerated abuse, Reade was unrepentant. In 1870 he wrote to the *Pall Mall Gazette* on 'How lunatics' ribs get broken':[77]

> Late in July 1858, there was a ball at Colney Hatch. The press were invited, and came back singing the praises of that blest retreat. What order! What gaiety! What non-restraint! Next week or so, Owen Swift, one of the patients, died of the following injuries: breast-bone and eleven ribs broken, liver ruptured.

Varney, a fellow patient, gave evidence against an attendant who Swift had annoyed, as Reade described:[78]

> Slater threw the poor man down, and dragged him into the padded room, which room then resounded for several minutes with a 'great noise of knocking and bumping about', and with the sufferer's cries of agony till these last were checked, and there was silence. Swift was not seen again till Saturday morning; and then, in presence of Varney, he accused Slater to his face of having maltreated him, and made his words good by dying that night.

After the accused walked free, Reade explained how attendants evaded discipline for physical abuse:[79]

The keepers know how to break a patient's bones without bruising the skin. The refractory patient is thrown down, and the keeper walks up and down him on his knees, until he is completely cowed. Should a bone or two be broken in the process, it does not matter much to the keeper: a lunatic complaining of internal injury is not listened to. He is a being so full of illusions that nobody believes in any unseen injury he prates about.

In his letter Reade offered a £100 reward to anyone producing evidence to convict whoever had killed a patient at Lancaster Asylum in 1863 (two attendants were imprisoned for seven years for manslaughter). Yet the impact of *Hard Cash* was not so much in raising concern at the treatment of patients, but in contributing to public fears of wrongful detention. This was an issue that dominated lunacy policy in the mid- to late nineteenth century. To the consternation of Lord Shaftesbury, the focus shifted from care of patients inside, to protection of people outside.

Shades of brown

Perhaps the only benefit of the swollen asylum population was the opportunity it created for classification of patients. There was no standard nomenclature for the various types of insanity, but by the mid-nineteenth century alienists were using similar categories in their reports, with diagnostic tables typically including:

* mania (acute or chronic)
* melancholia (acute or chronic)
* general paralysis of the insane
* dementia (primary, secondary, organic or senile)
* amentia (with or without epilepsy)
* epilepsy (acquired).

A typology of moral and physical causes was also applied, with differing indications for treatment. Physical aetiology included intemperance, privation, fever, sunstroke, head injury, epilepsy and idiocy; prognosis depended on the degree and permanence of the bodily insult. Moral insanity, a term first used by Bristol physician James Cowles Pritchard in his 1833 *Treatise on Insanity*, was a disorder of the passions often without impairment to the intellect. Monomania, whereby the sufferer presented madness in one faculty only, epitomised alienists' therapeutic optimism in the early years of the asylums. As explained by Samuel Tuke at The Retreat,[81] this partial form of insanity was fully reversible by moral management, but such a regime was becoming less feasible in the county asylum. Nonetheless, about one-third of patients with first episodes were discharged within a year; in the absence of specific medical interventions, probable factors in spontaneous recoveries were respite from a stressful situation, and the orderly asylum routine.

In staking their claim as medical experts, asylum doctors sought more effective physical methods of treatment. The pharmacopeia at this time was sparse, with no drugs of any lasting benefit. Natural substances such as opium and cannabis began to be replaced in the 1860s by chemical agents such as bromide of potassium and chloral hydrate. However, bromides required an increasing dosage to maintain the sedative action, causing confusion, and disturbed patients emerged from a fug with their delusions intact. The more powerful hyoscine, which could be injected for rapid action in a frenzied patient, was prescribed sparingly due to its toxicity. Crude sedatives were prescribed sparingly, as indicated by the Lunacy Commissioners' report at Colney Hatch in 1882, stating that merely thirteen male and fifty-one female patients in a population of over 2,000 were sedated at night, and only two men and seventeen women in daytime.[82] Drugs gradually became more prominent in asylums, as doctors experimented with various plant extracts and reported their findings in the *Journal of Mental Science*. Following the invention of the dynamo by Michael Faraday, electrical power was harnessed as a potential treatment, Turner Jones at Denbigh Asylum purchasing a galvanic shock machine in 1850.[83] In the 1860s, impressive results with the Turkish bath were recorded by Edgar Sheppard at Colney Hatch. The temperature for this prolonged bathing was adjusted for calming or stimulating effect. From 6 a.m. to 8 p.m., relays of six patients were taken to the bathing suite; thus half of the male population could be treated in one day.

The category 'dementia' (literally loss of mental faculties) included patients who would now be diagnosed as schizophrenic, for whom prospects were poor. The monotonous asylum regime was coloured by the delusional idiosyncrasies of such patients, as in this remarkable case described in the medical report for 1870 at Fishponds Asylum in Bristol:[84]

> Among the deaths was that of one of the celebrities of the Asylum, known to the Visitors as the 'Man with the Wheel'. He had been an inmate from the first opening of the establishment in 1861. His delusional ideas related principally to his having a wheel perpetually working within his body, the revolution of the wheel giving him no rest night or day so that he had not slept for many years. He said, 'Tomorrow at ten o'clock the wheel will stop and I shall be in Heaven'. As the Asylum clock was striking ten the following morning his Spirit took its flight.

Epileptic patients presented considerable management problems for attendants. Longitudinal records maintained by RG Rose at Colney Hatch revealed that in one year the 300-plus epileptics suffered an astonishing average of eighty *grand mal* fits daily (excluding nights when no records were made).[85] Leather caps were worn to prevent head injury during a convulsion. At Fishponds, medical superintendent Henry Stephens conducted a trial of concentrated juice of heathbed straw, a common plant that some French alienists had promoted as a cure for insanity; only one of the six epileptic patients showed any improvement.[86] Bromides could reduce the frequency and severity of epileptic seizures, but withdrawal effects were hazardous. With a minimal night watch, sometimes patients suffocated from a seizure in bed. *Status epilepticus*, a continuous series of major seizures, was a common cause of death in asylums. Physical labour was believed to be particularly important for epileptic patients, whose behaviour was unpredictable and sometimes violent, as in this medical commentary:

> Of all the various classes of cases found in our County Lunatic Asylums, none give so much trouble and annoyance, and have so little interest connected with them as the Epileptic Maniacs. If a black eye is given, it is sure to be by an Epileptic – if two patients fall to fisty-cuffs, the chances are, one or both Epileptics. If furniture is broken, the probability is, an Epileptic has been the cause of the mischief. Joined to this they are irascible to a degree, always dissatisfied, quarrelling, and fighting; they half fill the list of wet and dirty cases; they cannot be trusted day or night without fear of some contretemps occurring. Purgatives only relieve them for a time; anodynes are worse than useless; no remedy has ever been brought forward that has been productive of any permanent benefit.[87]

With a relentlessly rising population, medical superintendents argued that many patients were inappropriate for a lunatic asylum. Most undesirable was the suspected or convicted criminal, who could be removed to an asylum if believed insane. The Lunacy Commissioners frequently expressed concern about the impact of criminal patients on the therapeutic *milieu*, and in the House of Lords in 1852 Lord Shaftesbury proposed a state institution similar to Dundrum Central Criminal Asylum in Ireland. An Act was passed and in 1863 Broadmoor State Asylum opened for male and female criminal lunatics. Although necessarily built for security, with barred windows and inspection slits in the doors, no mechanical restraint was used. Moral management, however, faltered after several escapes and an attempted murder of the medical superintendent, who was struck by a large stone in a sling while attending the chapel with his family, inflicting a severe head injury.

Among the incurable patients in asylums were those with congenital mental defect, known as 'amentia'. The Lunacy Commissioners were concerned about mixing of mentally defective children with adult lunatics, and recommended special institutions for their care. Inspired by the work of French physician Édouard Seguin, philanthropic campaigners in the mid-nineteenth century believed that mentally defective children could be educated to live with a *modicum* of independence, In 1848 an idiot asylum was opened at Highgate in London by Reverend Andrew Reed, who was impressed by a training institution for 'cretins' (persons with mental and physical underdevelopment caused by an inactive thyroid gland) at Abendberg in Germany. About seventy 'pupils' were accommodated, with fees paid by their families, and a similar number were supported by charity at Essex Hall, a disused hotel nearby. The Highgate branch moved to a magnificent purpose-built institution with 500 beds at Earlswood in Surrey in 1855. Charitable institutions for the mentally defective of private and pauper classes were planned on a regional basis. In 1859 Essex Hall moved to become the Eastern Counties Asylum at Colchester; this was followed in 1864 by the Royal Albert Asylum for

Idiots and Imbeciles of the Northern Counties in Lancaster, and the Royal Western Counties Institution in Exeter; in 1866 Dorridge Grove Asylum near Birmingham catered for the Midlands.[88] The Scottish National Institution for the Education of Imbecile Children at Larbert in Stirlingshire opened in 1862. These institutions were primarily intended for children, but as few patients were discharged, adults soon accumulated. Meanwhile large numbers of mental defectives remained in lunatic asylums.

The Lunatic Asylums Act 1845 had given counties power to build separate asylums for chronic cases, and eventually two institutions of this type were built in London. The Metropolitan Poor Act 1867 made the maintenance costs of asylum inmates chargeable to a single body instead of the thirty boards of guardians in the city. The Metropolitan Asylums Board (MAB) was established to provide institutional care for incurable cases deemed inappropriate for workhouses but not needing costly asylum treatment. Two matching institutions were built at Leavesden to the north and Caterham to the south, each with a capacity of 1,600. They were designed on the pavilion plan, with three-storey ward blocks connected by corridors and overhead walkways; this layout allowed better classification, hygiene and ventilation.[89] Initially Caterham and Leavesden received a large number of patients from existing asylums: Colney Hatch offloaded 491 chronic cases. Although officially known as Metropolitan imbecile asylums, their intake was mixed. Of the 448 admissions to Caterham in its second year of operation, 137 were idiots or imbeciles, and 263 had dementia; more than half of admissions were aged over fifty.[90] Medical superintendent James Adam complained of parish officers often bringing in debilitated elderly people at death's door. For example, in 1875 a man aged seventy-six was sent by the Wandsworth and Clapham Union, only to die within a week.[91] The cemetery was filling fast. Despite these challenges, the MAB asylums were praised by the Lunacy Commissioners: children were placed in the care of a schoolmaster and his wife, and half of the adults were usefully employed.

The austere MAB asylums rose from sylvan countryside, lacking any hint of ornament to relieve the drab expanse of chalk brick. Meanwhile the Lunacy Commissioners, in their periodically updated guidelines on asylum construction, advised architects that superfluous features would not be authorised. As a pragmatic decision, the maximum number of patients per acre was increased from four to ten. With only one in eleven patients deemed curable in the Lunacy Commissioners' reports, county justices saw the asylum as a poor return on investment, and they were no longer prepared to spend ratepayers' money on palatial pretensions and therapeutic idealism. In 1877 the first lunatic asylum exclusively for chronic cases was opened by the Middlesex authorities at Banstead in Surrey, diverting 1,600 patients from Hanwell and Colney Hatch. Comprising four male and seven female blocks on the three-storey pavilion plan, Banstead Asylum received faint praise in a *Middlesex County Times* report: 'The interior is cheerfully coloured in three shades of brown.'[92]

Table 1.2 Size of county and borough asylums[80]

Year	Number of asylums	Number of patients	Average number of patients
1850	24	7,140	297
1860	41	15,845	386
1870	50	27,109	542
1880	61	40,088	657

Degeneration

Asylum labour was cheap. Among the 130 subordinate workers at Caterham Asylum were attendants of first and second class, with men's annual salaries starting at £25 and women's at £15; a solitary night attendant was paid £28.[93] The male head attendant received £44 and his female counterpart £32. Matron Emma Mosely received a relatively high £160, £10 more than the assistant medical officer, as she was effectively in charge of the female department. The chaplain was paid £200, the house superintendent (in charge of the buildings) £300, and at the top of the tree was Doctor Adam, on £500.

By the mid-1880s Caterham Asylum had three doctors, thirty-four male attendants and thirty-nine female attendants during daytime, and a night staff of six men and seven women, but the inmate population had grown to over 2,000.[94] In all asylums the strength of the workforce was failing to keep pace with the increasing number of patients.

To attract good staff, the Lunacy Commissioners urged visiting committees to improve working conditions. The medical superintendent's residence in the main building was replaced by a comfortable villa away from the bustle. This also freed space for patients: at Sussex Asylum accommodation for one doctor was sufficient for a dormitory for sixty-one patients![95] In some asylums semi-detached houses were constructed for the head attendant and matron, and cottages were built on the edge of the grounds for married charge attendants and their families. Such expenditure was justified by the need to retain valued workers in an unattractive vocation, while also promising future employment to their offspring. Loyal service was rewarded by medical superintendents, who ensured that deserving attendants received a small pot of money on retirement. The Lunacy Commissioners related staff continuity to quality of care, as in their report at Denbigh Asylum in 1880:

> The attendants seemed to us to be kind to the patients, and evidently much good feeling exists between them, and we have much pleasure in recording that out of the 30 attendants on the male side, not one has seen less than 2 years' service, and 24 have been here for more than 5 years.[96]

Tight discipline was a major factor in the high staff turnover. Of 567 attendants in the employ of West Riding Asylum between 1860 and 1880, ninety-one were dismissed.[97] Typical reasons for dismissal were drunkenness, insubordination, brutality and theft. Petty pilfering was inevitable, as hungry young workers were tempted to forage in an institution with large stores of goods; black markets were created in tobacco and other comforts. Gender segregation was tested by illicit rendezvous before the 10 p.m. curfew. Lockhart Robertson at Sussex Asylum exclaimed: 'This house is a hospital for the treatment of disease not a matrimonial agency office!' Illustrating the unbending regime, his successor Samuel Williams sent this memorandum to nurse Annie Rolset in 1872:[98]

> In January last I posted a notice stating that any nurse found with her light burning, after 10.15 p.m. unless for a good reason would be required to resign the situation. Notwithstanding this, you are reported as having a light burning at 10.23 p.m. on 20th inst. You state that this was an accident, and I am willing to believe you, and so will not enforce any threat of requesting resignation, but as such accidents show carelessness, I fine you 2/-.

In his patriarchal role, the medical superintendent kept a moral hold on asylum life, deciding what was best for patients and staff. According to Lord Shaftesbury and some asylum doctors, intemperance was the foremost cause of insanity. Undoubtedly alcohol was causing major problems among the masses. In 1874 beer consumption reached a peak of 34.4 gallons per head (four times the level drunk today).[99] Intoxication temporarily relieved harsh realities but exacerbated poverty, and fears of consequent moral decline spawned the Temperance Movement. To rescue the poor from squalor and vice, evangelical campaigners lobbied Parliament against 'demon drink', achieving shorter public house opening hours, and resumption of tax on beer. Medical attitudes to alcohol were changing. Doctors had tended to prescribe alcohol for a plethora of symptoms, but scientific evidence undermined its use as a stimulant.

Meanwhile, it remained a dietary fixture in asylums (see Figure 1.1). When the Cumberland and Westmoreland Asylum opened in 1862, no beer was provided to patients. Initially sceptical, medical superintendent Thomas Clouston found this experiment successful. A decade later at Carmarthen, George Hearder was the first to withdraw alcohol from the diet of an existing asylum.[100] Some asylum doctors were wary of Temperance zealots, but a *Journal of Mental Science* editorial in 1881 declared that beer was 'quite unnecessary in county asylums'.[101] In 1884 Daniel Hack Tuke[102] conducted a survey of all 129 mental institutions in Great Britain and Ireland, finding that half had eliminated alcohol except for medicinal purpose. While supporting this trend, Tuke sympathised with the view of the Lunacy Commissioners that to deny a poor man of a lifetime habit was lamentable. At the recently opened Banstead Asylum, which housed patients with no prospect of discharge, the daily ration was three pints of ale. For a while ale continued as an inducement for working patients. However, total abstinence was necessary for alcoholic patients, and this was awkward when beer was in general supply. Drunkenness in staff was also a problem. Some medical superintendents feared that withdrawal would cause great dissatisfaction in the ranks, but many

TABLE XV.

PAUPER DIETARY.

	MALES.	FEMALES.
BREAKFAST. EVERY DAY.	Milk Porridge or Coffee, with 4oz. of Butter for 12 Patients .. 1¼ pt. Bread .... 7 oz.	Tea, Coffee, or Porridge............ 1 pt. Butter for 12 Patients 4 oz. Bread .... 6 oz.
DINNER. SUNDAY.	Roast Meat, free from Bone .... 6 oz. Bread .... 4 oz. Vegetables........ 16 oz. Beer............. ½ pt.	.... 5 oz. .... 4 oz. .... 12 oz. .... ½ pt.
MONDAY.	Australian Meat .. 5 oz. Bread .... 4 oz. Vegetables........ 16 oz. Beer .... ½ pt.	.... 5 oz. .... 4 oz. .... 12 oz. .... ½ pt.
TUESDAY.	Currant or Fruit Pudding .... 16 oz. Beer ... ... ½ pt.	Rice Pudding .... 12 oz. Bread .... 5 oz. Cheese .... 1 oz. Beer.............. ½ pt.
WEDNESDAY.	Meat, in pie, free from Bone .... 5 oz. Pie Crust .... 10 oz. Potatoes, sliced .. 12 oz. Beer .... ½ pt.	.... 4 oz. .... 8 oz. .... 8 oz. .... ½ pt.
THURSDAY.	Boiled Meat, free from Bone .... 6 oz. Bread .... 4 oz. Vegetables........ 16 oz. Beer .... ½ pt.	.... 5 oz. .... 4 oz. .... 12 oz. .... ½ pt.
FRIDAY.	Irish Stew ... ... 1¼ pt. Bread .... 6 oz. Beer .... ½ pt.	.... 1 pt. .... 5 oz. .... ½ pt.
SATURDAY.	Rice Pudding .... 16 oz. Bread .... 6 oz. Cheese .... 1 oz. Beer .. .. ½ pt.	 Currant or Fruit Pudding .... 16 oz. Beer .... ½ pt.
SUPPER. EVERY DAY.	Bread.. .... 6 oz. Butter for 12 Patients 4 oz. Tea .... 1¼ pt. or Bread with Milk Porridge .... 1¼ pt.	Bread .... 5 oz Butter for 12 Patients 4 oz. Tea .... 1 pt.

The Stew, made of Australian Meat, Potatoes, Vegetables, &c.
Beer, 14 Gallons to the Bushel.
A Salad once a week.
Tea or Coffee instead of Milk Porridge on Rice Pudding Days.
Regular Workers in the Garden, Laundry, &c. have, at 11 a m., Bread, 4oz.
Cheese, 1oz., Beer, ½ pint; at 4 p.m., Beer, ½ pint.
Seed Cake twice a week in lieu of Bread and Butter.

Figure 1.1 Diet table at Nottingham Asylum, 1874[103]

workers (particularly nurses) were willing to accept cash in lieu. By the end of the decade beer was completely withdrawn at most asylums, with milk, tea or oatmeal water served instead. In the aftermath few problems were reported by medical superintendents, who observed better conduct in patients and staff.

Alcohol had already been strictly controlled in Scottish asylums, where Calvinist tradition was evident in the strict rules governing staff behaviour, as in this puritanical notice displayed at the Murray Royal Asylum:

> No Attendant, Servant, or other Officer, shall dance with any other Attendant, Servant or Officer.[104]

While withdrawal of beer was presented as morally virtuous, it also demonstrated the changing power dynamics in the asylum. From the visiting committee's perspective, the brewery was a profligate operation with the expense of malt and the labour in producing, storing and distributing the fermented brew. Yet more importantly, by defining alcohol as a drug, doctors were imposing their professional authority, as they slowly but surely wrested control from their lay employers. Every aspect of the asylum regime became a clinical matter, including the issue of restraint. Publicly, alienists were keen to distance itself from punitive use of strong clothing, manhandling by attendants and the padded room, but David Yellowlees of the Glasgow Royal Asylum warned in *The Lancet* in 1872 against sentimental aversion to restraint, which he regarded as a necessary contingency for the safety of patients and staff.[105] While opposing mechanical apparatus, Marriott Cooke at Worcester Asylum justified use of seclusion:[106]

> I am sure that there are some cases, both curable and chronic, which are greatly benefited by being isolated for a few hours in the quiet of a single room. I believe also that it is far better, in the interest of the patient himself, let alone that of the staff, to place him, when he is very violent, for a short time in a padded room, rather than to keep him in the day-room fighting and struggling with four or five attendants.

In 1877 a commission appointed by *The Lancet* on care and treatment of the insane, led by Joseph Mortimer Granville, reported on county asylums in the London area. They had found Hanwell resting on its laurels, no longer the progressive institution of Conolly's time. Aware that cases of abuse were tarnishing the reputation of asylums, the commission drew attention to the quality and supervision of attendants. The medical officers at the Surrey Asylum in Wandsworth were praised for their vigilance in making unannounced visits to wards at night as well as in daytime. The message was that whenever attendants were left to their own devices, patients were at risk.[107] Surveillance, however, was not the only solution to the problem. This untrained body of men and women needed positive instruction.

Although lectures for attendants had been initiated at several asylums, the instructors themselves had no specific qualification in their field of practice. Of course, asylum doctors were trained in medicine, which had recently developed a professional framework with registration by the General Medical Council.[108] However, medical officers in asylums had little prestige, and the label 'alienist' reflected their marginalisation in the wider profession. In pursuing their claim as a rightful branch of medicine, asylum doctors clung to the coat-tails of clinical science. In 1865 their organisation was renamed the Medico-Psychological Association (MPA). The Certificate in Psychological Medicine was introduced, later accredited by the General Medical Council, although this was not an obligatory qualification. Meanwhile the *Journal of Mental Science* was favouring articles on pathology and treatment over philosophical musings. Medical superintendents attended professional meetings, such as James Crichton-Browne's renowned *conversaziones* at the West Riding Asylum, which drew audiences from near and far.

By the late nineteenth century the aetiology of insanity had crystallised into two prominent theories, with significant implications for the work of attendants. The first entailed dirt and germs, with the conjecture that insanity resulted from continual breathing of air polluted by miasma, which were putative substances emitted by sick people or putrefaction. As knowledge of pathogens advanced in the late nineteenth century, the culprit changed to microbes. Laboratories were established at many asylums, where medical officers studied samples of blood, urine and sputum by microscope. The Lunacy Commissioners recommended routine autopsies, and in post-mortem examinations of the brain, any abnormalities in size or shape of ventricles were recorded. For the Holy Grail of a pathological cause of insanity, no visceral organ was excluded in the search for a putative toxin or lesion.

Asylums dealt with the pauper class, and the snobbery of medical superintendents is often apparent in their attitude to 'the great unwashed', whose filthy homes and foul habits explained not only their disproportionate mortality in fever epidemics, but also the prevalence of lunacy. Many patients suffered from tuberculosis, which doctors speculated as a late manifestation of insanity.[109] Mortality from this contagious disease was far higher than in the general population, and with so many people in close contact, it became obvious that the asylum was contributing to the problem. The Lunacy Commissioners urged isolation of patients with infectious disease in an infirmary ward, but this was not always feasible. On all wards there was great emphasis on bathing, fresh air, purgatives and scrubbing of floors and walls.

The second theory of insanity gained momentum in the light of Charles Darwin's theory of evolution, as presented in *The Origin of Species* in 1859. It was known that many patients had a family history of mental disorder, but this was now placed on a scientific footing. Henry Maudsley, son-in-law of John Conolly and leading alienist of the late nineteenth century, asserted the deterministic nature of insanity:

> Multitudes of human beings come into the world weighed with a destiny against which they have neither the will nor the power to contend; they are like the step-children of nature, and groan under the worst of all tyrannies – the tyranny of a bad organisation.[110]

While positing no distinct line between sanity and insanity, Maudsley explained that in severe forms behavioural symptoms tended to arise long before the underlying corporeal fault was apparent, as in senile dementia, general paralysis or epileptic mania.

> No one now-a-days who is engaged in the treatment of mental disease doubts that he has to do with the disordered function of a bodily organ – the brain … Insanity is, in fact, disorder of brain producing disorder of mind.[111]

Hereditary theory had a dramatic impact on care of the insane, as it undermined the assumption of moral treatment that nurture was the key to recovery. Darwin's contemporary Herbert Spencer coined the phrase 'survival of the fittest', expressing his view that the State should not interfere with the process of natural selection. The incapacitated, therefore, should be left to die to preserve the health of the population. There was growing fear in the Victorian Establishment of the urban poor 'outbreeding' the educated class, thwarting the progress of society and potentially leading to degeneration of the human species. Maudsley hinted at the eugenic ideas that would dominate psychiatry in decades to come:

> We should not willingly select for breeding purposes a hound that was deficient in scent, or a greyhound that was deficient in speed, or a racehorse that could neither stay well or gallop fast. Is it right then to sanction propagation of his kind by an individual who is wanting in that which is the highest attribute of man – a sound and stable mental constitution?[112]

Daniel Hack Tuke, a descendant of The Retreat founders, continued to raise the banner for moral treatment among professional peers. In 1882 Tuke and Bucknill wrote *Psychological Medicine*, the standard textbook for asylum practice, which reinforced the original ideals of the asylum system. However, therapeutic optimism was overturned by the pessimistic law of destiny. Moral treatment was a reasonable strategy for managing patients and encouraging desirable behaviour, but if character could not be changed, it was naive to expect insanity to be cured by kindness. The falling cure rate had demoralised asylum doctors, but now they had an important role in social betterment. Only segregation could arrest the trend of evolutionary reversal, and this became the primary function of the asylum.

As public attitudes hardened, stigma towards lunacy increased. The asylum placed the mad out of sight and out of mind, and its workforce was itself stigmatised. As Erving Goffman discovered a century later, nurses and attendants responded to this social adversity by pronouncing the distance between themselves and the patients. This was perhaps illustrated by their perpetuation of the legendary link between the Moon and madness. Such belief persisted in popular imagination – and among workers from rural shires steeped in folklore.[113] Eminent alienist Forbes Winslow[114] was intrigued by the insistence of the matron of his private asylum that patients were more agitated at full moon, and he considered the possibility that for a manic patient, a moonlit night could exacerbate restlessness.

In a crowded dormitory, other patients could have been provoked by an agitated insomniac. Most doctors, however, dismissed the notion outright. Here can be seen a sharp contrast between the scientific pretensions of asylum doctors and the cultural norms of attendants.

In our story so far, first-hand accounts from attendants are like hen's teeth. Twentieth-century retrospect tended to portray these workers as an indolent, ignorant and subservient workforce, but historian Ann Digby admonished her peers for overlooking the hidden dimension of asylum care.[115] Scull and other sociological critics have viewed the organisation and management of asylums only as a means of social control, but such portrayals deny the benevolence and compassion in the system. Despite the adversities of asylum work, there is evidence of humane practice and positive relationships with patients. Some ambitious alienists may have been more interested in polishing their own and their institution's reputation than in raising the status of their underlings, but undeniably attendants were the backbone of the asylum, and myriad reports applaud their sterling service. A major omission, however, was the views of attendants themselves. Approaching the turn of the century, their voices would soon be heard.

Notes

1 Crossley FH (1949): *The English Abbey* (3rd edition).
2 Knowles D (1969): *Christian Monasticism.*
3 Bailey MD (2003): *Battling Demons: Witchcraft, Heresy, and Reform in the Late Middle Ages.*
4 Broedel HP (2004): *The Malleus Maleficarum and the Construction of Witchcraft: Theology and Popular Belief.*
5 Ball P (2006): *The Devil's Doctor.*
6 The brain, according to Aristotle, existed to cool the blood and passions; it had no role in thought processes.
7 Borde A (1542): *A Compendious Rygment or a Dyetry of Helth.* Quoted by DH Tuke (1882): *Chapters in the History of the Insane in the British Isles.* 27. Andrew Borde was an English physician, traveller and writer (c1490–1549).
8 Andrews J, Scull A (2001): *Undertaker of the Mind: John Monro and Mad-Doctoring in Eighteenth-Century England.*
9 Skultans V (1979): *English Madness: Ideas on Insanity 1580–1890.*
10 Andrews J, Scull A (2001).
11 The most famous member of the Clapham Sect was Sir William Wilberforce, abolitionist of slavery.
12 Digby A (1985): Moral treatment at the Retreat, 1796–1946. In *The Anatomy of Madness: Essays in the History of Psychiatry; Volume II: Institutions and Society* (eds WF Bynum, R Porter, M Shepherd).
13 Foucault M (1967): *Madness and Civilization: a History of Insanity in the Age of Reason.*
14 Custodial ideas were spatially apparent in Stafford, where the asylum was built next to the gaol.
15 The visiting committee of the Surrey Asylum, for example, included a man of the cloth, a banker and brewer. See Ian Lodge Patch (undated, c1985): *Springfield: a Short History.*
16 Jones K (1993): *Asylums and After: a Revised History of the Mental Health Services: From the Early 18th Century to the 1990s.*
17 Jones K (1972): *A History of the Mental Health Services.* 76–77.
18 Haslam J (1809): *Observations on Madness and Melancholy* (2nd edition). 26.

19   Hammond JL, Hammond B (1939): *Lord Shaftesbury.*
20   Ellis WC (1838): *A Treatise on the Nature, Symptoms, Causes and Treatment of Insanity, with Practical Observations on Lunatic Asylums.*
21   Smith LD (1988): Behind closed doors; lunatic asylum keepers, 1800–60. *Social History of Medicine.*
22   Lodge Patch I (c1985).
23   Ellis (1838). 194.
24   Kent County Mental Hospital (1927): A retrospect 1828–1927. In *A History of Oakwood Hospital 1828–1982.* 5–6.
25   Ellis (1838). 149.
26   Ellis (1838). 195–196.
27   Conolly J (1847): *On the Construction and Government of Lunatic Asylums and Hospitals for the Insane.* 117.
28   Hanwell Asylum. *Rules and Regulations for Keepers.* Appendix in Ellis (1838).
29   Browne WAF (1837): *What Asylums Were, Are, and Ought to Be: Being the Substance of Five Lectures Delivered Before the Managers of the Montrose Royal Lunatic Asylum.* 151.
30   Lodge Patch I (c1985). 7.
31   Eager R (1945): *The Treatment of Mental Disorders (Ancient and Modern).*
32   Ellis WC (1838). 275
33   Gardner J (1999): *Sweet Bells Jangled Out of Tune: a History of the Sussex Lunatic Asylum, Haywards Heath.*
34   Michael P (2003): *Care and Treatment of the Mentally Ill in North Wales 1800–2000.*
35   Michael P (2003). Nichols saw the responsibilities as too onerous and was replaced by Shaw, an older nurse who ran the female side for fifteen years.
36   Michael P (2003).
37   *Asylum Journal* (1854): Suicide of Dr Grahamsley, Medical Superintendent of the Worcester County and City Pauper Lunatic Asylum.
38   Crammer J (1990): *Asylum History: Buckinghamshire County Pauper Lunatic Asylum – St John's.*
39   Nolan P (1993): *A History of Mental Health Nursing.* 57.
40   Berthier M (1863): Qualifications of attendants upon the insane. *Journal of Mental Science.* 57.
41   Spratley VA, Stern ES (1952): *History of the Mental Hospital at Hatton in the County of Warwick 1852–1952* (2nd edition).
42   Palmer E (1854): Description of the Lincolnshire County Asylum. *Asylum Journal.* 74
43   Robertson CL (1861): Some results of night staffing at the Sussex Lunatic Asylum. *Journal of Mental Science.*
44   Eager (1945).
45   Hunter R, Macalpine I (1974): *Psychiatry for the Poor: 1851 Colney Hatch Asylum – Friern Hospital 1973: a Medical and Social History.* 364. Farm figures for 1st January 1856.
46   *Quarterly Review* (1857): Lunatic asylums. 364
47   Hamlett J, Hoskins L (2013): Comfort in small things? Control and agency in county lunatic asylums in nineteenth- and early twentieth-century England. *Journal of Victorian Culture.*
48   *Quarterly Review* (1857). 365.
49   *Quarterly Review* (1957). 365.
50   Somerset County Asylum (1852): *Fourth Report of the Somerset County Asylum for Insane Paupers 1851.*
51   Hall P (1991): The history of Powick Hospital. In *The Closure of Mental Hospitals* (eds P Hall, IF Brockington).
52   Hunter R, Macalpine I (1974).
53   *Quarterly Review* (1857). 375.
54   Lockley D (2011): *The House of Cure: Life within the Leicestershire Lunatic Asylum.* 21.

55 Walton J (1981): The treatment of pauper lunatics in Victorian England: the case of Lancaster Asylum 1816–1870. In *Mad Doctors and Madmen: the Social History of Psychiatry in the Victorian Era* (ed. A Scull).

56 Matthew. *Holy Bible*, vii:12.

57 Hawkins H (1870): *Work in the Wards*. 11.

58 Etchell M (1863): *Ten Years in a Lunatic Asylum*. 292. A fictional but faithful account of the experience of madness and the asylum, from the perspective of the genteel class.

59 Buckinghamshire County Pauper Lunatic Asylum (1866): *Twelfth Annual Report on the Buckinghamshire County Pauper Lunatic Asylum*.

60 Robertson CL (1860): A descriptive notice of the Sussex Lunatic Asylum. *Journal of Mental Science*.

61 Russell D (1997): *Scenes from Bedlam: a History of Caring for the Mentally Disordered at Bethlem Royal Hospital and the Maudsley*. 51.

62 Hunter R, Macalpine I (1974). In 1861 the head attendant was given a new title in the asylum hierarchy: 'inspector'.

63 *The Builder* (15 July 1865): Lunatic asylums.

64 A term coined by Michel Foucault, whose historical work *Madness and Civilisation* attributed institutionalisation to society's inability to cope with unreason.

65 Scull A (1979): Museums of Madness: the Social Organization of Insanity in 19th Century England.

66 Jones K (1972).

67 Showalter E (1987): *The Female Malady: Women, Madness and English Culture, 1830–1980*.

68 Commissioners in Lunacy (1859): *Twelfth Annual Report of the Commissioners in Lunacy for England and Wales*.

69 A pitiful existence recalled in Jennifer Worth's *Shadow of the Workhouse: the Drama of Life in Post-War London*. Workhouses were deterred from providing more fruitful occupation as this would threaten local employment.

70 Bartlett P (1998): The asylum, the workhouse, and the voice of the insane poor in 19th-century England. *International Journal of Law and Psychiatry*.

71 Until 1871, when Poor Law guardians were given statutory powers to detain any workhouse inmate.

72 *Quarterly Review* (1857). 354

73 Hunter R, Macalpine I (1974).

74 Robinson ADT (1989): Dorothea Dix: when will we see your likes again in Scotland? *Psychiatric Bulletin*.

75 Commission of Lunacy for Scotland (1859): *Report of the Commission of Lunacy for Scotland 1857*.

76 MacCammond I (1963): *The Argyll and Bute Hospital 1863–1963*.

77 Reade C (1899): *Hard Cash: a Matter of Fact Romance*. London: Chatto & Windus. 623–624.

78 Ibid.

79 Reade C (1899). 625. The term 'keeper', while officially discarded, may have lingered among staff.

80 Jones K (1993). 116.

81 Tuke S (1813/1964): *A Description of The Retreat: an Institution near York for Insane Persons of the Society of Friends* (revised edition).

82 Hunter R, Macalpine I (1974).

83 Michael P (2003). Shocks were applied to the body, not the head as in the later development of electroconvulsive treatment.

84 Early DF (2003) *'The Lunatic Pauper Palace': Glenside Hospital Bristol 1861–1974*. 14–15.

85 Hunter R, Macalpine I (1974). .

86 Early DF (2003).

87 Duckworth Williams SW (1864): *On the Efficacy of the Bromide of Potassium in Epilepsy and Certain Psychical Affections*. 4

88 Digby A (2013): Contexts and perspectives. In *From Idiocy to Mental Deficiency: Historical Perspectives on People with Learning Difficulties* (eds D Wright, A Digby).
89 As at St Thomas' Hospital in London, a design approved by Florence Nightingale.
90 Metropolitan Asylum District (1872): *The Second Annual Report of the Committee of Management of the Metropolitan Imbecile Asylum, Caterham, Surrey 1871–72.*
91 Malster R (1994): *St Lawrence's: the Story of a Hospital 1870–1994.* A more resilient patient was Samuel Gibson, one of the last survivors of the Battle of Waterloo, who had sustained permanent brain damage on being struck by a French hussar's sabre, died in 1891 at the remarkable age of 101.
92 Quoted by Cowper-Smith F (1977): Banstead Hospital. *Nursing Times.*
93 Metropolitan Asylum District (1872).
94 Malster R (1994).
95 Gardner J (1999).
96 Quoted by Michael P (2003). 86.
97 Russell R (1988): The lunacy profession and its staff in the second half of the nineteenth century, with special reference to the West Riding Lunatic Asylum. In *The Anatomy of Madness: Essays in the History of Psychiatry; Volume III: The Asylum and its Psychiatry* (eds WF Bynum, R Porter, M Shepherd).
98 Gardner J (1999). 215.
99 Best G (1979): *Mid-Victorian Britain 1851–75.*
100 McCrae N (2009): Beer in mental institutions: a historical perspective. In *Beer in Health and Disease Prevention* (ed. VR Preedy).
101 *Journal of Mental Science* (1881): Asylum reports for 1879.
102 Tuke DH (1885): On alcohol in asylums, chiefly as a beverage. *Journal of Mental Science.*
103 Nottingham Asylum (1875): *Nineteenth Annual Report of the State of the United Lunatic Asylum for the County and Borough of Nottingham, 1874.* 33.
104 Murray Royal Asylum (1869): *Special Regulation anent Dancing.*
105 Andrews J (1997): A failure to flourish? David Yellowlees and the Glasgow School of Psychiatry, part I. *History of Psychiatry.*
106 Cooke EM (1895): A review of the last twenty years at the Worcester County and City Lunatic Asylum, with some conclusions derived therefrom. *Journal of Mental Science.*
107 Granville JM (1877): *The Care and Cure of the Insane: Being the Reports of the Lancet Commission on Lunatic Asylums 1875-6-7, for Middlesex, the City of London, and Surrey, and a Review of the Work of Each Asylum.*
108 The register for practice was introduced by the Medical Registration Act 1858.
109 Koch discovered the bacillus in 1882.
110 Maudsley H (1870): *Body and Mind: an Inquiry into their Connection and Mutual Influence, Specially in Reference to Mental Disorders.* 43.
111 Maudsley H (1874): *Responsibility in Mental Disease.* 226.
112 Maudsley H (1874). 276.
113 McCrae N (2011): *The Moon and Madness.*
114 Winslow FB (1867): *Light: its Influence on Life and Health.*
115 Digby A (1985).

2 Professionalisation, or organised labour

The Devil made work for idle hands. As attendants waited to be posted to the new male ward blocks at the Bristol Asylum at Fishponds, they ruminated – and conspired. Their temporary redundancy was caused by a strike by the builders, and when the wards belatedly opened, the attendants decided to take their own action. They withdrew their labour, but were swiftly dismissed, leaving only the head attendant and one man who had been off sick. Replacements were appointed, and life went on as before. In his annual report, the medical superintendent regretted the incident as a uniquely troubling experience.[1] This was late-Victorian Britain, and as the working class began to assert itself as a political force, there would soon be more 'trouble at t'mill'.

Colonies of confinement

While society showed little interest in conditions in asylums for either patients or staff, there was much concern about wrongful detention. In 1884 the case of Georgina Weldon caused a storm. Weldon was an eccentric, litigious lady who sued Forbes Winslow for false imprisonment when he sent her to an asylum. Aided by the secretary of the Lunacy Laws Amendment Association, she overturned her detention and won damages. The judge highlighted the folly of a system where any person could make an order for any other person, supported by two doctors who might have no experience in lunacy, but who would happily sign and collect their fee. Riding on public opinion, Lord Milltown proposed a motion in the House of Lords to ensure nobody could be committed to an asylum without a legal judgment. Lord Shaftesbury vehemently opposed this, fearing that early treatment would be deterred. After fifty-six years as a Lunacy Commissioner he resigned in 1885. When the Billwas withdrawn he reverted to his role, and died later that year still at the helm. Nobody had worked harder or achieved so much for people afflicted with mental disorder, but the tide had turned.

The year 1890 is stamped on asylum history. The Lunacy Act, which would prevail for seven decades, was passed towards the end of a dramatic century when Great Britain had emerged as the most powerful and advanced country in the world. In a cast-iron social hierarchy, this statute cemented the role of the asylum as a place of confinement. With Social Darwinism to the fore, institutional segregation was a means of preventing procreation of tainted stock. A pronounced boundary was drawn between the sane and insane, the latter regarded as suffering from a permanent rather than reversible malady. Whereas previous lunacy law arose from concern at the plight of the mentally disordered, the 1890 Act appeared primarily to protect society. In a legalistic system, certification required a magistrate's order, supported by medical evidence. After so many cases of people being wrongfully 'put away', the admission procedure was tightened to leave little doubt that anyone sent to an asylum was truly mad. The 1890 Act increased the administrative burden, as observed by medical superintendent TA Chapman at Hereford Asylum:

> The effect of recent legislation has been to insist on a large increase of certificates, reports, signing and countersigning of orders, checking and counterchecking everything in an elaborate system of book-keeping, more time being taken in recording and certifying what you have done than there is time left to do it in.[2]

The Lunacy Act was not intended to increase admission to asylums, but the deluge of insanity continued. In 1844, the year before statutory provision of county asylums, there were 20,893 registered insane persons in England and Wales, from an overall population of 16 million (a rate of 1.27 per 1,000). By 1890 this had increased to 86,067 certified lunatics in a population of 29 million (2.93 per 1,000). At the beginning of the twentieth century the rate was rising towards 4 per 1,000.[3] Most of the original county asylums had doubled or trebled in size. The relatively small asylums in agricultural counties, where unemployment had become a serious problem, were inundated by the flood of insanity. The Wiltshire Asylum in Devizes, which had opened in 1852 and had 289 patients by the end of 1854, had grown by 1899 to a population of 863. The Devon Asylum, originally built in 1842 for up to 400 patients, was extended several times; in 1884, following erection of blocks containing 200 beds, the register of inmates lengthened to 832. A plan to build an asylum for northern Devon was rejected, but there was some reprieve on the opening of Plymouth Asylum in 1891. Soon, further extension was forced upon the county council, and completion of several new blocks in 1907 raised the population over 1,000.

To the chagrin of medical superintendents, asylums were being used for the least desirable recipients of Poor Law administration: 'the dying, the demented and the dangerous'.[4] Yet despite the impersonal and degrading conditions, people were kept alive who might otherwise have perished in slums. Alongside increasing admissions, the number of patients was growing due to their greater longevity. Boarding out contracts were made by asylums with no more room to spare in stairwells or corridors. Patients were sent to the cheapest destination, sometimes hundreds of miles away, inhibiting contact with families. Lunacy Commissioners and asylum administrators could see no light at the end of the tunnel.

Architecture of segregation

The Local Government Act 1888 passed control of lunatic asylums to the new county and borough councils, and membership of visiting committees passed from magistrates to elected councillors. The London County Council (LCC) faced a Sisyphian task in containing metropolitan lunacy. Existing institutions were taken over: Hanwell, Colney Hatch, Banstead and the planned asylum at Claybury from the justices of Middlesex; and Cane Hill from Surrey.[5] Clearly these five asylums were insufficient. The Lunacy Commissioners urged immediate attention to this pressing concern: at Colney Hatch they passed from one ward to another through galleries filled with additional beds. Meanwhile the Lancashire Asylums Board, with its five massive asylums at Rainhill, Whittingham, Prestwich, Lancaster and Winwick, was planning its sixth institution at Whalley. The Glasgow Lunacy Board, serving the rapidly expanding second city of the Empire, was in dire need of accommodation. Completed in 1897, the Glasgow City Asylum at Gartloch was an awesome red sandstone structure of the Scottish baronial style, its lofty twin towers piercing the north-eastern horizon.

Having purchased land at Bexley Heath in Kent, the LCC Asylums Committee engaged leading asylum architect George Hine. Asylums of the mid-nineteenth century onwards had been built on the echelon plan, with a staggered succession of blocks projecting outwards from the administration block, served by a lengthy zig-zag corridor. This layout, like a broad arrow, was exemplified at the huge Menston Asylum in Yorkshire. To limit the distance from the central facilities and for the medical superintendent, head attendant and matron on their daily rounds, the ward blocks were built close together, but this created in a brick maze. Deficiencies in asylum architecture had been compounded by repeated extensions that starved wards and airing courts of fresh air and sunlight. Following in the footsteps of his father TC Hine, whose designs included a grand private asylum in Nottingham, George Hine's first commission had been for the Nottingham Borough Asylum at Mapperly. At Claybury Asylum, commissioned by Middlesex but opening in 1893 under LCC, he first applied his novel plan for the construction of pauper asylums. This compact design, utilitarian and sparing of ornament, resulted in his appointment as consulting architect to the Commissioners in Lunacy.

Hine's layout comprised double-decked ward blocks on a crescent arching around the administrative and ancillary core, circumnavigated by a curved corridor. The needs for segregation and surveillance were fulfilled while affording each ward fresh air and an unimpeded view of the grounds. The symmetrical design was slightly distorted by extra blocks on the more populous female side. A birds-eye view would confirm female territory by the positioning of the laundry, while the workshops, boiler house and water tower were located within the male quadrant. The kitchen, dining hall and recreation hall were located centrally. Modest stonework was afforded for the administration building, but overall the structure was a monotonous expanse of red brick and barred sash windows, relieved by yellow brick patterning. Three-storey wards were deemed too imposing, and after Claybury were generally avoided. Tunnels followed the course of corridors above, housing the heating and water pipes, and later the electrical wiring. At Claybury, the tunnels totalled ten and a half miles in length. Complying with the Lunacy Commissioners' guidelines, the chapel was positioned away from the main buildings, with a pleasant aspect near the main drive. Wards were intended for no more than fifty patients.

After Bexley Asylum opened, pressure continued to mount on the LCC Asylums Committee. At Cane Hill, blocks for an additional 900 patients were erected. In 1896 LCC purchased the Horton Manor estate at Epsom, a site of over a thousand acres fifteen miles from London. In haste a cluster of corrugated iron units was installed around the old Manor House for 400 harmless female patients. These buildings were approved by the Lunacy Commissioners on a temporary basis only, initially for seven years (they remained in use until the hospital closure a hundred years later). Cheap construction, however, could be hazardous. At Colney Hatch a temporary building of wood and iron was erected in 1896 to house 320 women. The Lunacy Commissioners warned of the combustibility of this structure, and were vindicated in 1903 when the building caught fire. Fifty-one lives were lost – the worst disaster in British asylum history. Patients were 'charred to embers, not one of the corpses being recognisable'.[6] Apparently some had resisted rescue attempts. No nurses were badly hurt, and their courage in saving 269 patients was acknowledged.

The first substantial asylum to be built on the Epsom site was Horton. In a visit to North American asylums, an entourage of LCC had been impressed by an institution in Maryland, which mostly comprised separate villas connected by open corridors. Horton opened in 1902 mostly to Hine's standard design but with villas for five hundred patients, and corridors walled on one side but open to the gardens (the damp and chilly air of Epsom was not appreciated and the corridors were later enclosed in brick). Meanwhile, a new type of institution was being built on the northern edge of the site, through patients' labour.

A priority of asylum design at the turn of the century was classification. Detached villas were built at asylums old and new, separating working and convalescent patients from those with acute or chronic mental disturbance. Housed in buildings of domestic design, patients of the farm or laundry villa were rewarded with extra food rations and relatively comfortable facilities. Many of the most productive patients were epileptic. The West Sussex Asylum in Chichester opened in 1897 with a male epileptic block of fifty-four beds, and a female block of sixty-six beds (amounting to a quarter of the total);[7] such patients were expected to contribute to the upkeep of the institution. LCC made use of the physically agile and stabilised epileptic men for the construction of their third institution at Epsom. Ewell Epileptic Colony opened in 1903 as a series of forty-bedded, single-storey units, each run by a married couple, with a central dining and recreation hall. Working on a large farm to serve the whole estate, the 326 colonists were warned that breach of discipline or idleness would result in their transfer to a less desirable institution.[8] Two more conventional asylums were later built: Long Grove opened in 1907; West Park was nearing completion in 1914 but was abandoned in wartime and did not eventually open until 1924. A sixth asylum

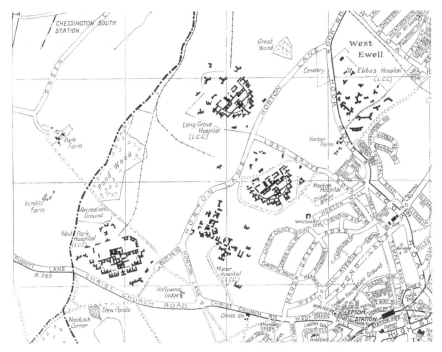

Figure 2.1 The Epsom Cluster[9]

never left the drawing board. At its peak, the Epsom Cluster housed 10,000 of London's mental patients (see Figure 2.1).

Cure rates had plummeted since the mid-nineteenth century, and as the asylum became a permanent residence for the majority of patients, a more homely environment was urged by the Lunacy Commissioners. In Hine's heyday, in 1897 a deputation from the Edinburgh District Lunacy Board toured mental institutions in France, Germany and England to inform the design of a new institution for the city. While admiring some features of the recently built asylums at Cane Hill, Claybury and Menston in Yorkshire, they found the enormous block-and-corridor structures oppressive. A better impression was made by Alt-Scherbitz in Germany, where domesticated units were spaced widely apart, with gardens instead of exercise courts, and lanes rather than connecting corridors. The visitors observed a soothing effect on patients, contrasting with the colossus of Claybury:[10]

> The collection of so many lunatics together under one roof has a somewhat terrifying effect upon the visitor. It may well be imagined that it has a similar effect upon the patients. The day-rooms, the airing yards, the dormitories, are all crowded. In the wards for quiet patients there are 106 in one room. All the blocks are upon the locked or closed plan, little freedom of ingress or egress being permitted to the patients.

The Edinburgh authority subsequently built Bangour Village, the first large mental institution in Britain of wholly villa layout. In England, the core structure was retained in new asylums, but it was accepted that for the cure rate to improve, new cases must not be contaminated by the refractory wards. At Netherne in Surrey, and the East Sussex Asylum at Hellingly, the admission block was placed away from the main block, with several villas scattered around the estate.

Meanwhile the older asylums with their unplastered walls, open fires and limited ventilation, were gradually upgraded – largely thanks to the perseverance of the Lunacy Commissioners on their annual inspections. The custodial appearance was softened by replacement of iron-framed windows with wider wooden sashes. Ernest White, on becoming medical superintendent at the City of London Asylum at Dartford, wrote of major structural improvements to bring the institution up to date: unnecessary walls were dismantled and wider windows were installed. Believing that dimly lit, confined living space contributed to agitation and violence, White remarked:[11]

> We have realised that the more glass you have in an asylum the less you have broken.

Electrical lighting and internal telephone lines were installed, and a gas central heating system offered great improvement over the existing fires, as explained by the Committee of Visitors at Hereford Asylum:

> The abolition of open fires would certainly have many advantages. Apart from the coal saved, which might go far to reduce or even meet the cost of new apparatus, the saving of mess and dirt in the woods would be an almost incalculable blessing. We are supplied with a very dusty coal, and the wards are often thick with the flying ash, and everything is densely covered by it. The danger of open fires to patients by setting fire to their clothes, &c, is by no means trivial; an accident of this sort occurs in some Asylum or other every year, so far our turn has not yet come.[12]

The introduction of electric light, central heating and the telephone were significantly labour saving for nurses, who had hitherto tended the fires, lit and extinguished the many gaslights on each ward, and made frequent errands to relay information. Due to inadequate sanitation in wards, general bathrooms were installed on male and female sides, each fitted with several baths and showers and walls of white–glazed brick. An operating theatre was installed in some institutions, particularly where the local general hospital refused certified patients for surgical operation. Yet as the asylum was being modernised, the sheer weight of numbers reduced care to a dehumanising economy of scale. The continued expansion required a growing workforce of nurses and attendants.

Brain over brawn

In 1895 medical superintendent Marriott Cooke reflected on how the standard of attendants had improved since the opening of Worcester Asylum:

> The general tone and capability of the attendants and nurses has been decidedly raised during the past twenty years. As a whole, they are more intelligent, more suited to bear responsibility, of better physique, and are more attentive and considerate to their patients. These improvements have been brought about because a better class of persons have been attracted to the service, by the extension of leave of absence, by the consideration shown for their comfort in the way of food and accommodation, and in the providing of good cottages for the families of the married men, by a more complete system of training, and by the increase that has been made in the number of the staff in proportion to patients.[13]

A major contribution to the progress of mental nursing was the *Handbook for the Instruction of Attendants on the Insane*. In 1884 the MPA had commissioned four of its members to produce this hardbound volume, which became popularly known as 'the Red Book'. Its first part covered basic anatomy and physiology, first aid, hygiene, physical diseases, and the principles and practice of nursing care. The second half focused on mental nursing: basic psychology, mental disorders and symptoms, nursing care of the insane and general duties in the asylum. Throughout its sixty-four pages the book emphasised unquestioning obedience to medical authority.

In 1889 the MPA appointed a committee to devise a course of training for attendants, with a curriculum based on the handbook. This would be the first national qualification for nurses in Britain. After two years of training, an examination was sat for the award of the Certificate of Proficiency in Nursing the Insane. For the first examinations in May 1891 there were thirteen candidates from Birmingham Asylum and six from nearby Rubery, and a total of sixteen from Scotland (eight from Stirling District Asylum, five from the Royal Asylum in Perth, and three from Kirklands in Boswell).[14] From then onwards, examinations were held in May and November at whichever asylums put candidates forward. Nurses and attendants were examined in three stages: a written paper, an oral paper and a practical examination, all marked by the medical superintendent and an external assessor from the MPA.

The MPA qualification was promoted by medical superintendents keen to educate and improve the quality of care. Acknowledging that most attendants had never sat a written examination, Alfred Miller at Hatton Asylum directed them first to the oral examination of the St John's Ambulance Association, whose first aid manual was known in asylums as the 'Black Book'. Miller persuaded the visiting committee to award an annual supplement of a sovereign to those gaining the MPA certificate, and by 1896 forty of the nurses were qualified, including all but one of the charge attendants.[15] By 1899 almost every asylum was participating in the scheme, and each year about six hundred certificates were awarded, to a roughly equal number of men and women.[16]

As well as their heavy practical duties, attendants and nurses were now expected to be nimble with the pen. However, in most asylums there was no tangible reward for passing the MPA examination; nurses attended lectures in their own time, with textbook and examination fee at their expense. The MPA certificate was not necessary for promotion, which depended on years of service. Few members of the nursing staff sat and passed the examination at Devon Asylum; the medical superintendent attributed this to workers being of the 'uneducated class', and also poor retention: in 1892 merely forty-nine of the ninety-two nurses and attendants had worked there for more than two years.[17] To increase the number of trained nurses, more suitable recruits were needed.

The MPA appointed a registrar to maintain a record of certificate holders, and to strike off any nurses dismissed for serious misdemeanour. A qualified nurse sent packing by the medical superintendent would thus be subjected to public disgrace, leaving no chance of their employment in another asylum. This is how professions maintain standards and public confidence, but at the time it may have appeared to nurses as an unnecessary ratchet to an already tight disciplinary framework. The first case reported to the registrar was a nurse from the Fife and Kinross District Asylum in Cupar sacked by Doctor Turnbull:

> Lillian Ames passed the Attendants' Examination in May last and obtained the usual Certificate but has since been discharged from service here on account of Becoming inefficient in her work and having behaved roughly to one of the patients. I understand that such a circumstance ought to be reported to you in order that such notice of it may be taken on the Register as you may find necessary.[18]

In the 1890s matrons and nurses in general hospitals were striving for professional status. Florence Nightingale had introduced nurse training in 1860 at St Thomas' Hospital, but nurses who had gone to the trouble of gaining the certificate were disillusioned by the lack of reward. The British Nursing Association, initiated in 1887 by Mrs Ethel Bedford Fenwick, had a primary objective to gain state registration of nurses. When this body introduced its own register as an intermediate step, mental nurses did not want to be left out in the cold.

Mindful of the adverse working conditions and educational deficits of asylum staff, in 1895 two medical officers and head nurse Laura Evans at Berrywood Asylum in Northampton founded an association for attendants and nurses. Also involved was writer and ex-nurse Honnor Morten, who described the aims of the Asylum Workers' Association (AWA):[19]

1   To improve the status of asylum nurses and attendants
2   To secure the sympathy and co-operation of all those interested in institutional work and efforts, and
3   To provide a home of rest and nursing for those engaged in asylum work

The first president Sir Benjamin Ward Richardson proclaimed in his opening address:

> We want to improve the attendants: many of them have not been properly trained. We want them to be masters of their own work.[20]

Among the doctors on its council was Sir James Crichton Browne, a prominent member of the MPA. At a meeting of the Royal British Nurses' Association (now with royal patronage) in 1895, Crichton Browne persuaded the quorum to pass a resolution to incorporate MPA certificate-holders on a separate part of the proposed register. This caused a furore. According to Mrs Bedford Fenwick, who had not attended the meeting, 'no person can be considered trained who has only worked in hospitals and asylums for the insane'; furthermore, 'considering the present class of persons known as male attendants, one can hardly believe that their admission will tend to raise the status of the association'. [21]Today some general nurses continue to express scepticism about whether the work of the casually-dressed mental health nurse is 'real nursing', but in the late nineteenth century the contrast between mannered middle-class women in prestigious teaching hospitals and the uneducated asylum attendant was stark. Furthermore, the general hospital nurses' cause was associated with the Suffragette movement. [22]

Ironically, mental nursing had beaten general nursing to introduce a national training scheme, and the argument that asylums could not teach physical care was mistaken, as trainees spent time in an infirmary ward and nursed sick and paralytic patients. However, mental nurse training had weaknesses. The MPA qualification was achievable within two years, a year less than in general hospitals. Some asylums continued to issue their own certificates for nurses and attendants. At Berrywood Asylum a three-year course had been instituted in the 1880s, and Laura Evans saw this as superior to the relatively short and superficial MPA training:

> So long as the Medico-Psychological Association is satisfied with the present system of training, so long will such Associations as the British Nurses' sneer and look down upon the Mental Nurse, and I am not surprised either, for I should certainly think twice before engaging some of those that have received its certificate.[23]

The MPA appealed for uniformity. For equity with general hospital nurses, three-year training became standard, and the few remaining independent courses were discontinued. Alienists were proud of their achievement: a national qualification for nurses under medical control. Training was transforming asylum nursing, according to William Bevan-Lewis, medical superintendent of the Wakefield Asylum, although he raised the old adage that 'a little learning is dangerous'.

> The nurse, instead of being the modest handmaiden of science, becomes obtrusive in her desire to exhibit her knowledge … This tendency to fussy

prattling places her at a great disadvantage when contrasted with the calm, self-controlled, silent behaviour of the accomplished nurse, who is ever ready to afford information when requested.[24]

Asylum workers unite

By the late nineteenth century, the working class was gaining collective strength through trade unions, which represented a tenth of the male adult workforce. Having plenty to complain about, asylum workers would have taken interest in conflict elsewhere, such as the Great Dock Strike of 1889, and a mass walkout by young women at a match factory. Unlike other large bodies of workers, however, nurses and attendants had no union to fight their corner. Working conditions were onerous, and discipline unforgiving. With fourteen-hour shifts, six days a week, nurses had little leisure time. The day off was often spent in bed due to exhaustion. Living quarters were hardly amenable to anything but sleep: typically a small, windowless room shared by two nurses, who used the patients' basins and lavatories at the end of the ward. Working a shorter shift, the night staff had only one day off in a fortnight. Their life was governed by the telltale clock, which allowed the medical superintendent to see at a glance whether hourly rounds of the wards had been completed.

To leave the institution a pass was required. Attendants handed their keys to the hall porter, and went to the front or rear lodge gate where their time of departure was recorded. The asylum was prohibitive for romance or sexual liaison. As fastidious matrons showed as much interest in the behaviour of their nurses as of the patients, courting was a continuous obstacle course. Every night couples gathered alongside the perimeter wall; nurses stole a few minutes embracing their lovers but did not push their luck too far. To return after the ten o'clock curfew risked summary dismissal. A sympathetic gate porter would allow some leeway, but by ten past ten the gate was shut for the night. An intrepid nurse might scale the wall or find a gap in the fence and sneak into the building, but would need to retrieve his or her keys in the morning.

Gender segregation was pronounced, as in rules issued by the Berkshire Asylum Visiting Committee:[25]

> No male Attendant, Servant, or Patient, shall be allowed to enter the female side. Any Attendant or Servant transgressing this rule, unless a satisfactory explanation be given to the Superintendent, shall be immediately dismissed. No male person, excepting the Medical Officers, Engineer, and Chaplain, shall at any time have keys admitting them to any of the female wards.

Many probationers changed their minds on a career in mental nursing due to the restrictions placed on their personal lives. Nurses found to be pregnant were dismissed; these may have included probationers who did not know that they had conceived at time of appointment, but it is also possible that clandestine couplings occurred within the institution. Women were barred from marriage. Men could marry with permission of the medical superintendent, but this was normally limited to charge attendants, who were then eligible for a cottage in the asylum estate (where available). The temptation of intimacy was not always heterosexual. On the female side an occasional sacking offence was sexual relations between nurses; Gittins[26] suggested that mental nursing may have attracted lesbian women at a time when homosexuality was taboo.

Despite a growing membership, the AWA was an underpowered vehicle for improving working conditions. Its bulletin *Asylum News*, launched in 1897, presented an upbeat view of asylum life. There were news items; series such as Biblical references to insanity and practical tips on nursing care; lists of nurses awarded the MPA certificate; appointments, retirements and obituaries; reports of cricket and football matches, concerts and fêtes; and correspondence. Constrained in tone, *Asylum News* tended to support the establishment, with editorial comment that 'discipline is as essential for the organisation of the asylum as that for an army'.[27] In 1898 it featured the presidential address by Sir James Crichton Browne. Describing himself as an 'asylum worker' with over thirty years of experience, Crichton Browne advised members that medical guidance was necessary for the stability of the organisation, and to prevent degeneration into trade unionism.[28] Dismayed by the course demeanour of fellow attendants, a reader complained that values espoused by the bulletin were not always evident:[29]

> Would it not be advisable to try to alter the state of affairs as regards conversation or language among some attendants themselves which points to this Christian spirit being sadly lacking? ... It is anything but edifying!

While never a radical publication, *Asylum News* maintained pressure for a nurses' pension, and it provided a forum for debate (see Figure 2.2). Contributors raised issues such as the excessive hours of duty:

> It is to my mind unreasonable that a man or woman should be compelled to work for 80 hours a week in the company of insane people. Yet, I am told that in many places the hours worked exceed that number, the weekly leave being, in a few cases, half a day weekly and a full day once a month, which means that on average 87 hours are worked.[30]

The convention that applicants for promotion be trained in general nursing was criticised, some senior nurses having been appointed with no experience in caring for the insane.[31] George Robertson, medical superintendent of the Stirling District Asylum at Larbert, drew rancour for introducing female nurses to male wards to care for bedridden, paralytic and epileptic patients on the basis that men lacked the caring skills.[32] Letters from male attendants portrayed this as the thin end of a wedge, threatening men's jobs (female nurses were cheaper). A medical superintendent in another asylum reported that a similar scheme had been abandoned, but no reasons were given in *Asylum News*[34] (as well as resentment, perhaps there was fraternising among staff).

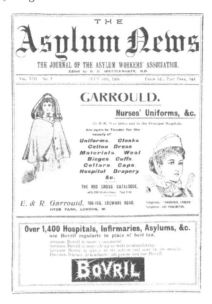

Figure 2.2 An edition of *Asylum News*[33]

Fearing the spread of labour disputes to asylums, the MPA and visiting committees approved of the AWA, whose activity could be contained. With a committee dominated by doctors, ladies and clergy, the AWA had good intentions, but it was a paternalistic rather than truly representative organisation, as illustrated by this comment by an associate member in *Asylum News*:

> The Asylum Workers' Association has always kept before its members the fact that by no other means than by unswerving loyalty to the authorities, self-sacrificing interest in their work, and a full appreciation of all that is implied by the word 'status', can they ever hope to gain their proper place amongst the bands of workers who are performing valuable service to the community.[35]

The AWA was ineffectual against pennypinching local authorities, and it failed to secure a pensions clause in Lunacy Bills in Parliament in 1899 and 1900. Disillusioned by a paltry membership of three thousand, an attendant at an Irish asylum appealed for greater participation of asylum workers in the work of their representative body:[36]

> It is not very creditable to Asylum Workers to allow the excellent work that has been done to lag for lack of membership. There are supposed to be 20,000 Asylum Workers in the United Kingdom and if this little army were to band themselves together and join with one voice for the demand of the many reforms urgently needed, and for the elevation of those to whose care are entrusted the nursing of the insane, victory would be in sight.

Staff grievances were not readily heard in a hierarchical regime where each member of staff from laundress to medical superintendent knew their place. The latter, as stated in the Berkshire Asylum rules, 'shall have paramount authority in the Asylum, subject to that of the Visiting Committee',[37] Medical superintendents needed a strong character to run their institution efficiently, and little tolerance was shown for underperforming or insubordinate workers. Indeed, discipline was the main cause of the high staff turnover at asylums. The Scottish Board of Commissioners in Lunacy reported that of 2,292 staff leaving asylums in 1906, 1,248 were dismissed for misconduct. In that year Horton Asylum was embroiled in a public scandal. Nine men were sacked for theft of asylum goods, including the chief clerk, who was the highest-paid officer after the medical superintendent; he and three others were found guilty at the Assizes. The court expressed the view that the asylum was grossly mismanaged, and Doctor Bryan was forced to leave by the visiting committee.[38]

Always alert

As patients were classified by behaviour rather than by disease or prognosis, the asylum was not run like a hospital: this was moral rather than medical management. Compliance was rewarded, while truculent patients were sent to the noisiest and least comfortable wards, where staff ruled by brute force. Instances of physical restraint were carefully recorded for inspection by the Lunacy Commissioners on their annual visits, as in this example in the Wiltshire Asylum Report for 1891:

> Four women have been restrained by gloves or sleeves for medical reasons for 2487 hours, and on 488 occasions; and 2 men and 3 women have been wet packed on 3 and 13 occasions, and for 31 and 74 and-a-half hours respectively.[39]

Nurses bore the brunt of violence. In their annual report for 1906, the Lunacy Commissioners reported a nocturnal rebellion in a ward accommodating some dangerous male patients.[40] A noisy patient had been moved to a side room but continued to disturb the others, causing much agitation. The assistant night inspector rang the emergency bell and his superior came to his aid. The offending patient enticed his peers to direct their aggression at the attendants, using their chamber pots as weapons. In a *maelstrom* of projectile pottery, the inspector's left arm was broken, and two attendants who had been raised from their sleeping quarters sustained severe cuts to their heads. The riot was eventually quelled without any patients being hurt. Sometimes doctors and inspectors were attacked. In 1901 the *Asylum News* reported an attempted murder of a Lunacy Commissioner:[41]

> In course of an official visit to the London County Council Asylum, the Heath, Bexley, a patient in Ward J2, who had secrete d the broken blade of a table knife, apparently with a view to attacking a member of the Visiting Committee to whom he had taken a dislike, struck Mr Urmson with this

weapon, inflicting a would some two inches in length over the jaw. Happily Mr Urmson had just turned his head, and so the blow was prevented from falling upon the neck as the assailant had intended.

Drugs were increasingly used to maintain order. Campbell Clark, medical superintendent of Lanark County Asylum, described various options for calming the restless patient:[42]

(1) Opium is a certain hypnotic; but it is not one to be trifled with. It disturbs secretory and digestive functions where pushed indiscriminately. Given in moderate doses, it quickens mental activity, unless the patient discourages thought and allows himself to fall into a passive state which paves the way for its soporific action.

(2) Chloral is also a certain hypnotic, but here also great care requires to be exercised, especially in weakness of the heart, respiratory disease, and disease of the blood vessels. It may produce headache, drowsiness, sickness, loss of appetite, and disorder of the liver, but it is safer than opium.

(3) Bromide of potassium is a very safe hypnotic; it rarely disturbs the digestive and hepatic functions, but given alone it is physically depressing if continued for a long time, as the dose requires to be increased. When sleeplessness is acute, and accompanied by excitement, a combination of bromide of potassium with chloral is a much more effective hypnotic.

(4) Paraldehyde, but for its offensive taste and smell, would be a favourite hypnotic, and it is especially indicated where cardiac or general weakness contra-indicate the exhibition of depressing remedies. It is best administered in drachm doses with *Tr Aurantii*, which helps to mask its most unpleasant taste and smell.

(5) Sulphonal has been much in favour for a time, but after the novelty of its use wore off, it fell rather into disrepute. The chief reasons assigned to this were its insolubility, its irritant effects on the gastro-intestinal tract, and the occasional occurrence of haemato-porythrinuria after its use. I have still faith in sulphonal, and if caution is manifested in its use, it will be found both safe and reliable. As it does not dissolve well, its action is necessarily slow. It is best given after mixing with boiling milk, which is afterwards allowed to cool a little, or it may be given in alcohol. The urine should be examined frequently, and the faintest tinge of red, or a darkening of its colour, should be taken as a warning to stop the medicine.

(6) Hypodermic treatment – morphia, hyoscyamine, hyoscine, have been tried. In ordinary practice, as in relieving pain in order to procure sleep, morphia is an excellent expedient, but the injection must be given by the doctor himself. In the treatment of acute mental excitement, the hypobromate of hyoscine is prompt and reliable.

For extremely disturbed patients, the anaesthetic agent chloroform was sometimes used.[43] Patients were simply 'knocked out' by these drugs, which had no lasting benefit.

Perhaps the most effective guard against violence was occupation. Around half of the patients were put to work, many in the farm and gardens. In the past, farming was second nature to male patients, many of whom were agricultural labourers, but in an increasingly urban, industrialised society, fewer patients were experienced in this work. Nonetheless, every morning large gangs of patients assembled to toil in the fields or tend livestock. Recreation was another means of pacifying the inmates. Articles in *Asylum News* promoted music for patients, with remarks on how blank faces came to life in response to an air of Bach or a popular music hall song. Concert programmes suggest competitiveness in the range and difficulty of tunes performed by the asylum band. No expense was spared on the decorative outfits of bandsmen, who would not have looked out of place at a military parade. The most notable asylum musician, albeit before he found fame, was Edward Elgar. Son of a Worcester church organist, in 1879 Elgar became bandmaster at Powick Asylum, where he conducted public concerts on Sunday afternoons, and was paid for each composition of a polka or waltz (later known as 'the Powick Pieces'). Elgar later acknowledged that 'the experience of writing for a haphazard and often unpredictable combination of instruments was a valuable discipline for an aspiring composer'.[44]

Preventing escape was a priority of nurses and attendants. Most patients who succeeded in fleeing the asylum were returned on the same day, but if a lunatic could remain at large for the statutory period of fourteen days, certification was rescinded. Nurses were punished for such lapses, as noted in a Wiltshire Asylum Report of 1900:

> One male patient escaped during the year, and was absent sixteen hours. Though the patient was aided by a fog, his attendant, in charge of a small working party, contributed to his escape by want of supervision, and, as a punishment, he was called upon to pay the expenses attending the recapture.[45]

Despite the threat of pecuniary loss, nurses could not always prevent a determined quest for freedom. Harald Hewitt described his successful escape from the Dorset County Asylum in 1914, after the medical superintendent had denied his request for discharge:

> Decided to make the attempt to escape this evening if circumstances were favourable. For two days past I had secreted bread and butter, put it in my pocket during the meal, and then later wrapped it in paper. I commandeered a towel and some blind cord, and tied this in the towel, in a neat bundle. The window of a room off the corridor had a thick belt of laurels immediately underneath it. On pretext of going to the washroom, which was at the end of the corridor, I covered this bundle with a loose towel taken from my room, went quickly into the room which was then empty, and threw the bundle out

of the few inches open at the bottom of the window into the laurels, noting which window it was, so that I could find it after dark.

So many attendants about that I had no chance till quarter to seven. Went down to the washroom with a small bundle under my coat. I slipped quickly across the corridor to the coal locker opposite (this was usually locked). The bottom part of its small window was locked like the other windows, to open only a few inches. But the top part of the window, though working very stiffly, opened further, as I had noted when I was able to get into the locker, unobserved, once before. I just had room to struggle out of it with my bundle. A kind of patient who is allowed a lot of freedom, and helps in the garden, unfortunately, was just passing at the moment. 'Hi, where you going to?' he shouted two or three times.[46]

Hewitt was not to be denied.

A wild rush through a thicket of laurels, down a steep hill, over an iron fence, over a fallow field, through a gap in the hedge, over a gate into a field of rather thin wheat; ran 30 or 40 yards out into the wheat and then lay down flat. Seven o'clock struck after. The alarm was soon given, and I saw two or three attendants in pursuit. They passed round the edge of the field where I was lying, but fortunately they had not seen me. It was after nine when I heard some attendants returning. I remained lying down till I heard the asylum clock strike ten. At ten I got up and went half-way to the buildings. Again hearing voices I crouched on the fallow a little longer.[47]

At nightfall Hewitt continued with his meticulous plan.

At 10.30 a drizzle of rain came on, and I went into the grounds, and to the summer house. I went towards the building to the boot room to try to get my boots. I had to escape in indoor shoes; as a precaution we were not allowed boots inside. But there was a light on in one of the attendants' rooms not far from it on the ground floor, shining out across the lawn. I had to wait till this light went out, sheltering in the summer house till after eleven o'clock. The window of the boot room only opened a few inches at the bottom. When we came in from exercise I had seen that it was not bolted. I had put my Burberry coat on a peg close to the window, and had previously bent the iron peg down so that it would slip off easily. My boots, fastened together, were under it on the seat. I managed to reach both with my arm, without using the stick I had taken from the croquet lawn. Then in drizzling rain to the window, out of which I had thrown the towel containing bread and butter. Dived into the thick laurels and found it, the old clergyman in the next room singing and shouting to himself. Back to the summer house, put boots on. Very glad of the Burberry, as it was raining steadily. Through the plantation belt, over the iron fence, down two or three fields, waded across a good-sized stream, as I could find no bridge, and got to the Sherborne Road about midnight. I walked about forty miles, and by six the next evening I reached the house I was making for.[48]

Evading capture until his certification became null and void, Hewitt then sailed to Canada, leaving his attendants to count the cost in deductions from their wages.

Patients were regularly visible to people living in the vicinity of the asylum. The gentry of Epsom in Surrey, horrified by the multiple mental institutions in their midst, were regularly confronted with their new neighbours. Walking parties of patients, led by attendants with peaked cap and whistle, trudged along the lanes, often visiting a local public house on their way back. After several incidents of drunkenness, nurses were admonished and there would be no more pitstops at The Cricketers. At Horton Asylum there was an embarrassing incident with a young German woman. Married with two children, her husband rarely visited and in 1905, a year after her admission, the patient escaped, only to be returned to the asylum three hours later. Six months on, she was found to be pregnant. She refused to divulge the imminent father to an interpreter brought from Colney Hatch Asylum. The baby was immediately handed to Camberwell Board of Guardians, who demanded maintenance payment from LCC. After the birth, the patient admitted to a brief sexual liaison with an unknown man on Horton Lane.[49]

Tainted stock

By the late nineteenth century it was obvious that the existing system for treatment of mental disorder was ineffective and unsustainable. Prominent alienists such as David Yellowlees of the Glasgow Royal Asylum began to argue for a division of mental institutions into a well-equipped hospital for acute cases and a less costly depository for the incurable. The latter already existed at Caterham, Leavesden and Banstead, and Lancashire Asylums Board built Winwick Asylum specifically for chronic cases. In 1903 the MAB opened Tooting Bec Asylum for the elderly insane, with a small number of mentally defective patients deployed as ward workers. Certification could be avoided for people with senile dementia, while reducing demand on LCC asylums. With a suburban location near the new underground line, Tooting Bec was convenient for visitors, but Poor Law credentials were manifest in its forbidding multi-storey blocks.[50]

The idea of a hospital for acute mental illness was encouraged by visitors to the psychiatric clinics of Germany and Austria. Attached to university medical schools, these clinics were centres of postgraduate training for psychiatrists and neurologists. Many cases were assessed and treated as outpatients. Significantly, the doctors decided who was admitted – not lawyers. Henry Maudsley, the leading name in psychological medicine in Britain, saw the German model as the future of psychiatry. Then in private practice in London, Maudsley pledged funds for a modern hospital for treatment of acute mental disorder. A condition was to locate this within a four-mile radius of Charing Cross, for close links with teaching hospitals and to encourage research. In 1908 LCC approved his plan and a site was chosen opposite King's College Hospital at Denmark Hill. By 1915 construction was complete, with six wards and a total of 144 beds, although the original purpose was temporarily waylaid by war.

A Postgraduate Diploma in Psychological Medicine was introduced in 1911 (this qualification did not become a requirement until the 1930s), but to genuinely improve their professional status, asylum doctors needed to develop their theory and practice. The search for a pathological cause of insanity was boosted by the opening of a central laboratory for the LCC asylum service at Claybury. Meanwhile, diagnostic practice advanced as British asylum doctors became aware of the work of Prussian psychiatrist Emil Kraepelin. Despite the efforts of Daniel Hack Tuke and others in the late nineteenth century to instil a standard nosology, diagnoses remained vague and inconsistent, and the term 'mania' was liberally applied. Kraepelin delineated two primary forms of insanity: manic-depressive psychosis and dementia praecox. A clear division was made between reactive states (neurosis) and severe insanity (psychotic disorders): whereas the former was potentially reversible, the latter was less fertile territory. As laboratory research had failed to identify a responsible pathogen, conditions such as dementia praecox were increasingly attributed to hereditary fault.

As well as intractable cases of mental disorder, asylums accommodated people with all kinds of social or physical problems. Medical superintendents expressed concern at the influx of alcoholic, epileptic, petty criminal and feeble-minded patients – all certified lunatics but not necessarily insane. Yet while the asylum was being used indiscriminately, the need for institutionalisation of such people was not doubted. The popular idea that women were admitted to asylums simply for bearing an illegitimate child may be exaggerated, but certainly there were female patients of low intellect who had been sexually exploited and unable to care for children born out of wedlock. Such women were blamed for spreading venereal disease, and for contributing to degeneration of the human stock.[51] Medical superintendent CS Morrison at Hereford Asylum commented on the need for certified institutions for these damsels in distress:[52]

> Early segregation and colonisation of imbeciles, weak-minded criminals and moral perverts, are expedients earnestly advocated, to largely control reproduction of their kind. It is, therefore, a short-sighted economy to encourage or to too readily acquiesce in weak-minded mothers shuffling off Union premises only again to re-enter later for the same reason … There appears to be given, in the opinion of the Commissioners of Lunacy, sufficient discretion, in the form of certification under the Lunacy Act 1890, to prevent the hapless mother going on indefinitely in her hapless way.

Eugenics pervaded Establishment thinking: it was feared that as the least fit members of society had the most offspring, soon they would become the majority. By 1906 there was an estimated 149,628 mental defectives in England and Wales, and this was seen as a major social problem.[53] An important development in the history of institutional care was separate provision for people with congenital mental defect. Despite the regional network of institutions established in the mid-nineteenth century, thousands of mentally defective people were housed in asylums. Although the Idiots Act 1886 had distinguished mental deficiency from insanity, the Lunacy Act 1890 defined a lunatic as 'an idiot or a person of unsound mind'.[54] The presence of young physically and mentally disabled children in institutions for the adult insane was criticised by medical superintendents and Lunacy Commissioners alike.

In 1904 a Royal Commission on the Care and Control of the Feeble-Minded was established, chaired by the Earl of Radnor. In its report four years later, the Radnor Commission recommended that mentally defective persons of all grades should be provided with lifelong care. The model for institutional care was the Gheel Colony in Belgium, where groups of people lived in separate villas under supervision but with minimal medical input: this was a social institution. Early institutions of the colony type, opened by Poor Law authorities, included Monyhull Colony near Birmingham and Stoke Park in Bristol (opened in 1908 and 1909 respectively). The Radnor Commission recommended that the mental institutions of the Metropolitan Asylums Board be transferred to LCC, including Caterham, Leavesden and Darenth Training Schools in Dartford; this sounded the death knell of the MAB.[55]

The Radnor Report led to the Mental Deficiency Act 1913. Poor Law Guardians became legally responsible to provide guardianship or institutional care for any mentally defective person who was neglected or without means of support, or who was involved in crime, drunkenness or having given birth to a bastard child. Existing asylums and colonies for mental defectives became certified institutions in the terms of the 1913 Act.[56] The categorisation of idiots, imbeciles, feeble-minded and moral defectives from the Idiots Act 1886 was maintained. While insanity was mostly an affliction of adulthood, the Mental Deficiency Act applied to all ages; young children, particularly those classed as idiots or imbeciles, would now be sent to colonies. Such institutions were to provide moral and occupational training, if only for the betterment of patients within their institutional setting. Segregation saved a multitude from eugenicists' more drastic proposal of sterilisation.

As the inspection regime had expanded, the Act renamed the Lunacy Commissioners as the Board of Control. Unlike the older regional institutions such as the Northern Counties Institution in Lancaster, which had grown to 750 beds by 1915, the new colonies were smaller and of domesticated design. However, accommodation remained scarce in most parts of the country. The tardiness of authorities in fulfilling the terms of the Mental Deficiency Act was criticised by inspectors, and planning was interrupted by war. Ten years after the Act the North Wales Mental Hospital kept fifty mentally defective patients, including two boys aged six and seven who were sent to the female side where they were nursed as babies.[57] In the 1920s, when the upkeep of many country estates was no longer viable, sites were sold cheaply to local authorities. In its new role, the manor house became the administration block of a mental defective colony set in luxuriant grounds: like the original asylums, this was an impressive façade to incarceration.

Petition and protest

In December 1909 the AWA held a celebratory banquet at the Gaiety Restaurant in London.[58] With MPA support, AWA president and Liberal politician Sir William Collins had submitted a Private Member's Bill, which passed surprisingly smoothly as the Asylum Workers' Superannuation Act 1909. The *Asylum News* hailed the Act, but many attendants were angered by compulsory deductions from their wages for a pension worth no more than retirement benefits already provided by their county authorities. In 1910 Lancashire asylum workers petitioned for higher pay to cover the pension contributions, but this was refused. Martin Meehan, head attendant of Winwick Asylum, sent circulars to other Lancashire asylums for a meeting at the Masons Arms in Manchester to organise a genuine trade union. Meehan's day off was cancelled, but young attendant George Gibson attended instead, and he was elected honorary general secretary of the provocatively named National Asylum Workers Union (NAWU).

The third meeting of the fledgling union at Victoria Hotel in Rainhill was attended by delegates from other counties. Reverend Samuel Proudfoot, a socialist Tractarian minister, sent a letter to 30,000 asylum workers, signed by twelve Lancashire attendants, urging them to unite in their struggle against asylum boards. A permanent staff was appointed, mostly of workers sacked for union activities. Reverend HMS Blankart, chaplain at Lancaster Asylum, was elected as general secretary. Blankart was dismissed for posting NAWU notices on the chapel wall, and for spending a night away to attend a union meeting at another asylum.[59]

Bolstered by its pension campaign, AWA membership increased to 5,680 by the end of 1911. However, this remained a minority of the eligible workforce. To the consternation of the AWA, attendants and nurses were being drawn to the NAWU, which in 1911 already had 4,400 members in forty-four asylums. After initially ignoring the new union in the *Asylum News*, the AWA denounced the upstart. An assistant medical officer at Omagh Asylum acknowledged dissatisfaction in mental nursing, but warned against division in the workforce. The NAWU, O'Doherty opined, was pitting subordinate staff against officers:[60]

> How can asylum workers strike? Under no conceivable circumstances could a strike be called in an asylum. It would be illegal, it would be mutiny, and the participants would be liable to prosecution.

Whereas the AWA sought gradual improvement through dialogue, the NAWU demanded substantial amendments to the Superannuation Act. It obtained an election pledge from Lord Wolmer, MP for Newton in Manchester, a constituency with a large number of asylum workers, although the resulting Bill faltered. Regarded by many attendants as too compromising, the AWA began to shed members. In 1914, just 3,214 remained on the books.

Meanwhile, serious industrial unrest was brewing around the country. Despite the social reforms of Lloyd George's Liberal government, including the National Insurance Act and introduction of the state pension, the unions were flexing their muscles. Radical socialists, anarchists and Suffragettes threatened the entire social order. Encouraged by the miners and other militant workers, in October 1913 NAWU members at West Riding asylums were balloted for strike action. Noting an overwhelming majority in favour at Storthes Hall and Wadsley asylums, the AWA regarded such sedition as 'a grave error'.[61] One of the gripes at the West Riding asylums was a board decision to replace butter with margarine. Despite assurance that margarine was no less nutritious, this was seen as penny-pinching from an already meagre diet. Fortunately a large stock of butter was discovered, which was distributed to staff while patients were served margarine.

Another dispute arose at Cardiff City Mental Hospital.[62] This hospital, which the city council opened in 1908 after many decades of expensive boarding out, attracted a highly reputed doctor to the post of medical superintendent. Edwin Goodall, however, soon got into difficulties with the attendants, who took their complaints to arbitration at the Cardiff Trades and Labour Organisation. South Wales was a hotbed of industrial conflict; in the infamous Tonypandy miners' strike, Home Secretary Winston Churchill had sent troops to quell the strikers. Goodall was accused of threatening NAWU branch secretary Darryl Williams; three hundred attendants had left since the hospital had opened; and the quality of food was criticised (butter, suspected to be margarine, was sent by Darryl Williams for laboratory analysis in Birmingham). The enquiry found little substance to the complaints, but with pressure applied by local MP William Brace, who was also leader of the South Wales Miners' Federation, concessions were won. In 1914, food was the cause of the first actual strike by NAWU members. The management at Rainhill in Lancashire having replaced meat with porridge at breakfast, thirty-five attendants occupied the mess room and refused to go to their wards, before medical superintendent Doctor Cowan acquiesced.

The Great War

Industrial strife was interrupted by declaration of war on 4 August 1914. There was an immediate response to Lord Kitchener's great mobilisation, and many of the fittest asylum attendants stepped forward, some of whom were Army or Navy reservists. At the North Wales Asylum, nineteen men enlisted, including twelve attendants. To replace them, retired attendants were brought in on a temporary basis, but after conscription was introduced, only four attendants stayed in post. In doing their patriotic duty, these men risked losing pensionable service, although the prevailing belief was that the war would be over by Christmas. As the military campaign got bogged down in the trenches, the AWA successfully lobbied for an Act of Parliament to ensure that on reinstatement, years spent on active service would count towards the asylum workers' pension. Quantity and quality of staff deteriorated on the male wards, where only older men or those unfit for military action remained. As recruitment was almost impossible in wartime, female nurses were deployed on male wards.[63]

In 1915, with an enormity of casualties arriving on hospital ships from the Western Front, the War Office requisitioned institutions for use as military hospitals. Some 15,000 beds were ordered. Asylums were targeted, as patients could be transferred elsewhere with minimal fuss. At the converted Fishponds Asylum, there was little time to prepare the medical and surgical facilities. Forty-five male patients were retained for menial labour,[64] but all others were moved en masse to other asylums. The medical superintendent remained, and was given an officer rank; he was now in charge of Beaufort Military Hospital. In Birmingham, Rubery and Hollymoor Asylums became the First and Second Birmingham Military Hospitals. The most significant structural alteration was to install operating theatres, but also temporary wards were constructed. At Hollymoor, the previous capacity of 640 steadily increased to 946 beds. In a busy week, 800 hundred wounded soldiers were received from the Western Front. By 1922, when Hollymoor reverted to a mental institution, 21,280 military casualties had been treated.[65] At the West Cheshire Asylum, a 320-bed annexe recently built for acute cases was used instead for patients transferred from Winwick Asylum near Warrington, another institution commandeered by the War Office.[66]

Overcrowding reached new extremes in the war. Patients decanted from other asylums slept in stairwells, corridors or day-rooms, and the recreation hall became a dormitory for incomers. Asylums reached a peak in population around two years into the war, before numbers began to fall. There were fewer admissions in wartime, but the main reason for the decline was a dramatic increase in mortality. At the relatively small Buckinghamshire Asylum, the resident population from 1910 to 1914 averaged 675, with an annual average of 67 deaths. After receiving large numbers of patients from Norfolk and Northamptonshire, on 1 January 1916 the asylum population reached 820, but during that year 110 died. At the beginning of 1918 there were 763 patients, but the death total for that year was a startling 257 – a mortality rate of over a third (in the 1920s it returned to an average of 10 per cent[67]).

According to detailed investigation of civilian mortality in the war,[68] over 100,000 lives were lost to starvation, but some sectors of society were particularly vulnerable. Food shortages worsened as the war went on, and inmates of mental institutions stood last in the queue. Each torpedo that struck an Atlantic convoy made another hole in the meagre asylum diet. At Hereford Asylum, where in 1918 porridge was withdrawn at breakfast, and the usual dietary table disappeared from the annual report, the Commissioner of the Board of Control commented on the ominous situation:

> Regular weighing of the patients should be instituted, especially as, owing to compulsory rationing, it is likely that their present diet may have to be curtailed in the near future.[69]

Cramped wards, malnutrition and poor sanitation were ideal conditions for the spread of infectious disease. Tuberculosis was a major killer in the war years, but in 1918 this was overtaken as a cause of death by the influenza pandemic. In the last year of the war a total of 18,330 asylum patients died, a high proportion having succumbed to Spanish influenza. In 1919 the number of deaths dropped to 11,317. After a heavy wartime toll, the resident population did not recover for many years. Overcrowding was alleviated as converted asylums returned to their original use, although some military hospitals continued in operation for two or three years after the Armistice. With the country on its knees from the war effort, patients were starving. In 1919 the average age at death at Hereford Asylum was forty-seven, down from sixty in the pre-war period; the total of seventy-three deaths in that year was the highest yet.

Many attendants never returned from the battlefield, and those who did were deeply affected by their experience. Public attitudes towards mental disorder softened after the Great War, which had left thousands of conscripts mentally wrecked by its horrors. Men with 'shell-shock' were typically mute or paralytic, but could also be excitable, sometimes screaming during the night. Psychological treatment by doctors trained in analytical methods, most famously by Colonel Rivers at Craiglockhart War Hospital in Edinburgh, was a passing phase. Frederick Mott suggested that the condition, while invoked by psychological stress, developed as lesions in the brain. Whatever the pathology, many of those afflicted were incapable of returning to civilian life and became long-term asylum patients, subjected to periodic examination by the Ministry of Pensions. The lunatic asylum seemed an unfortunate outcome for men who had suffered in the service of King and country.

Return to strife

After mass sacrifice in the Great War, society was restless for change. As well as social welfare, people expected better conditions in the workplace, a cause pursued by their trade unions. In 1918, the wartime 100-hour working week was imposed in asylums, and conditions of service had never been worse. The first official strike action by the NAWU was in Lancashire. In January 1918 the union presented a set of demands to the Lancashire Asylums Board, including a 60-hour week with 50 per cent extra pay for overtime, an award of £2 and 10 shillings on gaining the MPA certificate, and the right to post union notices in the mess rooms. In June the board granted a small pay award, but rejected all other demands without giving reasons. Consequently, in September 200 attendants walked out for a day at Prestwich, followed by 449 counterparts at Whittingham on the following day, with similar action by a smaller number at Winwick. The NAWU and the board agreed with the Ministry of Labour to seek arbitration, and although only modest concessions were gained, the reputation of the union was enhanced. Despite gaining pension rights for attendants on armed service, the AWA continued to lose members to the NAWU, and in 1919 it was disbanded.

NAWU membership reached 14,229 in 1919, at a time of a general surge in trade unionism in Britain. Substantial improvements were won, which in turn encouraged more claims. The number of female members rose to over a million in 1918, and they would no longer tolerate exploitation. In 1918 there was revolt at the Cornwall Asylum by female nurses, who complained of exhausting hours of duty, unpalatable food, lack of a bathroom, and being expected to sew material for uniform in their own time. Within two days of the appointment of Mrs Hawken, a nurse who had previously worked in the volatile atmosphere of Prestwich, sixty-two of the seventy nurses had joined the NAWU. In defiance they wore the union badge on their dresses. The ringleaders were sent packing by medical superintendent Doctor Dudley, but in solidarity their colleagues followed them out, and they struck for five days. Dudley sacked fifty strikers, but after negotiation with NAWU acting secretary Herbert Shaw, the visiting committee conceded to the nurses and accepted their trade union rights.

In 1919 control of the asylums passed from the Home Office to the new Ministry of Health. This move advanced the claim of psychiatry as a branch of medicine, and of mental nursing as part of the nursing profession. All asylums were to be renamed as mental hospitals, and attendants were to be known as nurses. Meanwhile the Nurses Registration Act passed in 1919 set up a national register under the General Nursing Council (GNC). The registration body reluctantly agreed to admit MPA certificate holders on a supplementary register, but insisted on producing its own entry qualification for mental nurses. In 1922, the first examination for the GNC certificate in mental nursing was passed by 161 nurses, of whom 113 were female.[70] The disproportionate female submissions to the GNC continued until the MPA examination ended after the Second World War.

National bargaining was introduced by the Ministry of Labour, with disputes to be settled by joint committees of employers and unions. Visiting committees joined the Mental Hospitals Association. Initially a separate industrial council for asylum workers was rejected by the government in favour of their representation on a joint council for local authority staff, but after a strike ballot by the NAWU with almost 8,000 (57 per cent of members) voting in favour, in 1919 a joint committee was formed specifically for asylums. Returning from military service, George Gibson warned that the MPA, which opposed the union's demand for shorter hours, was seeking a place on the Joint Conciliation Committee (JCC). Lay members of visiting committees regarded the JCC as a counterbalance to medical authority, and the MPA was refused.

After the NAWU secured JCC agreement to a 60-hour week (actually 48 working hours, taking account of meal breaks), in the early 1920s it continued to assert itself. A move to end medical superintendents' power of instant dismissal was obstructed by lunacy law, but right of appeal was won. At Stafford, the NAWU tackled the petty rule barring female nurses from using the front gate; they were forced to use the rear entrance, thus adding a mile to their journey into town. The threat of action was enough for the rule to be quietly forgotten.[71] Despite such gains the union lacked influence at national level. In 1920 its proposal for a new wage scale for male staff was broadly declined by mental hospital committees, and was not considered by the JCC. The union was a preserve of traditional gender attitudes. While some medical superintendents thought that female nurses provided better care to the sick and elderly, the NAWU argued that women should not be exposed to male patients who could be sexually inappropriate due to their illness. Reading between the lines, this was protecting men's jobs.

Industrial action by the NAWU reached its pinnacle at the 'Battle of Radcliffe'. In February 1922 the visiting committee at Nottinghamshire County Mental Hospital decided to cut wages and off-duty time, thereby exceeding the agreed maximum of sixty hours. On 10 April George Gibson, Herbert Shaw and the union solicitor attended a meeting nearby and agreed to strike action on the female side. The following day, female nurses occupied the wards. Inspired by their colleagues, the male nurses also withdrew their labour. All strikers were sacked with offer of reinstatement on signing an agreement of full obedience to their superiors. NAWU officers, barred from the hospital grounds, encouraged the workers to stand firm. On 12 April the strike ended when the clerk of the visiting committee and medical superintendent Dr Jones appeared at the barricaded wards with a force of bailiffs and plain-clothed policemen. After four hours of resistance the strikers were overcome and ejected from the hospital, with the concession of a maintenance grant until they found other work. The episode was covered sympathetically by the national press, but the *Nursing Times*, an organ of the College of Nursing, deplored the Radcliffe strikers.

Exposé

In 1921 a sensation was created by a book titled *The Experiences of an Asylum Doctor*.[72] Dedicated to 'all the insane poor in sympathy with their sufferings', this indictment of asylum care resulted from the author's stint as *locum tenens* at the large, antiquated Prestwich Asylum. Montagu Lomax described in dreadful detail the dilapidated and dirty buildings, the drab monotony, awful food and regular drugging and purging of patients. Lomax made scathing remarks on the quality of attendants, many of whom were lazy and tyrannical, although he blamed this on their abysmal treatment by management. Having also criticised the doctors, Lomax received little support from the medical profession. Articles in the *Lancet* and *British Medical Journal* dismissed him as a junior medical officer with little knowledge of mental hospital practice. A reasonable criticism was that Lomax had not made allowances for the deprivations of war, when many members of the medical and nursing staff had gone into military service. However, his outspoken dossier was widely reported in *The Times* and other newspapers, and could not be swept under the carpet.

In response to the Prestwich scandal, the government instructed a committee of two doctors and a member of parliament to investigate the administration of mental hospitals. Fearing victimisation of its members, the NAWU refused to participate, and consequently the scope of enquiry was limited to the size of mental hospitals and staff recruitment. In its report in 1923, the Cobb Committee concluded that Lomax had exaggerated his account, but accepted that conditions left much to be desired. Many buildings were no longer fit for purpose, although not all were old: twenty-two of the ninety-eight county and borough mental hospitals had opened since 1900, while at timeworn institutions such as Prestwich more modern blocks had been added. However, wear and tear had been exacerbated by overcrowding and lack of maintenance in wartime. As well as recommending various improvements to the wards and to the admission process, the report proposed that any new mental hospital should have a maximum of a thousand beds, with separate villas to allow more personal contact between nurses and patients. The Cobb Committee heard from medical superintendents that it was not in nurses' interests to reduce their working hours, as apparently they disliked the free time, preferring instead to be with their patients: this was a vocation, not factory work.

The voice of nurses was more accurately heard in another report resulting from the Lomax allegations. *Nursing in County and Borough Mental Hospitals*, published in 1925, was the product of the first official enquiry into mental nursing.[73] Data were presented from a comprehensive survey of all ninety-seven mental hospitals in England. Whittingham was the largest hospital with 2,838 beds, from an overall capacity of 108,646. Heading the nursing workforce of 16,949 were ninety-seven chief male nurses and ninety-seven matrons. Below the level of charge nurse was the large category of 'others', numbering 11,887; this included kitchen and laundry workers and servants as well as nurses. There was also a total of 2,045 night staff. On average there was a ratio of one attendant to nine patients on male side in daytime, and one in ten on the female side. The report described the wide-ranging duties of mental nurses, of whom just 1,588 men and 1,155 women held the MPA certificate. Many senior nurses lacked this qualification, and for such positions the report recommended training in both mental and general nursing. However, the authors concurred with Lomax, who they interviewed, that character of nursing recruits should take precedence over ability to pass examinations. Compassion could not be taught, and it was observed that some nurses were unsuited to the practice of caring. The report recommended a purpose-built nurse training school, lodgings set apart from the main buildings, and recreational facilities for off-duty staff. Although no immediate action followed, here was guidance for mental hospital management in attracting and retaining a higher calibre of nurses.

As dust settled on the Great War, there was some reprieve from overcrowding in mental hospitals, before the long-term rise in population resumed. At Graylingwell in Sussex, over 200 beds were vacant after it reopened as a mental hospital, and this situation was exploited. In 1922 contracts were made with Middlesex to take thirty women from Napsbury Mental Hospital at 35 shillings per week, and with Croydon Mental Hospital for thirty male and fifteen female patients.[74] However, once local admissions increased the guests were returned. Soon all was back to normal.

Fever and focal sepsis

Asylums were a breeding ground for contagious disease. In stifling, airless dormitories, nurses relied heavily on patient labour for the arduous cleaning and polishing routine. There was a pervasive odour of a combination of sweat, tobacco, boiled vegetables, floor polish and drains. Slop pails were used at night, and the faecal air was thickened on the day of the weekly purgative. Poor sanitary conditions produced waves of dysentery and enteric fever. Board of Control inspectors frequently expressed concern at the resulting mortality, and urged prompt detection and isolation of the afflicted. Built sporadically at mental institutions (often in reaction to a particularly deadly outbreak of fever), an isolation hospital became a standard feature. Infected patients (and nurses) were confined at a safe distance from the main block.

Due to improved laboratory techniques, cases of tuberculosis could be confirmed by microscopic examination of sputum. Caution cards were issued for consumptive patients, who were barred from working in the kitchens. Pulmonary tuberculosis was so rife in asylums that many doctors thought it must be linked to insanity. Frederick Mott, who conducted post-mortem examinations at Colney Hatch, found mortality from tuberculosis fifteen times higher in patients aged fifteen to forty-five than in the general population.[75] There was no known cure, but fresh air was beneficial. While affluent sufferers went to private sanatoria in Switzerland or English coastal resorts, local authorities were building fever hospitals and tuberculosis sanatoria for the working class. In mental hospitals, verandahs were installed on the south-facing walls of wards accommodating tubercular patients.

Apart from the spike in deaths in the Great War, mortality from infectious disease steadily declined in the early twentieth century (well before the advent of antibiotic drugs). In 1900, 16 per cent of deaths at Colney Hatch were due to tuberculosis, and 14 per cent caused by an outbreak of colitis.[76] Thirty years later, Board of Control data for all asylums showed that from an annual total of 7,857 deaths, 667 were due to pulmonary tuberculosis (8.5 per cent).[77] By the end of the 1920s, systemic conditions such as cardiac disease were a more common cause of death. However, the growing proportion of elderly patients contributed to an increase in mortality from pneumonia.

Anecdotal observations by asylum doctors suggested that febrile illness sometimes brought temporary respite in mental disturbance. Fever, indeed, would have its use. The first major breakthrough in treatment of insanity was in 1917, when Austrian psychiatrist Julius Wagner-Jauregg in Austria devised malarial treatment for general paralysis of the insane (GPI). There were three stages of the disease. In the first stage the patient displayed excitability, insomnia and grandiose delusions, and became unable to manage his affairs. The second stage was marked by drowsy torpor and weight gain. Severe mental and physical deterioration occurred in the final stage; the bedridden patient died miserably after three or four days of convulsions and paralysis. The link between this degenerative condition and syphilis had been suspected for some time, with strong evidence provided by LCC laboratory at Claybury. In 1906 German bacteriologist August von Wassermann devised a specific serum test to detect syphilis, and when this was first used at Colney Hatch Asylum in 1912, syphilitic infection was found in thirty-eight of forty suspected cases of GPI. This discovery explained the higher prevalence of GPI in urban asylums (agricultural counties had few cases). At the Plymouth Borough Asylum it accounted for half of mortality, such frequency being attributed to the maritime enterprise of the town and the frequent arrival of crews from distant shores.[78]

Wagner-Jauregg had experimented with fever treatment for insanity as early as 1887, but it was not until 1917 that he first tested malarial infection in GPI. Six of his nine cases improved or remitted. For this discovery Wagner-Jauregg was awarded the Nobel Prize in 1927. Malarial treatment began in Germany in 1919, and in 1922 it was introduced at a few British mental hospitals. A special treatment centre was established by LCC at Horton Mental Hospital, in collaboration with the London School of Hygiene and Tropical Medicine (later named the Mott Clinic). Almost all of the malaria used in British mental hospitals was sourced from a sick passenger disembarking at Tilbury Docks in 1925. Mosquitoes were initially bred on the Isle of Sheppey in Kent, until an insectarium at Horton supplied mental hospitals around the country. Individual patients sat in a netted area until they had sustained several mosquito bites. Within a few days the symptoms appeared and the patient's fever was monitored. The disease was then terminated by quinine. A high rate of remission was reported, as much as 75 per cent at Horton, although later results were less promising. Although not a cure, malarial treatment arrested the progress of the disease: by 1930 GPI fell to ten per cent of mental hospital mortality.[79]

Another pathological pursuit was focal sepsis theory. In 1923 Henry Cotton, medical director of Trenton State Hospital in New Jersey presented to the MPA his hypothesis that insanity was a generalised result of pus infection in the bowels, teeth and tonsils, which caused microscopic lesions in the cerebral cortex. These lesions, according to Cotton, disappeared on eradication of the septic tissue. A prominent exponent of focal sepsis theory was TC Graves, medical head of Birmingham mental hospitals. In 1920 Graves was appointed medical superintendent at Rubery and Hollymoor, and in 1922 a joint board of research was initiated with the University of Birmingham, with Frederick Mott as honorary director. At the new laboratory at Hollymoor, Graves began in earnest his programme of removing teeth and tonsils from patients, in the hope that this would produce remission of mental symptoms. In some cases the gall bladder (or other internal organs) was removed. Surgical procedure was augmented by ultra-violet light treatment to eradicate any lingering infection. Claiming impressive results, Graves visited other mental hospitals such as Powick to cleanse the inmate population.[80] While focal sepsis theory was not widely accepted, application of a biological hypothesis it drew psychiatry closer to medicine. It also emphasised the importance of hygiene; in reality, however, many mental hospital patients lacked a toothbrush. Epileptic and refractory patients were considered by medical officers to be better off without teeth, and visiting dentists did little other than radical extractions.[81]

Unlocking the doors

Following the Prestwich scandal, the Board of Control urged hospital authorities to improve conditions for patients. Inspectors praised initiatives such as craftwork, and noted the arrival of wireless radio and gramophone on the wards. Films had started in some asylums before the war; at the newly opened Severalls in Essex the first 'cinematographic entertainment' occurred on Boxing Day in 1914,[82] and this became a weekly feature in the 1920s. With live musical accompaniment, silent drama or comedy films were watched by male and female patients from separate sides of the recreation hall. Gangs of staff and patients laid many a cricket pitch, bowling green, tennis court and wooden pavilion. Patients' football and cricket teams were started, and motor coaches were hired for matches at other hospitals.

A radical change was the unlocking of wards at some mental hospitals. In 1922, doors were opened throughout Littlemore Mental Hospital in Oxford by medical superintendent Saxty Good, who saw tradition, hierarchies and routines as barriers to progress. His experiment was a guiding light for others. At the newly opened West Park in Epsom, four male wards and villas with cooperative patients were unlocked.[83] Another development was extension of parole, with graduation from corridor to grounds to town, and some patients allowed out for a whole weekend. In the 1927 report of Kent County Mental Hospital, 130 male and 300 female patients were in unlocked wards, while thirty-one male patients were on weekend parole.[84] Airing courts were made less custodial in appearance, with walls or railings lowered and masked by shrubs. At Upton Mental Hospital, formerly the West Cheshire Asylum, the high wall alongside the Liverpool Road was pulled down on instruction of the medical superintendent, who probably felt his share of stigma at this pronounced segregation from the outside world.

A reluctant profession

Trade unions began to merge in the 1920s to increase their bargaining power; for example, various labour bodies combined to form the mammoth Transport and General Workers' Union. The NAWU and the Poor Law Workers' Trade Union merged in 1921, but parted company in the following year.[85] In 1923, after the NAWU joined the Trades Union Congress, George Gibson led a delegation to meet government minister Neville Chamberlain, demanding improvements in pay, working hours, training, pensions and protection of staff exposed to contagious disease. In the General Strike of 1926 mental hospital workers were among a list that the TUC exempted from withdrawal of labour, although the NAWU wholeheartedly supported this mass action in sympathy for the miners.[86] By the late 1920s the influence of the NAWU waned, with membership hovering around 11,000 – less than half of a growing workforce. Hard lessons were learned from the aborted workers' revolution.

As militancy in mental hospitals faded, the College of Nursing, *Nursing Times* and *Nursing Mirror* encouraged nurses in all settings to maintain discipline and to wear their badge of registration with pride. Yet mental nurses were dragging their heels on the ascent to the sunny uplands of professionalism. They retained the outlook of a lay occupation. Articles in the nursing periodicals of the 1920s suggest more concern with working conditions than with patient care; concepts of mental disorder and treatment were uncritically accepted as medical matters.[87]

In the plethora of histories of mental hospitals published since their closure, authors found few nurses whose experience went back as far as the 1920s. The oldest interviewee in James Gardner's history of the original Sussex Asylum at Haywards Heath was Eileen Cruttenden, who left home in Port Talbot in Wales in 1924 to work in the kitchens. Arriving at the Brighton Borough Mental Hospital late in the evening, she was fed in the mess room and then guided by the cook to a room at the top of the main building, their path dimly lit by gas lamp (the hospital had no electricity):

> We walked through the dormitory, where the patients were in bed, to where I was to sleep. At the time I did not know that the nurses slept up there as well. I thought I was the only one. We got into this side room. She lit the gas jet there. It had bare boards, brick walls but they were painted in that awful dark brown …'Well, I'll leave you now. Be down in the kitchen by half-past six. In the morning, the night nurse will give you a call.' Next morning, I was dressed at 5 o'clock and so was already up when the nurse gave me a call. Then I opened the door and saw all these patients outside. Some were standing up with nothing on; some were dressing. They were all chattering to one another and calling out. It was all a jumble. I thought, I'm not going through there. I was too scared. So I went back into the bedroom, unlocked the door, then locked it. I waited there until the cook came and fetched me. She wasn't very happy. She had to come all the way up.[88]

Rich anecdotal material was gathered in the early 1990s by co-author PN, who interviewed eight male and four female nurses who had worked in the 1920s. One interviewee described his arrival at a mental hospital late on a winter evening, where he was met by a smartly uniformed porter who recorded his personal details and weighed him. After receiving two pieces of bread with margarine and cheese, he was shown to a small room next to a ward. He got into one of the two beds, but his reading was abruptly halted:

> At about ten o'clock, the lights went out and some minutes later the door opened and an attendant came in obviously the worse for drink. I discovered later that on his day off every month he got drunk. He started swearing and shouting at me and told me to get the hell out of his bed. I was so scared I jumped out of bed and just as I was settling down, I heard him collapse on the floor. When I awoke in the morning, he was fast asleep on the floor and had obviously spent the night there.[89]

Throughout the night his sleep was punctuated by shouts and screams of patients, presumably suffering from nightmares. In the morning he began duty on an admission ward for fifty men, where his first task was to scrub six side rooms. An attendant explained why the walls were plastered with faeces: the patients had received their weekly dose of 'white mixture'. A few days later he was summoned to the cricket field by the head attendant, but he failed to impress and was never asked to play again. He did not find his colleagues friendly, and took some time to fit in.

Gender differences were evident in Nolan's interviewees in their attractions to mental hospital work. In order of importance, men valued a secure job, companionship, and sporting and musical activities; women gained most satisfaction from caring for patients, relationships with colleagues, taking pride in their ward, walks with patients and the weekly dances.[90] Least appealing for both sexes was the regular scrubbing of floors and walls, poor food and public reprimands. While male nurses settled on a job for life, a third of female nurses left within their first year of service. For those who stayed, compensation for the monotonous ordeal was the opportunity for professional qualification. However, the training environment was not ideal, as this ex-attendant described:[91]

> In my group, there were four probationers, two males and two females. We used to meet in a corner of one of the admission wards, close to a cupboard which contained surgical instruments. We stood throughout the lecture, and there were times when I nearly dropped off; we had been on duty since 6.30 a.m. We never knew what the topic was going to be until we got there. The teacher would give a demonstration after which each of us would have the opportunity to practice. The evening would end at exactly 8 p.m.

By the end of the 1920s, due partly to the problems of recruitment, and partly to union agitation, nurses' conditions had materially improved. In 1921 a staff club was opened at Coney Hill Asylum in Gloucestershire, affording nurses a place to socialise. Supping ale after a long shift, nurses may have thought that life was not so bad. As working hours reduced, the mental hospital became a place not only of work and sleep, but also a modicum of social life.

Notes

1 Early DF (2003).
2 Hereford County and City Asylum (1896): Twenty-Fourth Annual Report of the Committee of Visitors of the Hereford County and City Asylum 1896.
3 Jones K (1993).
4 Early DF (2003). 28.
5 On the expansion of Greater London, Middlesex County Council took over the former Surrey Asylum at Springfield, while Surrey relied on its second asylum at Brookwood; accommodation in these counties later being supplemented by new institutions at Napsbury and Netherne respectively.
6 *Asylum News* (15 February 1903): The fire at Colney Hatch Asylum. Each asylum had its own fire brigade, mostly comprising male attendants. The maximum height of buildings was determined by the reach of water hydrants.
7 Hopper B (2011): *Better Court than Coroners: Memoirs of a Duty of Care* (volume I).
8 Cochrane DA (1985): *The Colonisation of Epsom: the Building of the Epsom Cluster by the London County Council in its Historical Context.*
9 Excerpt from *Street Plan of Epsom and Ewell.* GI Barnett & Sons.
10 Edinburgh District Lunacy Board (1897): *Report of Deputation from the Edinburgh District Lunacy Board Appointed to Visit Certain Asylums in France, Germany, and England, Recommended by the General Board on Lunacy.*
11 White EW (1900): The remodelling of an old asylum. *Journal of Mental Science.*

12   Hereford County and City Asylum (1893): Twenty-First Annual Report of the Committee of Visitors of the Hereford County and City Asylum 1893.
13   Cooke EM (1895). 394.
14   Nolan P (1993).
15   Spratley VA, Stern ES (1952).
16   Nolan P (1993).
17   Eager R (1945).
18   Quoted from the *Register of Attendants* in the Royal College of Psychiatrists library by Nolan (1993), 71.
19   Morten H (1897): Asylum attendants. *Nursing Notes*.
20   Morten H (1897).
21   Bedford Fenwick E (1896): On male attendants. *Nursing Record*, 2: 49.
22   Abel-Smith B (1960): *A History of the Nursing Profession*.
23   *Asylum News* (15 March 1904): Correspondence.
24   Bevan-Lewis W (1907): On the formation of character: an address to the nursing staff at the Retreat, York, delivered November 1st, 1906. *Journal of Mental Science*.
25   Berkshire Asylum (1903): *General Rules for the Government of the Asylum*. 18.
26   Gittins D (1998).
27   *Asylum News* (15 January 1901): Notes and news.
28   Crichton Browne J (1898): Presidential address. *Asylum News*.
29   *Asylum News* (15 March 1903): Correspondence.
30   'Veritas' (1906): How to improve the conditions of the asylum service. *Asylum News*.
31   *Asylum News* (15 February 1901): Notes and news.
32   *Asylum News* (15 June 1902): Correspondence.
33   *Asylum News* (15 July 1904).
34   *Asylum News* (15 October 1902): Notes and news.
35   Associate member (1909): *Asylum News*.
36   *Asylum News* (15 January 1907): Correspondence.
37   Berkshire Asylum (1903). 8–9.
38   *Journal of Mental Science* (1904): The management of the London County Council Asylums and the Horton Asylum scandal.
39   Wiltshire County Asylum (1892): *Report of the Committee of Visitors for the Year 1891 and Forty-First Annual Report of the Medical Superintendent of the Asylum for the Insane Poor of the County of Wilts*.
40   Commissioners in Lunacy (1906): *Sixty-First Report of the Commissioners in Lunacy*.
41   *Asylum News* (15 May 1901): Notes and news.
42   Campbell Clark A (1897): *Clinical Manual of Mental Disorders for Practitioners and Students*. 102–3
43   Kent County Mental Hospital (1927).
44   A recording was recently released. Elgar E (2014): *Music for Powick Asylum*. Quote from sleeve notes.
45   Wiltshire County Asylum (1900): *Forty-Ninth Annual Report of the Wilts County Asylum for the Year 1900 and Financial Statements for 1899–1900*.
46   Hewitt H (1923): *From Harrow to Herrison House Asylum*. Abridged quotation 55–8.
47   Hewitt H (1923) Abridged quotation 58–9.
48   Hewitt H (1923) Abridged quotation 59–62
49   Valentine R (1996): *Asylum, Hospital, Haven: a History of Horton Hospital*.
50   Firman C, Crump D (1985): Tooting Bec Hospital. *Nursing Mirror*. In 1926 the institution was extended to sixty-seven wards and a capacity of 2,400.
51   Thomson M (1992): Sterilisation, segregation and community care: ideology and solutions to the problem of mental deficiency in inter-war Britain. *History of Psychiatry*.
52   Hereford County and City Asylum (1912): Fortieth Annual Report of the Committee of Visitors of the Hereford County and City Asylum 1912.
53   Tredgold AF (1908): *Text-Book of Mental Deficiency*.

54 Jones K (1972). 112.
55 Malster R (1994).
56 A matching law was passed for Scotland. The first certified institution to open under this statute was Stoneyetts, built by Glasgow Parish Council in 1913.
57 Michael P (2003).
58 *Asylum News* (15 January 1910): Banquet in commemoration of the passing of the Asylum Officers' Superannuation Act.
59 Greene B (1975): The rise and fall of the Asylum Workers Association. *Nursing Mirror*.
60 O'Doherty P (1912): A plea for cohesion among asylum workers. *Asylum News*.
61 *Asylum News* (October 1913): Unrest in the West Riding Asylums.
62 Beech I (2013): *Butter, Bands, Bandages and Bolshevism: Care, Conditions and Culture in Cardiff City Mental Hospital before WWI.*
63 Michael P (2003).
64 Early DF (2003).
65 Crofts F (1998): *History of Hollymoor Hospital.*
66 Wall BA (1977): *A World of its Own: Chester's Psychiatric Hospitals 1829–1976.*
67 Crammer J (1990).
68 Dumas S, Vedel-Petersen KO (1923): *Losses of Life Caused by War.*
69 Hereford County and City Asylum (1918): Forty Sixth Annual Report of the Committee of Visitors of the Hereford County and City Asylum 1918.
70 Nolan P (1993).
71 Arton M (1998): *The Professionalisation of Mental Nursing in Great Britain, 1850–1950.*
72 Hopton J (1999): Prestwich hospital in the twentieth century: a case study of slow and uneven progress in the development of psychiatric care. *History of Psychiatry.*
73 Board of Control for England and Wales (1925): *Report of the Board of Control's (England and Wales) Committee on Nursing in County and Borough Mental Hospitals.*
74 Hopper B (2012): *Lest we Forget: Memoirs of a Duty of Care* (volume II).
75 Hunter R, Macalpine I (1974).
76 Hunter R, Macalpine I (1974).
77 Board of Control for England and Wales (1931): *The Seventeenth Annual Report of the Board of Control 1930.*
78 Pilkington F (1958): *Moorhaven Hospital, Ivybridge, South Devon: Historical Review 1891–1958* (2nd edition).
79 Board of Control for England and Wales (1931).
80 Hall P (1991).
81 Crofts F (1998).
82 Gittins D (1998). 100.
83 Johnson BCT (1969): *West Park: the First Sixty Years.*
84 Kent County Mental Hospital (1927).
85 Carpenter M (1988): *Working for Health: the History of COHSE.*
86 Farman C (1974): *May 1926: the General Strike: Britain's Aborted Revolution?*
87 Ramon S (1985): *Psychiatry in Britain: Meaning and Policy.*
88 Gardner J (1999). 290.
89 Nolan P (1993). 89.
90 Nolan (1993). Other ex-nurses were interviewed but the data were not reliable due to memory deficits or communication difficulties.
91 Nolan (1993). 92.

3   Shocks to the system

What makes a hospital? The derivation of the term is in a place of shelter or lodging, as in 'hospitality', but modern usage is confined to a building where the sick receive medical treatment. The asylums had been renamed 'mental hospitals', but the contrast with physical health care was stark. A hundred years since the emergence of psychiatry, there was no effective remedy for insanity. Except at the Maudsley Hospital and the City of London Hospital at Dartford, all patients were subjected to the stigma of certification by the 1890 Lunacy Act. Despite a fair proportion of cases discharged after a few weeks, many patients admitted in their youth went on to a lifetime of incarceration. There was no spectrum of mental health, but a dichotomy of the sane and insane. As hefty legal fees were incurred whatever the verdict, doctors assessing a person's mental state for a magistrate's Reception Order were wary of being sued for wrongful detention. This issue continued to make headlines, most notably the Hartnett case in 1924, when a Kent farmer was awarded substantial damages against a Board of Control Commissioner.[1] People in distress could not be admitted until they were exhibiting obviously irrational behaviour, when they would be taken away by burly men in suits, while neighbours peered through net curtains. The asylum continued to loom large in the public imagination.

In the aftermath of the Prestwich scandal, in 1924 the Ministry of Health established a Royal Commission on Lunacy and Mental Disorder, tasked with reviewing the laws and administrative machinery relating to persons of unsound mind in England and Wales. Chaired by lawyer Hugh Macmillan, the twelve members included Sir Humphrey Rolleston, president of the Royal College of Physicians, but there were no mental hospital doctors. Evidence was taken from administrative bodies, Poor Law officers, magistrates, medical superintendents, the MPA, British Medical Association and the fledgling Mental After-Care Association. Interviews were also conducted with patients and the National Society for Lunacy Reform, specifically on allegations of abuse. No nursing opinion was sought, except for interviews with one female probationer and one male attendant, both of whom had left mental hospital work; they gave contrasting accounts of the prevalence of mistreatment. The Macmillan Commission's report of 1926 was an enlightened call for radical change to a stigmatised system that deterred people from seeking help.[2]

Contrary to the accepted canons of preventive medicine, the mental patient is not admissible to institutions provided for his treatment until his disease has progressed so far that he has become a certifiable lunatic. Then and only then is he eligible for treatment. It is perhaps not remarkable in these circumstances that the percentage of recoveries is so low ... Certification should be the last resort in treatment, not the pre-requisite. Hence the necessity in our opinion not only of making all institutions available for the reception of voluntary uncertified patients, but also of making provision either in connection with existing institutions or by the provision of new institutions.

Mental institutions, therefore, were to become more clinical and less custodial. Existing legislation had been excessively concerned with preventing improper detention, and the Royal Commission rejected a tightening of admission process suggested by the National Society for Lunacy Reform. Instead, access to the mental hospital would be freed as much as possible from legal jurisdiction. A period of observation and treatment before certification was recommended. Two types of patient were identified for whom certification could be averted: first, mild, uncertifiable cases; second, people with certifiable illness who were willing to be admitted voluntarily. Instead of the archaic terms 'lunacy' and 'insanity', patients had potentially treatable 'mental disorder'. Brief episodes of active treatment were envisaged, with the earliest possible discharge.

The Macmillan Commission's report was mostly written into the Bill, which passed without major amendments as the Mental Treatment Act 1930. Undoubtedly, this was a turning point in the history of mental health care in Britain. The Act introduced admission on a voluntary or temporary basis for people with acute mental disorder who were likely to make a swift recovery. Thus, a mother with puerperal psychosis, for example, could now be treated without the stigma of committal under the Lunacy Act. Restrictions were placed on the voluntary patient's liberty: discharge could be requested in writing to the medical superintendent, but with a minimum notice of three days, and only within the first month of stay. However, magistrates were excluded from the admission process for such patients, as reception and care of such patients was to be decided on medical grounds alone.

Another milestone was the end of the Poor Law. Since the beginning of the century the parsimonious system of pauper relief had been gradually dismantled, but despite the establishment of the Ministry of Health in 1919, most mental hospital patients continued to be charged to their local Board of Guardians. This association with pauperism, heavily criticised by the Macmillan Commission, officially ceased with the Local Government Act of 1929. The Poor Law administrators were disbanded, their role taken over by local authorities. The mental hospital was thus brought into line with physical health care, open to all. However, in practice the administrative changes were merely symbolic. Patients previously of pauper status were simply relabelled 'rate-aided'. In cities, patients continued to be admitted via the observation ward of a former Poor Law institution or infirmary; such establishments were passed to local authority control, but performed basically the same role. In London the reception wards governed by the Metropolitan Asylums Board, which was disbanded in 1930, passed to the London County Council. As before, patients who did not recover in an observation ward were distributed to the archipelago of LCC mental hospitals on the periphery of the metropolis.

To fulfil the objectives of the Mental Treatment Act, county authorities knew that modern facilities were needed, away from the custodial atmosphere of the old buildings. Institutions of the turn of the century, such as Netherne in Surrey, had opened with a separate admission unit,[3] but at most mental hospitals, admissions continued to be received at the business entrance of a daunting edifice and sent wherever a bed was available. The experience of entering a mental hospital was greatly improved following a spate of building in the 1930s. New admission units, with their contemporary architecture not dissimilar to a school or light industrial unit, conveyed little hint of confinement. A person admitted for the first time was assured that he or she was not going to the notorious asylum but to a distinct hospital. Some may have felt duped on passing the gate lodge, but the admission building was indeed a physically and operationally separate entity. For example, Summersdale, which opened in 1933 at Graylingwell Mental Hospital in Sussex, had a splendid aspect over greenery fore and aft, and no railings. Pleasantly furnished with a polished pine floor, Summersdale had its own dining area and treatment rooms, and patients were allowed their own clothing. Nonetheless, a padded room was installed on each side, and there was no mixing of sexes.[4]

The declared role of the admission units was to treat nervous disease (some were labelled 'neurosis units'). In the heyday of Sigmund Freud and psychoanalysis, problems of the mind were to some extent normalised; one could be neurotic without the life sentence of stereotypical lunacy. People would often attribute anxiety or depressed mood to 'nerves', and the term 'nervous breakdown' entered common parlance.[5] Help became available without stepping inside a mental hospital, through a psychiatric outpatient clinic (introduced at many general hospitals in the 1930s), or private psychological therapy. Meanwhile, some institutions were renamed to reflect the changing clinical ethos: Colney Hatch became Friern Hospital for Nervous and Mental Disorders.[6] In 1937, the London County Council decided that 'mental' would no longer precede 'hospital'; thus by abbreviated titles Hanwell and Friern became indistinguishable from a general hospital.

Bed rest was standard on admission. Having single bedrooms, the reception units provided a suitable setting for prolonged narcosis, which was prescribed for conditions such as acute mania, suicidal ideation and hysteria. Sedated by heavy doses of sodium amytal, sometimes patients were kept asleep for a week or longer, being woken only for meals. This procedure required basic nursing care and vigilance for respiratory crisis or other medical emergencies. Meanwhile hydrotherapy, a ubiquitous treatment dating back to ancient civilisations, was in vogue in the early 1930s, and official openings of admission units typically boasted of a gleaming suite of baths. For up to several hours, patients lay in water regulated at a constant temperature, with a hole in the lid or canvas cover for the head. Several patients could receive the treatment simultaneously, under constant nursing observation. Cold baths soothed manic excitement or agitation, while melancholia responded best to warm immersion. As well as the immediate effects, it was speculated that continuous bathing removed toxins contributing to mental disorder, germ theory lingering in the psychiatric mindset.

An air of prestige was bestowed on nurses who worked in these centres of clinical promise. Traditional certainties of mental nursing in dealing with the pronounced insane were challenged by an influx of middle-class neurotic patients who were socially and intellectually superior to most of the nurses. The blunt nursing approach of the old block was deemed inappropriate for the genteel introvert needing to be handled with tact and sensitivity. Smarter nurses were selected, with preference to those with qualification in both mental and general nursing. Specific medical instructions were to be followed for each patient, and the nursing day was punctuated by regular monitoring and recording of pulse, temperature, nutritional intake, weight and sleep. The nurse was expected to listen to patients but not to overstep the mark by offering interpretations of their words or behaviour. Nurses observed, doctors explained.[7]

According to historian Joan Busfield,[8] the Mental Treatment Act transformed the role of the mental hospital from segregation to serving the community, but this did not happen overnight. Despite the emphasis on early intervention, it was not yet clear what was meant by 'treatment' as worded in the Act. The pharmacopeia remained primitive, and doctors rolled the dice with speculative, non-specific treatments such as ultra-violet therapy.[9] Other interventions such as deep sedation and hydrotherapy offered merely symptomatic relief. In reality, many patients did not recover quickly enough for discharge from the reception unit, which had a shortage of beds for new admissions. Patients with mild, reversible conditions went to convalescent wards or villas for perhaps a month to complete their recovery. Others were not so fortunate.

The 1890 Lunacy Act had not been repealed, and admission practice often defaulted to the assurances of certification. In some areas, the Board of Control found a lack of awareness of the Mental Treatment Act among doctors, Justices of the Peace and local authority officers. Five years after enactment, voluntary status accounted for 26.9 per cent of the total admissions in England and Wales, but there was great variation between hospitals. At the end of 1936 the voluntary share of the total mental hospital populace of 129,751 was only 5,655. Excepting 487 temporary patients, the remainder were certified.[10] Voluntary admissions were least frequent in the massive Lancashire; at Prestwich, where the exposé by Lomax had spurred legal reforms, the proportion remained as low as 5 per cent by the end of the decade. At Friern Hospital the resident population reached 2,654 in 1937, of which only twenty-five were voluntary and one of temporary status.[11] From a broader perspective, the Mental Treatment Act set in motion changes to the mental hospital system that would culminate in its demise, but in the 1930s the harsh regime prevailed: overcrowded wards, antiquated buildings and a stultifying institutional culture.

Life in the back wards

In his account *Inside the Asylum*, John Vincent described his voluntary admission to a mental hospital:[12]

> My wife and I boarded the bus which was to take us to the asylum. Was it to be our last journey together? As we alighted from the bus and walked along the drive every detail of the picture was indelibly printed upon my mind. An attendant in uniform came past us on a bicycle. A man was up a short ladder in the drive attending to the electric lights. Farther along the drive we met a company of what surely must have been some of the worst patients in the charge of an attendant. They were all old men with staring eyes. A moment later a large car overtook us, and I wondered whether the superintendent was in it. At last we were at the door. The great red brick building looked grim and forbidding.

Accompanied by his wife, Vincent was led to a waiting room to be interviewed by the medical superintendent, who finished by pressing a bell-push. An attendant came to escort him to a modern block at a distant corner of the grounds. On arrival he was asked to undress and don a nightshirt and pair of slippers for medical examination. Eventually taken to the dormitory, he learned that all new patients must to go to bed, although it was afternoon. Lonely and apprehensive, Vincent wanted to urinate but did not want to ask where to go as the whole ward would hear. After a period of inactivity, the silence was broken:

> An old man was walking up and down the ward. He carried cups and saucers and bed tables. When he came to my bed he stared at me out of glassy eyes. His mouth was drawn and twisted. He walked with a bad limp. At last he hobbled along with cup, saucer and plate, all bought separately. Then he came with an enamel jug and poured tea into the cup. Then he brought two slices of bread and butter covered with meat paste. The tea was nauseatingly sweet. But I was hungry and thirsty, and I ate and drank with gusto. Soon after he had finished, one of the men got out of his bed and went behind a curtain. I did not realise what he was doing until I smelt the horrible fetid odour. Then streams of men came walking up to the wash-basin near my bed. They took out their false teeth and put them in cups. The clock said five minutes to seven.[13]

For the occupants of the institutional hinterland, no benefits were derived from the Mental Treatment Act, as investment in new admission units arguably reinforced their hopelessness. Certified patients had a status of enforced dependency, as conveyed in this paternalistic statement in the Surrey County Mental Hospital rulebook for nurses (prepared one year before the Mental Treatment Act):

> Whether the patients belong to one section or the other, they are all equally held not to be responsible for their words and actions.[14]

Nihilism was illustrated by cursory entries in case notes: except for any physical illness, every six months a doctor would merely record 'no change'. Psychiatrist William Sargant[15] recalled the despairing scenes when starting as a locum doctor at Hanwell in 1934:

> Either I would find the patients semi-poisoned and doped with bromides, or else I might be immediately surrounded by a crowd of patients, dragging at my clothes and jealously hitting out at each other, the nurses doing their best to calm the pandemonium. At the end of the worst wards stretched a row of single cells. There was one whose occupant had not, it was said, emerged voluntarily for seven years. She often stood waiting for my visit with a large chamber pot in her hand ready to empty it over me as soon as the door opened. Other cells contained patients whose temper was periodically so uncertain that the nurse would unlock the door, push in a tin of food, and then quickly lock up again.

Abandon hope, all ye who enter here. A common utterance about asylums was that if you weren't mad when you came in, you certainly would become so. Without effective medication, many patients were stereotypically wild in appearance and behaviour, as in this personal account by JA Howard Ogdon, who described his stay at a county mental hospital in 1939:

> There were women whose natural charm and beauty could not be buried in an ugly, bag-like, Institution robe. And jostling them were screaming, blasphemous, bewhiskered old harridans, who might have stepped clean out of a Hogarth orgy. Well-set-up young men, in conjunction with the slobbering, tattered remnants of mankind. Some features they had in common. Their eyes were either dull, inert, and sunk in defeat – or they were bright with fear.[16]

In the 1930s the resident mental hospital population in Britain was rising by 2,000 each year. As well as the economic slump, a major contributory factor was the changing structure of society; as slum clearances and the wider availability of public and private housing encouraged the rise of the suburban nuclear family, people became less inclined to look after physically or mentally infirm relatives. The proportion of elderly patients was steadily increasing, including large numbers with senile dementia, whose eventide was endured in the mental institution because they had nowhere else to go.

The Royal Commission in 1926 had decreed that no new mental hospital should exceed 1,000 beds. However, when a large manor estate became available to the north of London, the Middlesex County Council saw a ready resolution to its problem of overwhelming demand. Alongside land set aside for a mental subnormality institution, the Middlesex authorities planned a new mental hospital of 2,000 beds. While described as a 'colony for rate-aided mental patients', the modern design of Shenley was lauded in a *Lancet* article.[17] Most patients were housed in separate villas, with access to the spacious, pleasantly landscaped grounds, but security was not abandoned. Large blocks of locked wards were placed centrally, surrounded by iron railings, with a total of fifteen padded rooms. Gender segregation was maintained throughout, with signs clearly delineating the boundaries of male and female parole. The self-contained reception unit had forty beds for each sex. Officially opened by King George V in May 1934, Shenley was rapidly filled by patients transferred from the other Middlesex institutions of Napsbury and Springfield, some of whom had been contracted out to provincial hospitals as distant as Hereford.

Elsewhere, new reception units relieved some pressure on the main block, but not all mental hospitals were able to provide this facility. In 1932 the Board of Control inspectors at Buckinghamshire Mental Hospital criticised an excess of sixty female patients over official bed capacity.[18] In response nineteen women were sent to the Cornwall Mental Hospital at Bodmin, over 200 miles away; another batch was sent to Littlemore. This was an unsatisfactory and costly arrangement. In 1934, after adjoining land was purchased, plans were agreed for a sixty-bed admission hospital, three fifty-bed villas and a nurses' home. However, the admissions unit, Beacon House, did not open until 1959. The Board of Control persevered in its drive for improvement, but county authorities paid more attention to sewerage than to mental patients, for whom expenditure had no political capital. Quality of care, comfort and hygiene inevitably declined; there were too many patients in the care of too few staff. Throughout the main block, corridors reverberated with an endless jangling of keys as doors were repeatedly unlocked and relocked.

The unbending institutional routine began early, around 6 a.m. Patients got up to wash in a sanitary spur at the end of the dormitory, where stable doors afforded little privacy and strips of newspaper served as toilet paper. Due to the inadequate facilities in wards, communal bathing blocks remained in use in most hospitals, as Ogdon experienced every Thursday morning:

> We were marched through a maze of corridors to the communal bathing centre … We were stripped in the vestibule and passed into the bathroom, with four baths separated by duck-boards. We stood in queues and bathed in turn – sometimes without change of water when time was running short.[19]

In co-author PN's study of nurses who started in the 1920s, a charge nurse likened the weekly bath routine to 'dipping sheep'.[20] Patients undressed in line, got into a bath vacated by the previous person, and had only a few minutes to wash themselves in the dirty water. There was often no soap and only a few towels for 80 patients. For the last patients the water was cold and the towels saturated. Some kindly nurses brought soap and razor blades for the patients to use. In her study of Severalls Hospital in Essex, Diana Gittins[21] was told by a laundress of communal bathing in the 1930s:

> As they went in, all they'd got on was a dress … and that was taken off and they were put under the showers, poor souls, and there they were with all the

water running down over their hair and everything else. And the nurses had big sponges and they did sponge them down after a fashion, but they weren't all that fussy about going in certain places, because sometimes they weren't all that clean. And then they wrapped themselves in these bath sheets and dried themselves as best they could, or the nurses helped them best they could – a bit on the rough side, some of them. It wasn't all as it should be. I saw rough handling … 'Oh, we've got this lot to do'. There was about I don't know how many on a ward – fifty, something like that. They've got a job to do, I know. But they didn't handle them gently. I've seen them pull them by the hair and all that sort of thin. And if they can't get their arms, pull their arms. I've seen them slap them and all that. And you didn't say anything about it, that was all taken for granted.

Smoking was not permitted before breakfast, so the porridge, 'door wedges' and lukewarm tea were rushed down. Working patients left the ward, although some stayed to perform domestic chores such as making beds, or polishing the oak floors with 'bumpers' (padded wooden blocks on a pole). Others were 'on draught' and allowed to lie down for an hour after their dose of a barbiturate or paraldehyde. As Ogdon described, the pleasure of a smoke in the day-room was abruptly terminated:[22]

> Near ten o'clock the charge-nurse shouted 'On to the courts! Boots!' and there was a scramble to change ward-shoes. Then we lined up along another corridor, being let out in file, and counted aloud as we passed by. One wag of a nurse used to get patients together by shouting, as a regular thing, 'Bring out your dead!'

Despite the benefits of exercise and fresh air, the airing courts were a deadening place. Pathetically, patients tottered around in the same direction under the vigilant gaze of nurses, positioned at various vantage points. Eventually a whistle was blown and patients were counted back inside. Only in the worst weather would sessions be suspended. Journalist Paul Winterton of the *News Chronicle*, whose book *Mending Minds* documented the day-to-day life of a mental hospital near London, described an enduring image:[23]

> The picture in my mind as I recall the last airing court I saw is one of brown-trampled earth, unrelieved by any green, and a few hard wooden benches; of a drab company of muttering, gesticulating, laughing or downcast men, shuffling on and on in a hopeless monotonous circuit.

Nurses were not allowed to converse on the airing court. Vigilance was required: a patient might try to escape over the fence, or commit suicide by climbing a tree; feeble-minded or psychotic patients might swallow stones or poisonous plants.[24] A retired nurse interviewed by co-author PN described the importance of these sessions in the mental hospital regime:[25]

It was common to refer to the practice as 'airing the patients'. The superintendent often used to ask 'Have the patients been aired?' It was widely believed that fresh air was good for people, particularly the sick and the mentally ill. The older staff used to tell us that bad smells and being cooped up inside drove people mad.

Back in the day-room, patients had another smoke. Recreational facilities such as billiards and board games were available but many patients simply retreated to chairs lined along the walls, staring vacantly as another monotonous day passed slowly by. Working patients' efforts were rewarded with extra rations in a mid-morning snack of bread and cheese. Ogdon was assigned to stamping ward numbers on clothes for male and female inmates. All patients' garments were made in the sewing room: calico underwear, moleskin trousers, tweed suits, canvas restraining jackets and shoes with tear-proof straps. The pooled attire was made to withstand heavy use, destructive tendencies of patients, and the hospital laundry. On admission Ogdon had received a set of clothing including a suit from the tailor's shop 'vile in quality and pattern'.[26]

The medical officers' ward round was completed by late morning. Lunch was announced by a hooter, and patients were escorted to the vast dining hall. The order of meals was that of the working class, with a two-course dinner in the middle of the day, and supper in the early evening. According to Ogdon the meals were 'unpalatably cooked and served. The worst dishes were the soups and rissoles: even the hungriest were deterred by the premonitory stench'.[27] Mental hospital cuisine was epitomised by the tripe barrel. Fresh vegetables and fruit were normally served, and the bland institutional diet was probably more nutritious than the average household, particularly in the hard times of the 1930s when families often went hungry until the next payday. After the checking of cutlery, patients were counted before returning to the ward. Able patients went back to work, while others spent a sedentary afternoon in the day-room, interrupted by another airing court session. The last meal of the day was a light supper of bread and jam, and sometimes cold meat, with a mug of tea. Apart from a warm milky drink before bed, it was a long wait until the next sustenance at breakfast.

Evenings were short, as patients adapted to a daily rhythm brought forward by two or three hours from working-class norms. This was for institutional convenience, but there was little reason to stay up in a comfortless environment. For Ogdon, winters stood out in memory because of the struggle against the elements. Unlike the bright, warm and well-equipped admission unit, 'the main blocks, where nearly 700 men were housed, were chilly, crudely and sparsely furnished, and badly lit. There was an inadequate open fire in the day-room, and a system of radiation that was never more than tepid.'[28] Nonetheless, a ward sister portrayed a merry scene as curtains were drawn on a typical day:[29]

> 4pm: a plain wholesome tea and the rest of the evening is given to recreation. We form a set for ping-pong and a whist party. Not much on the wireless

tonight, so we get Miss Brown to strike up on the piano, and dancing follows. 7pm: bedtime.

With no space for personal belongings, patients' clothes were tied together in bundles and placed under the bed. Few cared for a toothbrush; most patients had dentures, which were removed at night. Restless or disruptive patients received a sleeping draught from the night nurse, as another day ended.

The routine was punctuated by weekly events. On Sunday morning patients were taken to service in the chapel. Although it had lost its prominence in the mental hospital, religion was maintained in institutional ritual. John Vincent[30] perceived the weekly Anglican sermons as another form of discipline; patients were expected to listen attentively, while attendants chatted or read newspapers in the back pew and remained seated for hymns. Meanwhile entertainment kept up with the times. Cinematic apparatus, having been fitted in the recreation hall at the Kent Mental Hospital at Barming Heath in 1927, was converted to 'talkies' in 1933,[31] making the accompanying pianist redundant. Films were shown on one afternoon per week and were popular with patients and also members of staff, who often attended when off duty: as well as avoiding the vagaries of public transport to visit picture-houses in the nearest town, this was free entertainment. The privilege of the weekly film show could be readily withdrawn from an uncooperative patient. Tom Hopkinson, who applied to Rubery Hill Hospital in the late 1920s, impressed the medical superintendent in interview due to his previous experience as a projectionist. It became Tom's responsibility to cycle to Birmingham every Monday to return the previous week's film and collect a new one. Films were contained in as many as six cans and were very awkward to carry on a bicycle. Tom was adept at changing the reels speedily, but when the film spliced or the projector malfunctioned, he incurred the patients' wrath.[32]

The highlight of the week remained the patients' dance. Paul Winterton, entrusted with a master key by the medical superintendent to roam the hospital at will, began his narration in the main hall, where patients glided in time to waltzes performed by the hospital band of five male nurses. After fox-trotting with a pretty young female patient, Winterton enquired into her circumstances:[33]

> 'There doesn't seem to be very much wrong with her,' I suggested diffidently. 'No,' said the Superintendent, 'I'm glad to say she's made excellent progress lately and I think she'll be fit to go home in a few months.' 'She says she's had a nervous breakdown,' I remarked. The Superintendent smiled rather grimly. 'You can call it that if you like,' he said. 'She had domestic trouble and tried to cut her throat with a pair of scissors. You can see from the scar how nearly she succeeded. And not long ago she swallowed her tooth-brush and we had to operate to get it out. Still, we're very satisfied with her.'

Patients were not normally allowed to dance together: it was the nurses' job to go down the line and take partners. In a BBC documentary on Lancaster Moor,[34] an ex-patient told of the polished, sprung floor in the main hall, where it was reputed that after the lights were dimmed at the end of the dance, two figures could be seen dancing: this was a male and a female patient who had looked longingly at each other from opposite lines but had never been allowed to touch. Nonetheless, social events such as the weekly dance boosted patients' morale and created a sense of normality in the mental hospital. The Board of Control applauded the introduction of a hospital shop, enabling patients to spend their allowance on cigarettes or confectionery. Although personal clothing was the exception rather than the rule, some patients adorned themselves with items of their own making. An influential voice for the dignity and comfort of female patients was Dame Ellen Pinsent, a senior commissioner of the Board of Control, who had previously been active in reforming the care of people with mental deficiency. Dame Pinsent asserted the therapeutic value of hairdressing and decent attire, enabling women to take pride in their appearance.[35]

Christmas was traditionally celebrated with a pantomime and party. Patients and nurses alike looked forward to this climax of the mental hospital calendar, and much effort was put into preparations. In 1932, the Mayor of Brighton accepted an invitation to attend the patient's fancy-dress ball at the Brighton Mental Hospital in Haywards Heath, where several male nurses dressed as their female counterparts, and over half of the 340 patients in attendance were in costume:[36]

> To give anything but a vague description of the characters portrayed or the ingenuity of the patients in disguising themselves would be impossible but it was noticed that the women for the most part chose bright colours, while a large number of the men were resplendent in uniforms and deported themselves in true soldierly style. There were English, French and German soldiers, a Beefeater, a fireman, a footballer, two dudes complete with top hats, morning coats and walking sticks, a realistic Chinaman, many male and female French clowns with pointed hats, ballet girls, Victorian ladies, 'Buy British' and other advertising costumes, while one male patient, who represented a flower girl, bore the label 'Back to Eros'. The most prominent of all, perhaps, was a male patient who represented Gandhi. With his practically bald head, his spectacles and his white robes he was almost Gandhi's double. A huge block of salt gave a finishing touch to this impersonation.

Local people and relatives were invited to the summer fête, where they could purchase items of handiwork, and cheer as patients of all ages ran the circuit of the sports field, their ties or dresses flapping around them. Egg-and-spoon and sack races added to the jollity. Also in summer a charabanc trip was organised for each ward. Patients and their nurses spent the day at a coastal resort, relaxing on the beach, having fish suppers on the promenade and then stopping at a tavern on the way back for a glass of beer. In autumn the major event was the harvest festival, when the chapel was adorned with garlands of produce, and celebratory hymns were sung.

A parole system was established at mental hospitals in the spirit of the Mental Treatment Act. At Friern the grades were 'corridor', 'grounds', 'town' and 'special town'. The few trustworthy patients allowed freedom beyond the hospital gate signed 'an obligation to be of good character, not to pick fruit in the hospital orchards, post letters outside or help others to escape'.[37] Public houses were out of bounds, and the patient was to return before sunset. In progressive hospitals, unlocking of wards continued in the 1930s. Medical superintendent George Harper-Smith opened several wards on both sides of the Brighton Mental Hospital, and allowed some mixing of the sexes in exercise classes and entertainments. By 1939, 64 per cent of admissions to this hospital were voluntary.[38] Board of Control inspectors were impressed by the high proportion of unlocked wards at West Park in Epsom, where thirteen wards were open to the grounds and four to their own gardens.[39] For many patients, however, reprieve from the institutional gloom was limited to a weekly walking party. From the back wards, there was little opportunity to enjoy the green splendour of the hospital estate.

Black eyes and banter

The workforce at mental hospitals remained skeletal in the early 1930s. Typically, a medium-sized mental institution of 1,500 beds had a total medical staff of five: the medical superintendent, and chief and assistant medical officers on male and female sides. The nursing staff, headed by the chief male nurse and deputy on one side, and a matron and her deputy on the other, was much larger, perhaps comprising 200 nurses including probationers. However, this complement was spread thinly across the many wards, for day and night duty. Shortage of nurses was most acute on the female side, where there were more patients and higher staff turnover.

Reviewing mental hospital care in the early twentieth century, Hugh Freeman[40] contrasted the militaristic mode of male attendants with the Nightingale general nursing tradition on the female side. Transcending such differences was a distinct culture of mental nursing, with staff striving to maintain control in a challenging environment of overcrowding, understaffing and interminable routine. Nurses had little time or inclination for meaningful engagement with patients. Distance was preserved, as described in Vincent's account of his first interaction with a nurse:

> On the third or fourth day I suddenly became aware of a man standing beside my bed. He was wearing the blue suit of the male nurses with the addition of braid and gold trimmings. His eyes were deep and piercing. I said 'Good morning'. He made no remark and continued to stand and stare at me. I rolled over so that my back was towards him. Then he sat on the edge of my bed and asked me questions. His manner did not make me responsive. He seemed to be the symbol of authority, of the authority against which I had been a rebel all my life. Another senior nurse came in and asked me a question or two. He was a stern, unbending man, with no trace of soft humour in his face.[41]

Vincent observed that some nurses were unsuited to the care of vulnerable people:

> One nurse, when I asked what led him to take up his present work, replied with great candour that it was the certainty of exemption from military service. Some men were failures, not because they were inefficient, but because they lacked common humanity.[42]

While appreciating nurses' caring intent, Ogdon criticised their lack of sensitivity to patients' problems:[43]

> The average of psychological knowledge among the nursing staff wasn't worth a straw. Their skill in sick-nursing was correspondingly high. When the practical art was demanded, their enthusiasm and ability rose together. On the mental side there was little more than apathy. While I was in the Institution's big store, I found some old logs – day-books and night-books. Pitiable…did the Board of Control ever see them? Just a few cant-phrases, nearly run to death, the barest clichés of psychological jargon. Delusions. Everyone had delusions, and had them often.

George William Clarke, a young charge nurse at Bexley Hospital in the 1930s, had chosen mental nursing for a career after living near the perimeter of Colney Hatch in the 1920s:

> Very frequently, one of the inmates would try to escape, running from the Asylum grounds, with men in blue uniforms and key chains hanging in hot pursuit, the inmate running like a fox from the hounds. My immediate reaction was, what a way to treat human beings. I determined that I would try and improve the lives of these unfortunate people.[44]

In his enthusiasm for change, Clarke faced opposition from older, more experienced colleagues, who resented novices telling them how to do their job. Relaxations to the regime such as unlocking of ward doors and dismantling of airing court fences troubled nurses who would quickly speculate on worst-case scenarios. Yet flexibility was also evident in managing wards, as in the reciprocity described by a Prestwich nurse:

> You used to have favourites and we used to take little things in for them. Perhaps a couple of apples or oranges and give to them and they'd work their fingers to the bone, scrub the floors, do anything for you if you gave them an apple.[45]

Monitoring was a brake on abuse. As well as Board of Control inspections, each mental hospital's visiting committee made monthly visits to the wards, inviting comments and requests from patients, including appeals for discharge and any allegations of mistreatment. Medical examinations were performed every few weeks, potentially revealing bruises or other injuries. As well as the threat of dismissal, Section 322 of the Lunacy Act made anyone in charge of a mental patient liable to a fine or imprisonment on conviction of wilful neglect or abuse. The Macmillan Commission, despite hearing various allegations of cruelty, had praised the dedication and skill of nurses in caring for people ostracised by society.[46] In one instance, it had exposed sensationalism: an officer of the Wandsworth Board of Guardians had referred to a padded cell at Cane Hill as 'the Black Hole of Calcutta', but an unannounced visit to the specific room found this expression unmerited.

Nurses needed physical and mental strength to keep order on the ward, and prided themselves on their ability to do this without resorting to brute force. Tackling severely disturbed and aggressive patients tightened the bonds between nurses, who relied on each other for safety. A black eye was an occupational hazard, but there was danger of being severely maimed. Violence was particularly common on the female side,[47] as illustrated by a nurse on a refractory ward at Severalls in the 1930s:

> Here it could be rough and tough most of the time. Most patients were really violent, and one had to remember never to let anyone creep up on you from the back. Many a time you could be attacked for no reason at all, and end up on the floor with legs and arms flailing in all directions. Windows were smashed almost every day. We spent a lot of time sweeping up glass ... Quite a few had to be cared for in the side-rooms and padded rooms. I will never forget the first time I saw the patient in one of the pads. She just had a sheet over her shoulders – no other clothes, and when she was wet or soiled we just changed the sheet. She never moved and was fixed in a crouched position. At times we had outbursts of violence and had to call in the help of several staff. We often had our clothes torn from us, and it could be a hard time to get the patient in a side-room or one of the pads ... I did get used to this ward, but was not at all sorry to leave it.[48]

Inevitably some patients were manhandled, and not always with therapeutic purpose. Interviewing former nurses of the Bethlem and Maudsley Hospitals, David Russell[49] was told by those who had started their careers in the 1930s of frequent physical struggles with patients. One nurse told of being off sick through injury from a patient known as 'the Major'. On returning to work, he found that this patient had been moved to another ward, having sustained a broken arm in a suspected retribution by the interviewee's colleagues. A condition peculiar to mental patients was 'insane ear', whereby swelling led to a marked deformity; most common in general paralysis of the insane (GPI), mania and epilepsy, it may have been caused by repeated physical assault.[50]

Tools of the trade, albeit blunt, were found in the drug cupboard. Bromides had fallen from favour due to toxic confusion and skin inflammation. Newer barbiturate drugs such as sodium amytal were safer but at best a symptomatic intervention, controlling acute mental disturbance at the cost of debilitating drowsiness and dependence. The ace in the pharmacological pack was paraldehyde, which produced rapid relief of otherwise unmanageable symptoms. Normally administered orally in an aqueous solution, the substance had an unpleasant odour when excreted in breath and sweat. In emergency it was given by intramuscular route, causing much pain on injection. Despite its awful taste, paraldehyde was so addictive that patients would beg for more, reminiscent of Charles Dickens' Oliver Twist requesting more gruel in the workhouse. From the corridors, the reek of paraldehyde was a sure sign of where the most disturbed patients resided. Although drugs required medical prescription, in some cases they could be given on a *pro re nata* basis, and nurses may have been tempted to give fortified doses for a quiet night.

A major management problem for nurses was epilepsy. As well as the frequent seizures, nurses watched for the potentially dangerous event of *status epilepticus*, where an escalation of fits could lead to death if not rapidly terminated by injection of a hefty dose of bromide. As prophylaxis, drugs were of limited effectiveness, reducing the occurrence fits in some patients but making others worse. Due to the particular management problems, most large mental hospitals had wards for the epileptic insane. In his series on mental disorders for the *Nursing Mirror*, GWTH Fleming, deputy medical superintendent at the Dorset Asylum, described features of the epileptic personality, which was believed to result from many years of convulsions. The epileptic patient was typically 'cunning and deceitful, a potential criminal', with a tendency to shroud his faults in a cloak of piety:[51]

> He is religiose, that is he makes a great pretence of being religious, insisting on going to church on all possible occasions, walking about with a prayer book in his hand … He collects little personal affects and invests them with the greatest sanctity, and woe betide anyone who upsets the box!

A nurse at Severalls recalled her introduction to mental nursing in an epileptic ward in 1936:[52]

> The first ward I worked on was horrific: an epileptic ward with at least a hundred patients milling around. The noise was unbelievable – patients shouting, fighting and cursing each other. There were some wandering around with draw sheets tied round their necks because they dribbled so much – their mouths wide open – not a pretty sight. The dormitory was huge with four rows of beds and side-rooms along three sides of the room. The beds were only about a foot high for safety reasons, as all these people were prone to have fits at any time. The most difficult patients slept in the side-rooms – what a fight it was to push some of them in and get out quickly enough to get the door locked on them!

Another condition requiring much nursing attention was involutional melancholia, a depressive state arising in middle age, when physical vitality began to decline. Afflicted patients exhibited agitation and despair, and often suicidal ideation. Refusal of food was common in melancholic cases, to which nurses responded by force-feeding. Eggs, sugar, milk, cream, salt or fruit juice were administered in amounts of up to two pints, twice of three times daily. Brandy, aperients and sedatives were sometimes added to the mix.[53] A battle of wills was fought between patients who wanted to die and the nurses responsible for keeping them alive. A suicide caution card was issued by the medical officer,[54] and all nurses coming on duty confirmed by signature that they understood their responsibility:

> This Patient is regarded as being actively suicidal and must on no account be allowed out of observation. This Card must be shown and explained to every Nurse doing duty on the Ward, and each Nurse must acknowledge by his/her signature on the back thereof that this has been done.[55]

The nurse was never to let the suicidal patient out of sight, but this was a tall order. Amidst the bustle of the ward, momentary inattention could be tragic. While looking after a multitude of patients with minimal staffing, it was extremely difficult to monitor the suicidal and epileptic cases satisfactorily. This placed unreasonable burden on night staff: in the 1930s, compared to a national average of eleven patients per nurse in daytime, the nocturnal ratio was 53:1. In his thoughtful account of mental hospital life, Winterton[56] wrote positively of nurses as underappreciated but devoted personnel, hampered by the backwardness of their employing local authorities. Acknowledging the hardship, Ogdon remarked:

> Mental nursing is a bread-and-butter business, and there is not enough butter.[57]

Pay and perks

Historically, recruitment to mental nursing was so difficult that institutions accepted almost anyone who applied. However, in the global economic depression of the 1930s factories were forced to lay off workers, leaving 3 million unemployed to survive on minimal state welfare ('the dole') and many others barely feeding their families on part-time wages. Scores of men from the struggling industrial heartlands of central Scotland, south Wales and northern England arrived at the gate lodge of mental hospitals, seeking a stable job. For the first time, supply exceeded demand in mental hospitals, at least on the male side. In 1936, the 207 marchers who walked from Jarrow to the Palace of Westminster received vocal support, food parcels and overnight accommodation from some former workmates now nursing in various mental hospitals along their route.[58]

Mental hospital culture remained strictly hierarchical, with three distinct groups: the doctors, nursing staff and the patients. Medical officers instructed nurses on clinical and administrative matters, but social barriers did not permit informal conversation on or off the wards. Doctors dined separately in their oak-panelled rooms. On appointment, nurses submitted to absolute obedience to the medical superintendent, as detailed in the Surrey County Mental Hospitals rules:[59]

> All attendants and nurses render themselves liable to instant dismissal for any act of misconduct, such as great carelessness or neglect of duties imperilling the safety of the Institution; the welfare of the patients, or leading to the escape of any; roughness, harshness, or ill-treatment of any of the inmates in word or deed, or witnessing any and not endeavouring to prevent it, as well as to report it; immoral conduct, or intoxication, within or without the Hospital; dishonesty; gambling; receiving perquisites; bringing intoxicating liquors into the establishment; being absent without leave; found in the wrong division without permission; wearing clothing belonging to the patients, or to the Hospital, other than the uniform allowed; appropriating patients' provisions to their own use; insubordination, and refusal to obey Officers' orders.

Trade union membership was risky. In Gittins' study at Severalls, male attendants of the 1930s recalled the secrecy in joining and paying subscription fees to the Mental Hospital and Institution Workers' Union (so named after the NAWU merged with the Poor Law Institution Workers' Union). It was widely believed that if a member was discovered, he would be escorted off the premises. Men diverted from careers in the mines or foundries would have reinforced the camaraderie of a male working-class culture, but mental nursing was not ripe for a workers' struggle against the establishment. The Trade Union Congress (TUC) was courting nurses in the 1930s, but this was resisted by the College of Nursing, which asserted itself as the true representative of the profession, just as the British Medical Association did for doctors. From its *Nursing Times* podium, the College warned nurses of political exploitation.[60] The trade unions themselves feared infiltration by Communists, and the TUC urged unions to prohibit links to radical organisations. In 1934 the MHIWU rejected an application by the Colney Hatch branch to aid a local association opposed to Fascism and capitalism.[61]

While the MHIWU was a relatively weak union, mental hospital nurses were beginning to benefit from their inclusion in the wider nursing profession. In 1932 a *Lancet* commission drew attention to the adverse conditions of nursing; although the focus was on general hospitals, this influential report advocated for those who care for patients in any setting. Nurses were protected from the ravages of austerity. In 1931 the National Government led by Ramsay MacDonald imposed cuts in public service pay, reflecting depressed wages in industry. The MHIWU and MHA agreed to a temporary reduction of 2.5 per cent, but in some hospitals this was not implemented, and by the mid-1930s it was abandoned. Although curbs on union activity constrained the collective strength of the nursing staff, the authorities knew not to take their workforce for granted. The quality of nurses was unlikely to improve while the work was so arduous and poorly rewarded. In 1935 it was agreed to reduce the working week from 59 hours and 45 minutes to 54 hours, inclusive of meal breaks.[62] The long shifts continued, but with one half-day and two days off.

Wage recommendations by the Joint Conciliation Committee were not binding, allowing hospital authorities to set their own rates. In provincial mental hospitals in the early1930s male nurses started on around 34 shillings a week, with an increment of 2 shillings a week for each completed year of service.[63] Half of the pay was deducted for board, lodging and uniform. By the late 1930s male probationers in London County Council mental hospitals received 52 shillings per week – more than the starting rate for qualified nurses in the shires; there was no need to advertise. While male recruitment had improved, the situation was very different on the other side. Female probationers started on around 29 shillings a week, but a young woman could work in a factory for £2 to £3 a week, while preserving her friendships and freedom, with no residential compulsion or marriage bar. Opportunities for women had increased with the growth of service industries and clerical work. Throughout the 1930s the majority of recruitment advertisements by mental hospitals were for women. In this example in the *Nursing Mirror*, Croydon Borough Mental Hospital attempted to compete with nearby London institutions:

> Educated young women (18–25) wanted to train as nurses … Gross wages 35s 4d per week to commence, from which a charge is made for board, lodging, and washing, rising with increments and bonuses given upon passing examinations to 57s 9d per week. Two days' weekly leave and three weeks' annual leave.[64]

The discrepancy between male and female nurses' pay, although permitted by law, was becoming indefensible as recruitment problems on the female side worsened. As shown in Figure 3.1, in 1939 Graylingwell Hospital was offering local women a relatively generous remuneration in a market town with high employment.[65]

An unappealing situation for nursing staff was their accommodation, most nurses living in the main block. The shortcomings of these cramped barracks, often next to the wards, was appreciated by GWTH Fleming on his appointment as medical superintendent of the Hereford Mental Hospital at Burghill:

> To obtain and retain the services of good nurses it is absolutely essential to provide comfortable quarters for them. The present arrangement whereby 16 of them are housed in the old Isolation Hospital, 8 in the Laurels and the remainder in parts of the hospital is most unsatisfactory. We urgently need a Nurses' Home to accommodate some 45 nurses.[66]

Nursing periodicals in the 1930s were replete with articles celebrating openings of nurses' homes. Typically a flat-roofed block of three storeys, their modern, functional design contrasted with the Victorian labyrinth, liberating off-duty nurses from the sight, noise and smell of the wards. An exemplar was at Springfield Mental Hospital, officially opened by Princess Mary on 22 June 1931, which boasted parquet flooring throughout, single bedrooms (with fitted basin, wardrobe,

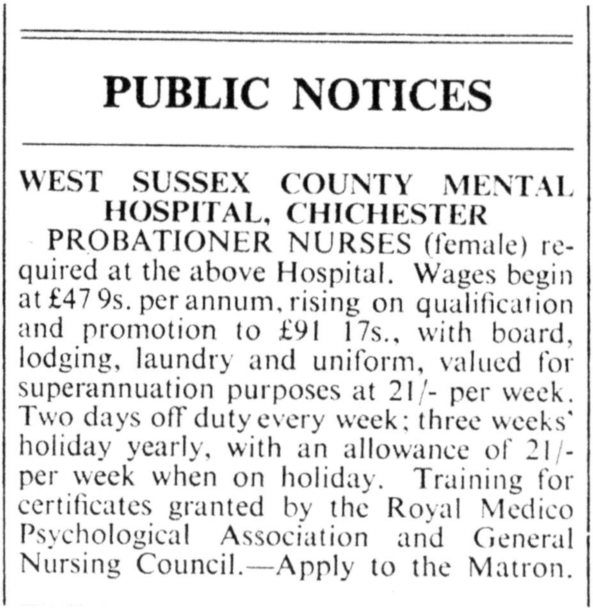

PUBLIC NOTICES

WEST SUSSEX COUNTY MENTAL HOSPITAL, CHICHESTER
PROBATIONER NURSES (female) required at the above Hospital. Wages begin at £47 9s. per annum, rising on qualification and promotion to £91 17s., with board, lodging, laundry and uniform, valued for superannuation purposes at 21/- per week. Two days off duty every week; three weeks' holiday yearly, with an allowance of 21/- per week when on holiday. Training for certificates granted by the Royal Medico Psychological Association and General Nursing Council.—Apply to the Matron.

Figure 3.1 Advertisement for nurses, Graylingwell

bed and armchair), a tiled kitchen, communal sitting areas furnished with piano, gramophone, writing tables and 'great vases of delphiniums'.[67] Spacious but barren sitting rooms were softened by rugs made in occupational therapy workshops. At Exeter County Mental Hospital, a *Nursing Mirror* reporter was impressed by 'a liberal-minded provision of cigarette and chocolate machines'.[68]

'Ladies first' was not so much gentlemanly as a pragmatic response to recruitment and turnover problems. At Plymouth Mental Hospital, a home was built in 1931 to accommodate fifty-two female nurses,[69] with appointment of a home sister to look after the girls, many of whom had left home for the first time. Recruits were informed that the home sister would look after them when sick, although this matriarch was unlikely to be sympathetic a mere cold or headache if wards were left short. In 1937, London County Council leader Herbert Morrison praised the new nurses' home at Friern Hospital, where all 117 rooms were provided for women (at the time, 270 of the 490 nurses were female).[70] By 1939 the Board of Control reported that one-fifth of mental hospital workers were still living in the main hospital blocks;[71] these were mostly male. At West Park in Epsom, a home was opened in 1938 for sixty-six female nurses, who had hitherto slept in rooms off the wards, but similar provision was not provided for men until 1959.[72]

At some institutions nurses were required to live in for their first five years. This was to inculcate an *esprit des corps*, while protecting younger staff from the distractions of life outside. Older nurses saw living in as a rite of passage for juniors. Yet as they were being built at all types of hospital, the nurses' home was seen by some in the nursing profession as a clipping of wings in a changing society, in which young women expected to be treated as independent adults and to enjoy a little freedom. The nurses' home maintained a captive workforce, but living in was also practically advantageous for mental nurses. As most mental hospitals were located away from public transport routes, travelling home would have added to the long daily ardour. A resident staff prevented shortages in bad weather, when the hospital might be marooned by snow.

Although married male nurses could live out, a few houses were normally provided on the perimeter of the grounds for these men and their families. With little to do on the hospital site off duty, many nurses preferred to work overtime.[73] Special permission was needed to attend funerals, weddings and birthday parties of close family members, and requests were often turned down. Nurses looked forward to visiting the local town on their day off to shop, meet friends, have a 'proper' meal and visit places of entertainment, but many became accustomed to spending their entire time in the hospital grounds, particularly as facilities improved.

Sport became more organised in the interwar period. Saturday afternoons were devoted to outdoor games, with inter-hospital tournaments established for football, cricket and hockey. Applicants were asked about their sporting abilities in interview: men who could contribute to the success of the football or cricket team were favoured. As noted by Cherry and Munting[74] in their study of sport in mental hospitals, some institutions attracted players of high standard. One of their informants, raised in the grounds of the Norwich Mental Hospital, recalled the football team, bolstered by former Norwich City players, winning a local league in the 1930s and gaining promotion to the Eastern Counties League; the cricket team boasted three current Norfolk county players. The mental hospital was an ideal training ground for Frank Close, a charge nurse at Banstead, who won a bronze medal at the 1936 Olympics in Berlin.[75]

Football and cricket tournaments were very competitive, with much pride at stake. From autumn to spring the hospital was represented by its football colours and in summer by flannels, caps and blazers adorned with the hospital crest. Sport was also a social leveller: while some medical superintendents assumed the captaincy of the cricket XI, football was more meritocratic. A memorable image was relayed to Cherry and Munting of Norwich medical superintendent McCulley in his football kit, holding an umbrella on the touchline in pouring rain, hoping for a game. According to Gardner,[76] superintendent George Harper-Smith at Brighton Mental Hospital never missed a football match, home or away. Sometimes hundreds of patients, staff and local people would assemble to support the hospital team, and busloads of supporters were conveyed to fixtures at other hospitals. As described by Kathleen Jones,[77] much was invested in the footballing representatives of the hospital:

> The team would be cheered off as the coach went down the long drive, and greeted with enthusiasm or commiseration on its return. Some long-stay patients could recite the scores from matches with this hospital or that over ten or twenty years.

Musical talent was also coveted. A male applicant of no use on the soccer field would yet appeal to the medical superintendent if he could play the cornet. Mental hospital bands performed to a high standard. Bandsmen had the privileges of time off for practice, extra food rations, and a bonus for public performances. The chosen few who played in the hospital band and football and cricket teams were excused from shifts, leaving others to cover. A 'lesser mortal' interviewed by Gittins[78] was forced to take his two days off on the Monday and Tuesday every week:

> Nearly all the charges had Sunday and Monday, or Saturday and Sunday. And then you come to the footballers – they had either Friday and Saturday, or Saturday and Sunday. And in the summer you had the cricket. And then the bandsmen had Wednesday and Thursday, because there was the band on the Friday and practice on the Tuesday. So Monday and Tuesday was left over … I went up to see Mr Markland and said 'Do you think I could have a change of days? My wife is sick and tired of seeing me wash day and ironing day'. So I had Wednesday and Thursday off for one sheet, which was three or four months. And then I went back to Tuesday and Wednesday. That was the set up, you see. And there was nothing you could do about it. 'If you don't like it, you know where the gate is!'

Transition in training

In the 1930s much progress was made in the training of mental hospital nurses. Typically an experienced female nurse was appointed to a combined role of home sister and tutor, with lecture rooms provided on the ground floor of the new nurses' home. Novices had a six-month probationary period on a ward, where they learned the routine. After one year they were allowed to attend lectures by the medical staff and matron, in their own time. At Barming Heath in Kent, where a new nursing school had opened in 1927, placements for trainees comprised six months in sick nursing, an admission ward, a ward for melancholic patients and an epileptic ward; and three months on tubercular, delusional and children's wards. Almost 100 lectures and practical demonstrations were given, the former by medical staff and the latter by the new sister-tutor or ward sisters.[79] Crammer[80] noted in his history of the Buckinghamshire Mental Hospital that one of the doctors stayed for only ten minutes of the lectures; he would leave with an instruction for trainees to open a particular chapter of the *Handbook for Mental Nurses*, and at the beginning of the next lecture he would check their reading with a few questions.

As an incentive for passing the preliminary nursing examination, nurses gained an extra 3s, and the same again for passing the final examination. In the 1930s the proportion of nurses gaining certificates in mental nursing increased steadily, reaching an average of 30 per cent by 1936. In London mental hospitals, where a nursing assistant grade had been instituted in 1928, probationers were required to complete training within five years or their contract was terminated.[81] However, in many provincial hospitals there was no requirement to take the nursing examination, and the pass rate was not high. A former nurse told of the tough RMPA examination at Severalls Hospital in the 1930s:[82]

> That day we sat there was thirty-one girls and twenty-four men – some men had failed a couple of times, but they played football or they were bandsmen, and they used to keep 'em. And up on the pass list was one woman and three – and they didn't give them away then. No, no.

The parallel training system continued. The General Nursing Council had decreed in 1929 that in future those gaining the Royal Medico-Psychological Association[83] certificate would not qualify for the state register, although this was not imposed by the Minister for Health. The College of Nursing asserted the right of the nursing profession to judge who could join its register,[84] but some medical superintendents insisted that only the RMPA had the necessary expertise to examine for the specialised work of the mental hospital. In favour of the RMPA examination was its lower fee, but this was not the only factor. While men tended to submit to the RMPA, holders of the GNC certificate were mostly female. Although there was little difference in the syllabus, the GNC set a more challenging examination. The GNC qualification was encouraged by matrons, who were doubly qualified in mental and general nursing.[85] Women may have identified more readily with the wider nursing body, while some men were reluctant to accept the label of nurse, despite its increasing official usage for both sets of staff. The inherent femininity of nursing was conveyed in its periodicals, with articles on skin care and advertisements for corsets. On the male side particularly, the RMPA was more representative of their interests.

For a nurse seeking promotion, the mental nursing certificate did not signify completion of training. In asserting a holistic view of physical and mental health, the Royal Commission of 1926 had recommended dual qualification for mental hospital nurses, which became a prerequisite of promotion to charge nurse. The need for this additional training was sometimes disputed, as it reinforced the perceived lower status of mental nursing. In 1937 the government appointed a committee chaired by Lord Athlone to enquire into the state of nursing. A subcommittee including George Gibson (General Secretary of the MHIWU), LT Felden of the MHA and Dr Masefield of the RMPA did not show favour to either RMPA or GNC training, but they were wary of the incursion of a general nursing culture.[86] By the end of the decade the RMPA route to qualification was in decline, but the core text remained its *Handbook for Mental Nurses*. As this was last updated in 1923, in 1937 the RMPA appointed a committee chaired by AAW Petrie, medical superintendent at Banstead, to revise the manual. Interrupted by war, the belated eighth edition did not materialise until seventeen years later.[87] Meanwhile the 'Red Book' was falling behind radical developments in mental health care.

Occupied minds

A repeated observation by Board of Control inspectors was of patients languishing in prolonged idleness in the day-rooms. This was a visible measurement of the quality of care, revealing a missed opportunity for nursing. From 1928 onwards the Board made a series of visits to Gütersloh in Germany, where Hermann Simon had initiated a scheme of therapeutic craftwork.[88] Positive results with the 'work cure' were also achieved at the Dutch mental hospital of Santpoort, where each of the 1,300 patients[89] was kept busy in some way; this was visited by several British delegations including the medical superintendent and staff of Chester Mental Hospital.[90] Nursing had traditionally being confined to basic necessities of care and containment, but forward-thinking authorities were keen to develop nurses' role in therapeutic endeavour. Among the first was Dorchester Mental Hospital, where occupational therapy was described as 'in full swing' in a *Nursing Mirror* article in 1930; instead of an assembly line producing prisoners' clothing for the Dorset gaol, patients were now busily crafting a diversity of articles through this 'curative and healing process'.[91]

For the role of occupation officer, mental hospitals began to send nurses for training at one of the new occupational therapy colleges. The first in England, Dorset House in Bristol, was founded by Elizabeth Casson in 1930. Casson had been inspired as a newly qualified doctor in a mental hospital by the tremendous boost to morale arising from the concerted effort of nurses and patients in making Christmas decorations; she realised that purposeful activity was integral to psychiatric treatment. Principal of Dorset House was Constance Tebbit, who had trained in occupational therapy in Philadelphia. Tebbit left to become occupation officer at Chester Mental Hospital in 1933, but resigned in the following year due to marriage.[92] A second school opened in London, in collaboration with the Maudsley Hospital. As the course at dedicated occupational therapy schools was long and fees high, some mental hospitals provided their own training. In 1933, the Warwickshire Mental Hospital at Hatton began two-month placements for every trainee nurse in its occupational therapy department.[93]

Intended as individualised treatment, occupational therapy could boost self-esteem and employment prospects. As well as promoting the recovery of mild cases, interest could be aroused in the listless and apathetic patients who would otherwise be abandoned to monotony. Nursing journals told of great pride taken by patients in the work, and of the dramatic change in atmosphere resulting from this enterprise. Winterton[94] described the industrious scene in the women's workshop:

> Anything like the popular idea of a mental hospital I cannot imagine. In one room, about forty or fifty patients were sitting, predominantly middle-aged, quiet, many of them dressed in gay colours, and having the outward aspect of perfectly sane people. Most of them were knitting, sewing, or crocheting, and the majority were completely absorbed. Some of the work they were turning out was magnificent – as good as handwork could be and far better than many sane people would be capable of.

Occupational therapy normally began on the female side, with work on a domestic scale. Articles entered at the Hospitals, Nursing, Midwifery and Public Health Exhibition in London in April 1936 were mostly made by women; among the many categories the Brighton Mental Hospital took prizes in embroidery and knitting.[95] Space could not be guaranteed in cramped hospitals: a weaving room used since 1924 at Bristol Asylum reverted to a dormitory in the 1930s.[96] To prepare men of an urban labour background for discharge and a return to gainful employment, purpose-built units with machinery were needed. At Netherne in 1933, charge nurse Starkey began teaching carpentry in the ward dining area, needing to clear away all materials after each session; three years later two rooms were set aside for this work.[97] Most progressive were the hospitals in Cheshire. At Macclesfield, where a male occupation officer was in post, a 170-feet pavilion was assembled with workshops for joinery, tailoring, upholstery, shoemaking, printing and bookbinding.[98]

In his book *Occupational Treatment of Mental Illness,* John Ivison Russell, medical superintendent of North Riding Mental Hospital, opined that mental nursing and occupational therapy were synonymous. He argued that nurses would gain more from additional qualification in occupational therapy than in general nursing.[99] Although the position of occupation officer did not require prior qualification in mental nursing, many medical superintendents believed that a nurse would have better understanding of the patients, although one might suspect that this was also to ensure medical control. Just as today drugs take the credit for patients' recovery rather than nursing input, occupational therapy was merely described by Maudsley psychiatrist Louis Minski in his *Nursing Mirror* lecture series as 'an adjunct to treatment'.[100] By contrast, in European mental hospitals the occupation therapist was regarded as a specialist. Nurses were not always able to fulfil the potential of occupational therapy, often reducing it to mindless piecework, not dissimilar from the inmate labour of the past. Much of the manufacture was for service of the institution: stools, brushes, mops and all kinds of clothing. A knitting class at Powick was observed by Board of Control inspectors as being held in enforced silence.[101] Some occupational therapy departments recruited from outside mental nursing, as doctors with a passion for this type of treatment saw more promise in bright and enthusiastic occupational therapists untainted by institutional culture.[102] Forming a national association in 1937, occupational therapy would emerge as a profession in its own right.

Clinical onslaught begins

The classification system devised at the turn of the century by Emil Kraepelin was meant to create order from chaos in diagnostic practice. Yet there was great variation between countries, between hospitals and between practitioners in the labelling of patients' problems. British doctors continued to apply the old concept of mania, which had much broader meaning than a state of extremely elevated mood. In 1930 at the North Wales Counties Mental Hospital, mania and melancholia accounted for over half of admissions (29.5 per cent and 22.7 per cent respectively). Just 5.6 per cent of admissions were for dementia praecox.[103] This condition had been renamed as schizophrenia by Eugene Bleuler, whose psychological formulation offered some chance of recovery. In British mental hospitals, however, diagnosis of this severe type of insanity was not made until ascertained by recurrent episodes of mania, and Kraepelin's term remained in use. As cases of dementia praecox usually became chronic, they accumulated to a high proportion of the resident populace.

Leslie Cook, in a presidential address to the RMPA,[104] recalled the situation at Bexley Hospital when he took charge of the female side in 1935. Responsible for eighteen wards in the main block and three convalescent villas, Cook found wards full of women with chronic schizophrenia, which he subdivided into three types: the 'burnt-out', harmless older cases; an apathetic, emotionally blunted type; and the excitable, noisy and destructive. Vast amounts of paraldehyde and chloral hydrate were used to sedate patients in the refractory wards, where an atmosphere of tension prevailed, with frequent eruptions of violence. Although some patients with melancholia recovered spontaneously, all but 2 per cent of patients overall, according to Cook, were doomed to spend the rest of their lives in the institution. According to the medical superintendent at Denbigh in 1937, of 1,359 patients, 1,308 were incurable; only ten men and eleven women were likely to fully recover.[105]

Wagner-Jauregg's dramatic discovery of pyrexial treatment for GPI had shown light at the end of the tunnel, but hubristic belief in its curative effects were not supported by results. A national evaluation by JA Sinton[106] at the special unit at Horton, which supplied mosquitoes for other mental hospitals as well as internal use, showed that less than a quarter of cases improved sufficiently for discharge. Most patients were treated at an advanced pathological stage, having incurred irreversible damage to the central nervous system. The breeding and handling of mosquitoes, inoculation of patients with a dangerously febrile disease, and careful monitoring of paroxysms before termination by quinine was a laborious process. Fever treatment prolonged the life of GPI sufferers, who had previously tended to due within three years, but it thus contributed to the accumulation of chronic patients.

As Shulamit Ramon[107] noted, despite the title of their professional body being the Royal Medico-Psychological Association, mental hospital doctors made scant reference to psychological theories in their writings. Insanity was considered not on a continuum of normality to abnormality, but as disease of suspected hereditary origin; eminent members of the profession were active in the eugenics movement. On these shores there was deep scepticism towards psychoanalysis, which was regarded as at best speculative, and at worst a dangerous adventure into disturbed minds. The Macmillan Commission[108] had heard little enthusiasm for such endeavour:

> Treatment for purely mental symptoms by psycho-analytical methods appears to have limited value because it requires the intelligent co-operation of the patient in a degree that few mental patients can give.

Few doctors were trained in these methods, yet Freudian influence was palpable. Until the 1920s the core text in British psychiatry, by Craig and Beaton, had focused on classification and symptoms. In a new manual of psychiatry in 1927,[109] David Henderson and Robert Gillespie applied the biopsychosocial 'reaction type' formulation of Swiss-American psychiatrist Adolph Meyer, which traced a navigable route between the determinism of Kraepelin and psychoanalytic conjecture. While the authors did not believe that insanity could be of purely psychological origin, they emphasised the influence of nurture, and the need for comprehensive assessment of the social background and life history of each patient. For Henderson and Gillespie, the treatment plan for psychosis entailed hospitalisation at the earliest opportunity, sedation, calming baths and tonics, and guiding patients towards an understanding of the cause of their illness. However, the hopelessly understaffed public mental institution was an infertile soil for talking therapy. There was little that mental hospital doctors could do to tackle the severe disorders that led to lifelong incarceration. Rudimentary drug treatment made patients more manageable but did not arrest underlying psychopathology. Psychiatrists desperately wanted a solution to the seemingly intractable problem of schizophrenia, the big beast of mental disorder. The call was answered by two simultaneous developments in the 1930s, which became known as 'shock therapies'.

The first revelation came from Vienna. Soon after its isolation by Canadian researchers Banting and Best in 1921, insulin drew interest from psychiatry. As the role of this hormone was regulation of glucose, it was initially tested for boosting weight in debilitated patients, but it was also found to have calming effects. Manfred Sakel, who had been using insulin to treat morphine addiction, observed that inadvertent coma had beneficial impact on patients with psychotic symptoms. He hypothesised a hypoglycaemic cure for schizophrenia, and treated his first cases in 1933. After intramuscular injection of insulin the patient became increasingly drowsy, before falling into deep coma after four or five hours. Impressive results were recorded, leading to the treatment being introduced at several psychiatric hospitals on the Continent.[110] After visiting Sakel's clinic in Vienna in 1936, Isobel Wilson of the Board of Control recommended insulin coma therapy in British hospitals.[111] It had already been initiated by Herbert Pullar Strecker at the Royal Edinburgh Hospital, supported by a Medical Research Council grant; he presented one of many glowing reports at the first international conference on shock therapy in Switzerland in 1937. Early results were reported in the nursing journals, Edward Larkin of West Ham Mental Hospital finding improvement in five of the six patients:[112]

> One walks into the ward, and sees perhaps five patients deep in a coma, gravely shocked, and finds at the same time the business of the ward carried on.

Despite a wave of interest in this apparently miraculous treatment, there were major obstacles to its implementation in the British context. Due to the mortal hazards, a special treatment unit was advisable, preferably on both male and female sides, for which there was little space in most mental hospitals. Insulin come therapy was labour-intensive, entailing daily treatments (with weekend respite) and medical attendance for several hours. A typical course entailed forty to sixty comas, but sometimes over 100. Groups of patients, fasted from the previous evening, received insulin at seven o'clock in the morning. The insulin dose was gradually titrated to a safe level to induce coma. The patient slipped into unconsciousness over a period of two to three hours. Hypoglycaemia was signalled by perspiration and restlessness; patients often freed themselves from their sheets and clothing, some requiring physically restraint to stay in bed.[113] Nurses watched patients carefully for signs of onset of coma, which a doctor confirmed by loss of corneal reflex. Once the first patient was comatose, continual medical monitoring was required, with two nurses in attendance for every six patients. Nurses recorded pulse and temperature on the treatment chart and reported any untoward events such as epileptiform seizures, which occurred in many cases. Deep coma was terminated after one hour (five hours after insulin was given) by a glucose solution via nasogastric tube. The patient stayed in bed for half an hour after waking.[114]

Although the treatment had remarkable effects on some patients, Sakel acknowledged that it had considerably less impact on chronic schizophrenia. A leading exponent in Switzerland reported full recovery in 73 per cent of early cases, and 50 per cent in cases of duration between six and eighteen months, but only 0.5 per cent in longer-term cases.[115] The mechanism of insulin coma treatment was unknown, various physiological and psychological actions being speculated. Illustrating how psychoanalytic ideas penetrated the walls of the mental hospital, William Sargant[116] recalled that 'one unit went so far as to recommend nurses with big breasts so that when the patient came out of his death-like coma, he was greeted on rebirth with this invitingly maternal sight'. Patients certainly received more attention from doctors and nurses, but perhaps most significantly they were exposed to a life-threatening situation, and their exhilaration on survival may have instilled a more integrated sense of self; it was observed that marked improvements were made by patients who had survived a protracted coma. Indeed, poorer outcomes were attributed to practitioners interrupting coma too soon.

Unquestionably, this was a perilous procedure. The London County Council limited the treatment to selected hospitals with suitable resources and expertise. Professor Edward Mapother, head of the prestigious Maudsley Hospital, initially barred insulin treatment, fearing litigation should a voluntary patient die during treatment; he eventually permitted it under supervision of a Swiss expert in November 1938.[117] Coma was interrupted early by intravenous glucose if there were signs of vasomotor collapse or respiratory distress. Nurses were expected to alert the doctor to such emergencies, as revealed by cyanosis or laryngeal spasms, but sometimes large doses of glucose failed to arouse the patient. At almost every mental hospital administering insulin treatment, patients succumbed to the catastrophe of irreversible coma. Proponents asserted that relieving morbidity of the many trumped mortality of a few. An empty bed; no more said.

The second of the new physical treatments was widely and rapidly introduced. Based on his thesis of biological antagonism between psychosis and epilepsy, Hungarian researcher Ladislas von Meduna devised a convulsive treatment for schizophrenia. Initially using camphor to induce seizures, he found a more reliable agent in a cardiac stimulant branded Cardiazol. Von Meduna claimed remission rates of up to 90 per cent in early cases, while chronic cases were also relieved. Again the Board of Control sent representatives to the originator's clinic, this time in Budapest.[118] The Cardiazol procedure required no special facilities, and in 1938 a Board of Control[119] survey showed that of ninety-two mental hospitals that responded, eighty-nine were using Cardiazol, compared to thirty-one performing insulin coma therapy.[120]

The standard Cardiazol course comprised twelve injections over a period of four weeks. Dozens of patients were treated simultaneously, each requiring a few minutes of medical input. Patients were fasted on the morning of treatment, and dentures were removed. A nurse held the supine patient's arm steady for the intravenous administration by the doctor, while a nurse opposite distracted the patient from the imminent chemical maelstrom. As producing a major epileptic fit depended on the substance reaching the central nervous system rapidly, a wide-bore needle was used. Almost immediately, the patient's face paled and stiffened. A peculiarity of Cardiazol convulsion was a sudden yawning spasm, when an attendant inserted a gag to prevent biting of the tongue. In a successful administration, seizure occurred within ten seconds.[121]

As with insulin coma therapy, Cardiazol appeared to produce best results in early cases of schizophrenia, but it was safer than Sakel's treatment. Ten deaths from 3,531 cases (0.3 per cent) were reported in a Board of Control survey,[122] considerably less than the 1.3 per cent mortality with insulin. Most adverse events were directly related to the severity of seizure, and the extreme stress on the musculoskeletal system often resulted in joint dislocations and long bone fractures. To prevent bone injuries, nurses applied pressure on the patient's hips and shoulders, although some doctors believed that limb restraint curtailed the therapeutic action. Afterwards patients were kept in bed for an hour, nurses recording pulse and responsiveness as they recovered consciousness. The toxicity of the analeptic agent caused confusion, and vomiting was common. Once alert, the patient was given a light meal and observed intermittently until bedtime.

The major problem with the treatment, as acknowledged by Thomas and Wilson of the Board of Control[123] was the terror experienced by patients between injection and seizure. Although patients had no recollection of the fit itself, they often recalled overwhelming alarm during the preceding aura. Based on patients' accounts, one exponent[124] described a feeling of bewilderment on injection, with steadily building apprehension as the drug circulated, causing sensations of burning and flashing lights. Articles in the *Journal of Mental Science* candidly portrayed desperate efforts to escape the injection, with patients scaling walls and in some cases attempting suicide. A patient at Holloway Sanatorium remarked: 'the very thought of it makes me shrink with horror'[125]. Reflecting on Cardiazol as 'mediaeval torture'[126], psychiatrist Henry Rollin told of reluctantly administering the treatment at Narborough Mental Hospital, and the 'unseemly and tragic farce of an unwilling patient being pursued by a posse of nurses with me, a fully charged syringe in my hand, bringing up the rear'.[127] For nurses, gathering patients for their next treatment was no easy task. Hostility was particularly expressed by patients whose injections had not culminated in seizure, a traumatic experience occurring in around a third of administrations; subconvulsive doses resulted in a confusional twilight state lasting for several hours.

Doctors claimed that the treatment made wards more manageable for nursing staff, but AJ Bain[128] warned against judging success by compliance. He described a patient, considered to have improved, who had previously pestered doctors for his discharge. On closer examination he had simply lost interest in his future, having been crushed by the volley of repeated convulsion treatments. Some commentators suggested fear as the therapeutic agent, thus likening Cardiazol to the surprise baths and swinging chairs of previous centuries. In the opinion of sociologist Andrew Scull,[129] shock therapy was a device of social control masquerading as medicine.

By the end of the decade, sober evaluation from longer-term studies showed that while the two shock treatments had equivalent impact on acute schizophrenia, insulin generally produced more lasting effects. It appeared to work best in catatonic excitement and in paranoid cases, the latter subtype of schizophrenia proving resistant to Cardiazol and least amenable to spontaneous recovery. Convulsive therapy transpired as most effective in states with depressive symptoms.[130] Here was an example of the 'therapeutic discipline' described by Joel Braslow,[131] a tendency for psychiatrists to redefine illness by whatever behaviours respond to treatment. Upside-down logic applied: shock therapy acted on schizophrenia, so patients were treated as schizophrenic. Insulin coma and convulsive therapies were empirical: their modus operandi was a mystery, but this did not detract from their enormous impact. While shock treatment conflicted with the prevailing caution of British medicine, mental hospital doctors believed that failure to grasp these opportunities would condemn patients to a miserable life of chronic illness and incarceration. The exciting advances provoked lively discussion at the annual gathering of the RMPA in 1938, which Sir Laurence Brock, chairman of the Board of Control, described as one of the most memorable meetings in the history of the association.[132] Psychiatry in Britain was being transformed from its erstwhile role as governors of a stultifying institutional regime to a discipline befitting its status as medicine. Meanwhile other methods were abandoned. When Runwell Hospital opened in Southend in 1937 its ultra-violet and plush hydrotherapy facilities were mothballed.

While the 'Red Book' predated shock therapy, articles in nursing periodicals, mostly written by doctors, described the nurses' contribution to these procedures. Their support for patients was regarded as a vital component of insulin coma treatment.[133] Psychiatric literature was dominated by the new treatments, but there was no journal specifically for mental nursing, and opportunities to attend conferences were scarce. A new textbook published in 1938, *Modern Mental Nursing*, included a mental nurse, Walter Salway Mayne, among its four authors.[134] The other three were Douglas Scott, a physiology lecturer; Jessie Masterton, a general nurse who was sister tutor at the Royal Edinburgh Hospital for Nervous and Mental Disorders; and Mildred Hainsworth, a tutor in nursing of sick children. Despite a praising foreword by Professor Henderson, physician superintendent at the Royal Edinburgh, the book could have been written for general nurses. Little guidance was given on the particular care needed by psychiatric patients, the book implying that mental disorders were to be treated no differently from physical disease.

There is scant detail on how nurses perceived the onslaught of physical treatments. Most historical perspectives present a positive view of this development, as it assimilated mental nursing to the technical practice of general nursing. Referring to the introduction of fever treatment for GPI at the North Wales Mental Hospital, Pamela Michael commented:[135]

> For the nursing staff this one breakthrough had a significant impact on their outlook and approach to their own role in the hospital. They began to identify themselves more closely with the mainstream nursing profession as it increased their general faith in scientifically grounded progress towards conquering mental illnesses.

Yet there is danger here of a Whiggish notion of progress. Arguably, the coercive use of physical treatments reinforced the custodial identity and practice of mental nursing. As nurses cemented their role as agents of control, their subservience shifted from a hierarchy based on social class, with the physician superintendent as 'lord of the manor', to a new order of medical hegemony. Shock therapies supplanted patients' potential for recovery with reliance on medical expertise, to which mental nursing was a mere accessory.

Taking stock

Towards the end of the decade, a fresh spate of mental hospital building looked inevitable. A few more hospitals had opened in the 1930s. The historic Bethlem Royal Hospital moved from its Lambeth premises[136] to a green site at Monks Orchard, in the Kentish fringe of Greater London. Conventional county mental institutions built in the 1930s were the aforementioned Shenley and Runwell, the Borough of Swansea opened its own hospital in 1932, and on 3 May 1939 Laurence Brock officially unveiled Barrow Hospital in Bristol. For many years the old Bristol asylum at Fishponds had been seriously overcrowded. The new hospital, planned for 1,150 patients, followed the now customary villa design. In the opening brochure,[137] former Fishponds medical superintendent E Barton-White lauded the design: as well as the treatment centre to which all new patients would be admitted, there were villas for either sex labelled 'parole', convalescent', 'semi-convalescent', 'able-bodied unemployed', 'non-parole' (a euphemism for locked ward), 'infirm and senile', and 'voluntary nerve'. Meanwhile the counties of Kent, Essex and Lancashire all had plans at advanced stages for new hospitals.

Sites had already been found at Lathom Park in Lancashire and at Margaretting Hall in Essex. The case for a third mental hospital for Kent was underlined in 1936, when the original asylum at Barming Heath received its highest annual figure of 496 admissions, and the resident population was over 100 in excess of capacity.[138] With war imminent, these plans were postponed indefinitely, and Barrow proved to be the last of the large public mental hospitals to open in Britain.

Unlike the sudden calamity of 1914, outbreak of war in 1939 had been long anticipated, and air raid precautions were a regular feature in nursing journals. Bomb drill at the Brighton Mental Hospital was described by Gardner:[139]

> In the autumn of 1937, all the asylum staff were given instructions on air raid precautions by a Home Office official. By October 1938, almost a year before the outbreak of war, 1000 gas masks were already in store at the hospital, each carefully marked with the patient's name. Coverings for the black-out were made, sandbags were put in place, wire netting was fitted on certain windows, and anti-shatter paint was also used on some of them although it was later discovered to be ineffective. The asylum chapel was rendered gas proof and was used to house the wives and young children of staff called on duty during an air raid. A decontamination and demolition squad was trained and equipped with steel helmets and protective clothing and gas masks.

At the Devon County Mental Hospital at Exminster, two teams were formed to deal with a possible gas attack.[140] At Barming Heath in Kent, the admission hospital Northdown House was opened by Minister for Health Walter Elliot in May 1938, with as much attention at the opening ceremony to preparations for war as to treatment facilities: on prominent display were air raid precautions, gas masks and decontamination suits.[141] Indeed, the new unit was commandeered by the Ministry of Health before it could receive its intended patients.

Ironically, British psychiatry owed its emergence from a clinical backwater to German psychiatrists. In the university clinics of Berlin, Heidelberg and Vienna, teaching and research were readily applied in practice, thereby strengthening the professional standing of psychiatry, unlike the isolated institutions in Britain. However, Germany's position as the international seat of psychiatry faltered after 1933, when Adolf Hitler swept to power, and immediately began his programme of racial cleansing. The Law for the Restoration of the Professional Civil Service removed Jews from professional practice. Hundreds of psychiatrists emigrated, many of whom came to Great Britain, where they were allowed entry as a 'distinguished person' but were required to renew their medical qualification.[142] Among the earliest arrivals in 1933 were Wilhelm Mayer-Gross, Alfred Meyer and Erich Guttman, who formed a research group with Aubrey Lewis at The Maudsley, focusing on neuropathology and genetics. Away from the intellectual environment of The Maudsley and the Royal Edinburgh Hospital, the émigrés were dismayed by the insularity and paucity of practice in county mental hospitals, while the RMPA seemed little more than a club for medical superintendents. Keen researchers, many of the newcomers had an orientation towards biological psychiatry;

others had an existentialist bent, although such philosophical discourse had little resonance in Britain.[143] However, dozens of eminent psychoanalysts also fled to Britain, most notably Sigmund Freud, whose move ensured that English replaced German as the language of psychoanalysis.[144] As well as their skills in academic organisation, research and teaching, the migrants also propagated new treatment and technology; for example, in 1937 Samuel Last, previously of the *Nervenklinik* in Bonn, introduced diagnostic assessment with the electroencephalograph at Runwell.

As war was declared in September 1939, the clock stopped on a decade of progress in the mental hospitals. From the Mental Treatment Act of 1930 to the widespread introduction of physical treatments, this was a time of significant change in the care of people with mental illness. Historical accounts of mental hospital nursing, mostly written by psychiatrists, have a tendency for simplistic 'dark ages' retrospect, yet at the time the nursing press issued platitudes about modern treatments and erasure of stigma. To some extent this was propaganda, challenging stereotypes to present mental nursing as an exciting and rewarding career. Willing outmoded practice to the past denied the uncomfortable truth of life in the wards. Fundamentally, the social world of the mental institution remained much the same. Interviewing former nurses of Prestwich Hospital, Hopton[145] was struck by the discrepancy between progressive developments in law, policy and philosophy of care, and the reality of conditions decried by Montagu Lomax that persisted at Prestwich and other mental hospitals. Why was the institutional regime so resistant to change?

The 1930s saw a burgeoning of sociological and psychological research on occupational and organisational behaviour. The 'human relations school' was a reaction to the scientific management of FW Taylor, which had encouraged production line piecework and a mechanistic regard for employees as links in the chain. Experiments by Elton Mayo and colleagues at the Hawthorne plant of the Western Electric Company in Chicago showed that organisations are not machines but cooperative communities. The most important finding was that workers are not primarily motivated by self-interest, as believed by Taylorites, but instead by membership of a social group; people are as much emotional as rational beings.[146] Sociologists had not yet subjected the mental hospital to analysis, but here was a community ripe for study.

While their treatment in the mental hospital was officially under medical direction, patients knew that their daily lives were controlled by nurses. The intransigence of institutional practice may be interpreted through the important work of social psychologist Kurt Lewin, whose field theory presented a method of analysing causal relations in social settings.[147] Lewin explained that human systems tend towards equilibrium, maintained by a 'force field' of competing pressures; individuals, groups and organisations alike exist in a 'system in tension' whereby behaviour is driven by positive and negative forces. In Lewin's biological analogy, organisations continually interact with their environment, gradually adapting and diversifying. However, the mental hospital remained a closed institution. In its attitude to patients and its traditional order and hierarchy, mental nursing

Table 3.1 Forces for and against change

Facilitators	Barriers
• Voluntary patients • New admission units • Early, treatable cases • Physical treatments and clinical procedures for nurses • Increase in qualified nurses • Occupational therapy	• Understaffing • Overcrowding • Challenge of maintaining order with inadequate medication • Engrained custodial mindset • Traditional hierarchy and discipline • Inadequate monitoring • Limited contact with outside world

changed at a glacial pace. Applying force field theory to the mental hospital, it can readily be seen that change faced powerful counteracting defences (see Table 3.1).

Nursing practice was undoubtedly affected by the Mental Treatment Act and the introduction of shock therapy, but the impact on doctors was more significant. Psychiatry, still more commonly known in Britain as psychological medicine, had at last gained credibility as a medical specialty, albeit of relatively low status. The Diploma in Psychological Medicine, was embedded as obligatory specialist training for medical officers. A persuasive case was made for mental hospital doctors to be paid on the same grading as their counterparts in general hospitals. Despite the powerful influence of eugenics, which emphasised the social function of mental institutions, mental disorder was now a clinical-somatic domain: in its conceptualisation as illness rather than as a state of being; in admission on basis of medical rather than legal criteria; and in its treatment by physical methods rather than by moral management.

The more medicalised the mental hospitals became, the less the authority of the Board of Control, whose recommendations could be sidelined by clinical judgment. Arguably, this was a loss for nurses, for whom the inspecting body had often advocated. Patient care may have provided a source of satisfaction for nurses, but the system did not afford them a genuine therapeutic role. In the tension between the intended role of caring for people with mental health problems, and maintenance of order, the latter prevailed. Nursing occupied a low rung of the hierarchy and was unable to chart its own destiny. Perspectives of nurses on the radical developments of the 1930s were scarcely considered in professional literature and in the management of the institution. Yet patients continued to depend most on those who watched over them, day and night.

Notes

1 Although this was reversed on appeal due to misdirection of the jury.
2 Royal Commission on Lunacy and Mental Disorder (1926): *Report of the Royal Commission on Lunacy and Mental Disorder.* 18–19.
3 Welch JC, Frogley G (1993): *A Pictorial History of Netherne Hospital.*
4 Hopper B (2011).
5 A peculiar condition of the 1920s and 1930s was encephalitic lethargica, which was initially believed to be caused by a microorganism in the nervous system, but as with chronic fatigue syndrome today, no pathology was found.

6   *Nursing Mirror and Midwives' Journal* (13 February 1937): Friern Hospital for Nervous and Mental Disorders: a new home for the nurses.

7   Chung MC, Nolan P (1994): The influence of positivistic thought on nineteenth century nursing. *Journal of Advanced Nursing.*

8   Busfield J (1986): *Managing Madness: Changing Ideas and Practice.*

9   Ultra-violet treatment was subject of a rare clinical trial report by nurses. Fisher and Lee were permitted by the medical superintendent at City of Nottingham Mental Hospital to present results from fifty patients with various disorders including dementia praecox, who received twenty exposures of around five minutes. The positive outcome was weight gain, and the writers promoted the 'tonic properties' of this treatment. Fisher RA, Lee JA (1930): Artificial light treatment in mental disease. *Nursing Mirror and Midwives' Journal.*

10 Board of Control for England and Wales (1937): *The Twenty-Third Annual Report of the Board of Control 1936.*

11 Hunter R, Macalpine I (1974). 154.

12 Vincent J (1948): *Inside the Asylum.* London: George Allen & Unwin. 22.

13 Vincent J (1948). 23.

14 County Council of Surrey (1929): *Rules for the Guidance of the Nurses, Attendants, and Servants in the Service of the Surrey County Mental Hospitals at Brookwood and Netherne.* 3.

15 Sargant W (1967): *The Unquiet Mind.* 12–13.

16 Ogdon JAH (1947): *Kingdom of the Lost.* 138–139.

17 *Lancet* (1934): Shenley Mental Hospital.

18 Crammer J (1990).

19 Ogdon JAH (1947). 131–132.

20 PN's records.

21 Gittins D (1998). 142.

22 Ogdon JAH (1947). 130.

23 Winterton P (1938): *Mending Minds: the Truth about our Mental Hospitals.* 149.

24 Nicoll J (1907): Mental nursing. *Asylum News.*

25 Nolan P (1993). 92.

26 Ogdon JAH (1947). 127.

27 Ogdon JAH (1947). 133.

28 Ogdon JAH (1947). 128.

29 *Nursing Mirror and Midwives' Journal* (9 July 1938): The charge nurse describes her day in a mental hospital.

30 Vincent J (1948).

31 Procter G (1982): Oakwood Hospital 1928–1982. In *A History of Oakwood Hospital 1828–1982.*

32 PN's records.

33 Winterton P (1938). 14–15.

34 BBC Radio 3 (December 1999): *Taking Over the Asylum.*

35 Hartley C (2003): *A Historical Dictionary of British Women* (2nd edition).

36 Gardner J (1999). 258.

37 Hunter R, Macalpine I (1974). 159.

38 Gardner J (1999).

39 Johnson BCT (1969).

40 Freeman H (2010): Psychiatry in Britain, c1900. *History of Psychiatry.*

41 Vincent J (1948). 34.

42 Vincent J (1948). 54.

43 Ogdon JAH (1947). 140.

44 Clarke GW (1985): 'Having a keen desire to take up mental nursing'. *History of Nursing.*

45 Hopton J (1999).

46 Royal Commission on Lunacy and Mental Disorder (1926).

47 An observation that continues to be made by nurses on intensive care or forensic units today.
48 Gittins D (1998). 139.
49 Russell D (1997): An oral history project in mental health nursing. *Journal of Advanced Nursing.*
50 Hare EH (1985): Old familiar faces: some aspects of the asylum era in Britain (part 1). *Psychiatric Developments*, 3: 245–255.
51 Fleming GWTH (1931): Some notes on mental disorder: epilepsy. *Nursing Mirror and Midwives' Journal.*
52 Gittins D (1998). 138.
53 Minski L (1936): Lectures on mental nursing XI: treatment and nursing. *Nursing Mirror and Midwives' Journal.*
54 Sewart M (1930): The suicidal patient. *Nursing Mirror and Midwives' Journal.*
55 Early DF (2003). 26.
56 Winterton P (1938).
57 Ogdon JAH (1947). 142.
58 Stevenson J, Cook C (2009): *The Slump, Britain in the Great Depression.*
59 County Council of Surrey (1929). 22.
60 *Nursing Times* (30 October 1937): Trade unions as we understand them. The College of Nursing received royal patronage from King George VI in 1939.
61 Arton M (1998).
62 Nolan P (1993).
63 In the pre-decimal system, there were 20 shillings to the pound.
64 *Nursing Mirror and Midwives' Journal* (19 November 1932). Although nurses' homes did not appear at most mental hospitals until the 1930s, the progressive Metropolitan Asylums Board erected a separate block for nurses at the Caterham Asylum in 1889. Scottish District Lunacy Boards built some fine nurses' homes in the late nineteenth century, as at the Lanarkshire Asylum.
65 *Chichester Observer* (5 August 1939).
66 Hereford County and City Mental Hospitals (1934): *Sixty-Second Annual Report of the Committee of Visitors of the Hereford County and City Mental Hospitals, 1934.* Building of the nurses' home at Burghill was delayed by financial constraints and then by war.
67 *Nursing Mirror and Midwives' Journal* (4 July 1931): Springfield Mental Hospital: Princess Mary opens the nurses' home.
68 *Nursing Mirror and Midwives' Journal* (15 September 1934): Devon Mental Hospital, Exminster: the wonderful year. Cigarettes were regularly advertised in the nursing journals in the 1930s.
69 Pilkington F (1958).
70 *Nursing Mirror and Midwives' Journal* (13 February 1937).
71 Board of Control for England and Wales (1939): *The Twenty-Fifth Annual Report of the Board of Control 1938.*
72 Johnson BCT (1969).
73 The term 'off-duty', still common parlance for the shift rota, made more sense in the past, when most of nurses' time was spent on the wards.
74 Cherry S, Munting R (2005): 'Exercise is the thing'? Sport and the asylum c1850–1950. *International Journal of the History of Sport.*
75 Cowper-Smith F (1977).
76 Gardner J (1999).
77 Jones K (1993). 146
78 Gittins D (1998). 178.
79 Kent County Mental Hospital (1927).
80 Crammer J (1990).
81 *Nursing Times* (4 September 1937): Long Grove Hospital, Epsom: the work of the male nurse.

82 Gittins D (1998). 179–180.

83 The MPA received royal patronage in 1926.

84 *Nursing Times* (17 June, 1939): The mental nurses' register. Mental nurses taking the GNC examination were not 'State registered', but joined a supplementary part of the register.

85 *Nursing Mirror and Midwives' Journal* (25 January 1930): Severalls Mental Hospital.

86 Arton (1998). The full report was never published due to outbreak of war.

87 Royal Medico-Psychological Association (1954): *Handbook for Mental Nurses* (8th edition).

88 Board of Control for England and Wales (1931).

89 *Nursing Mirror and Midwives' Journal* (27 March 1937): Mental nursing in Holland.

90 Wall BA (1977).

91 *Nursing Mirror and Midwives' Journal* (15 March 1930): Occupational therapy in a mental hospital.

92 Wall BA (1977).

93 Spratley VA, Stern ES (1952).

94 Winterton P (1938). 153.

95 *Nursing Times* (4 September, 1937). Report.

96 Early DF (2003).

97 Welch JC, Frogley G (1993).

98 *Nursing Mirror and Midwives' Journal* (25 January 1936): Cheshire County Mental Hospital: occupation and recreation at Macclesfield. Such enterprise was later renamed 'industrial therapy'.

99 Russell JI (1938): *The Occupational Treatment of Mental Illness.*

100 Minski L (1936).

101 Hall P (1991).

102 Clarke L (1997): Joshua Bierer: striving for power. *History of Psychiatry.*

103 Michael P (2003).

104 Cook LC (1958): The place of physical treatments in psychiatry. *Journal of Mental Science.*

105 Michael P (2003).

106 Sinton JA (1938): *Report on the Provision and Distribution of Malaria Therapy in England and Wales.*

107 Ramon S (1985).

108 Royal Commission (1926). 125.

109 Henderson D, Gillespie RD (1936): *A Textbook of Psychiatry for Students and Practitioners* (4th edition).

110 Wortis J (1959): The history of insulin shock treatment. In *Insulin Treatment in Psychiatry* (eds Rinkel M, Himwich HE).

111 Wilson IGH (1936): *A Study of Hypoglycaemic Shock Treatment in Schizophrenia.*

112 Larkin E (1937): Insulin shock treatment of schizophrenia. *Nursing Times.*

113 At Sakel's clinic in Vienna, metal cages were fitted to the beds.

114 Ingram ME (1939): *Principles of Psychiatric Nursing* (2nd edition).

115 Wortis J (1959).

116 Sargant W (1967). 55.

117 Sargant W (1967).

118 Thomas RW, Wilson IGH (1938): *Report on Cardiazol Treatment and on the Present Application of Hypoglycaemic Shock Treatment in Schizophrenia.*

119 Board of Control for England and Wales (1939).

120 Believing that spontaneous fits during insulin treatment were beneficial, some practitioners administered Cardiazol during coma.

121 McCrae N (2006): 'A violent thunderstorm': Cardiazol therapy in British mental hospitals. *History of Psychiatry.*

122 Board of Control (1939).

123 Thomas RW, Wilson IGH (1938).

124 Good R (1940): Some observations on the psychological aspects of Cardiazol therapy. *Journal of Mental Science.*
125 Gillespie JEON (1939): Cardiazol convulsions: the subjective aspect. *Lancet.*
126 Valentine R (1996). 80.
127 Rollin HR (1990): *Festina Lente: a Psychiatric Odyssey.* 69.
128 Bain AJ (1940): The influence of Cardiazol on chronic schizophrenia. *Journal of Mental Science.*
129 Scull A (1995): Psychiatrists and historical 'facts', part one: the historiography of somatic treatments. *History of Psychiatry.*
130 McCrae (2006).
131 Braslow J (1997): *Mental Ills and Bodily Cures: Psychiatric Treatment in the First Half of the Twentieth Century.* 34.
132 Royal Medico-Psychological Association (1938): Discussion at annual meeting. *Journal of Mental Science.*
133 Larkin E (1937).
134 Scott DH, Masterton JF, Hainsworth M, Mayne WS (1938): *Modern Mental Nursing.*
135 Michael P (2003). 131.
136 Now the Imperial War Museum.
137 Bristol Mental Hospital Visiting Committee (1939): *Opening of Barrow Hospital by Sir Laurence Brock, CB (Chairman of the Board of Control), May 3rd 1939.*
138 Proctor (1982).
139 Gardner J (1999). 262.
140 Pearce D (2011): Evacuation and deprivation: the wartime experience of the Devon and Exeter City Mental Hospitals. *History of Psychiatry.*
141 Proctor (1982).
142 Sharf A (1964): *The British Press and Jews under Nazi Rule.*
143 Peters UH (1985): *Anna Freud: a Life Dedicated to Children.*
144 Peters UH (1996): The emigration of German psychiatrists to Britain. In *150 Years of British Psychiatry* (volume 2): *The Aftermath* (eds H Freeman, G Berrios).
145 Hopton J (1999).
146 Midgley G (2000): *Systemic Intervention: Philosophy, Methodology and Practice.*
147 Lewin K (1952): *Field Theory in Social Science: Selected Theoretical Papers.*

4 Interregnum

Developments before, during and immediately after the Second World War changed not only the course of British psychiatry, but also the form and direction of mental nursing. While wars are wasteful and destructive, they can nonetheless be a powerful means of exploring and purging the national *psyche*, transforming people and organisations so that outcomes are achieved which, under normal conditions, would not have been possible.[1] Lessons are learned in crisis, and the sheer volume of psychiatric morbidity caused by the Great War had created unanticipated demand for treatment. Shellshock, it seemed, did not arise only from individual weakness, but from the monstrosity of trench warfare.[2] Assumptions about insanity as a hereditary disease, and pejorative notions of malingering, were undermined. Nonetheless, casualties were disposed to county mental hospitals, where staff had little idea of how to relieve their suffering.[3] While soldiers and their families faced an uphill struggle for justice from the bureaucratic labyrinth of the Ministry of Pensions, many psychological casualties of the fight for king and country languished in the asylum wastelands. As war loomed again over Europe in 1939, the British government planned a better response to a predicted whirlwind of mental trauma. The terrible force of modern weaponry having been demonstrated in the Spanish Civil War, the War Office predicted high levels of mental illness, with the civilian population as likely to be a target as military personnel and installations. The country was preparing for the worst.

The home front

As German troops massed on the Polish border in the summer of 1939, mental hospital superintendents were ordered to prepare for emergency, including evacuation at short notice. Fire drill was practised regularly, and each patient was given a gas mask and ration book. Thousands of windows were fitted with blackout blinds, and at hospitals most vulnerable to bombing, top floors were emptied, ground floor windows were sandbagged, and blast walls were built. Expecting a multitude of casualties, the War Office organised the requisition of mental hospitals, in part or whole. At Friern Hospital 624 beds were lost on handover of twelve wards to the Emergency Medical Service, staffed by doctors and nurses from St Bartholomew's Hospital.[4] Where whole hospitals were commandeered, patients were distributed to other institutions. In his reminiscences of West Park Hospital, Johnson described the mass influx of patients from nearby Horton, which had been converted for Emergency Medical Services use:[5]

> In two days over 400 female patients were transferred to West Park, and one remembers very well the orderly chaos of admitting, documenting, classifying and accounting for the property of such a throng of bewildered patients, let alone the problem of finding physical space to accommodate them.

A high proportion of male nurses and medical staff volunteered, perhaps fearing that waiting for conscription would imply cowardice and harm their employment prospects once war ended. Immediately after declaration of war, the Devon Mental Hospital lost forty-two staff to the armed services, including twenty-five nurses and two doctors who stepped up as reservists.[6] Many of the female staff left for the munitions factories or 'land army'. Although the staffing crisis was partly relieved by refugee nurses, and recalling of women who had left mental nursing on marriage, the gaps could not be filled and so patients were deployed in a wide range of care tasks. In 1941 the government passed the Mental Nurses (Employment and Offences) Act, which made it a crime for nurses to leave their jobs without permission. Under the 'Standstill Order', an absconding nurse could be sent to a prison for one month.

The period from late 1939 to early 1940 was dubbed the 'phoney war', when the country braced itself for invasion. As a precaution for aerial bombardment, The Maudsley Hospital was evacuated to two sites on the fringe of the metropolis. Led by Louis Minski, the medically orientated Maudsley psychiatrists moved to Sutton Emergency Hospital at Belmont. This former workhouse was adapted to treat an anticipated flood of casualties from the inevitable bombing of London. In reality, although the *Blitz* wreaked by daily and nightly air raids was tumultuous, the 800 Belmont beds were left empty, as collective hysteria failed to materialise. The hospital was used instead for neuropsychiatric treatment of military casualties, alongside its ongoing curative endeavours in schizophrenia and other mental disorders. For William Sargant,[7] a leading proponent of physical treatments, this was real doctoring. The other half of The Maudsley team went to Mill Hill Emergency Military Hospital, a converted boarding school in Middlesex, where the analytically orientated psychiatrists created a very different therapeutic atmosphere.

In May 1940, with the British Expedition Army retreating from its aborted campaign in northern France, batches of military casualties began to arrive at converted mental hospitals. In June the mass aerial bombing campaign that preceded an anticipated German invasion brought mortal danger to mental patients and their carers, with daily (and later nightly) disturbance of air-raid sirens, the fearsome drone of enemy bombers, anti-aircraft batteries, and shattering explosions. The father of Tim Mosses,[8] a charge nurse at Bexley during the war, took turns at fire-watching from the water tower; at various points on the horizon were the towers of other institutions, forming a vast visual field. At Fishponds, the war was on the doorstep:

Fire-watchers on the administration building watched the city burn whilst high explosives burst all around and 'Purdown Percy', the anti-aircraft gun on the nearby Purdown hill was deafening in its barely reassuring cacophony. The medical superintendent became more and more anxious and caused patients to be brought down to the basements when the air raid alert sounded. Morale was not improved by the nightly trudge to the cellars, which were lined with service pipes and gloomy in the extreme.[9]

Elsewhere, stray bombs and stricken aircraft fell on mental hospital estates near targeted towns and cities. Belmont was struck several times in the aerial barrage, and in one direct hit in September 1940 a block of three wards, one above the other, was destroyed. Sixteen patients were found dead, with many others critically injured. According to Sargant there were heroic efforts by staff and patients to dig out survivors from the rubble and human debris, as severely neurotic patients temporarily abandoned their symptoms in pursuit of a common cause.[10] In 1941 five villas at Friern were damaged or destroyed, with the loss of thirty-six patients and four nurses.[11] The strain on accommodation at West Park Hospital increased as evacuees arrived from the bombed wards of Hanwell and Friern Hospitals. Pearce[12] described an incident at the Devon Mental Hospital in April 1942:

> Four high-explosive bombs hit the hospital shortly before midnight. The floor of one psychiatric ward collapsed onto the infirmary below, together with two-thirds of its patients. The west walls of two of the Emergency Hospital wards were blown out, and the ceiling of one collapsed on the patients below. In spite of the blackout precautions and the loss of telephone contact with the outside world, all the survivors were brought about by 2 a.m. The patients were said to have coped extremely well, and casualties were mercifully confined to 14 patients killed and 25 patients and staff injured.

Patients contributed to the war effort as occupational therapy switched from production of hospital clothing and furnishings to priority materials such as camouflage netting. Manicured bowling greens and cricket pitches were dug up for growing crops, as mental institutions played their part in the 'Dig for Victory' campaign. Doris Bishop, who began her nursing career at Brighton Borough Mental Hospital, found the blackout oppressive:

> On night duty with all those bodies, and not a breath of air … All stairs had large Tate & Lyle treacle tins screwed to the walls with a candle burning in each, and a nurse patrolling every hour on every ward and dormitory. You were lucky you got ten minutes before you started off again.[13]

John Greene's story

There has been little research on the experience of nursing in the mental hospitals during the Second World War. However, co-author PN spent many an hour with nurses who started their careers in the 1940s or earlier, and one of his most enlightening contacts was John Greene.[14] A native of County Clare, like many young Irishmen, John sought work in England. In 1935, when aged nineteen, he responded to an Irish newspaper advertisement for junior nurses at Laverstock House near Salisbury. On appointment at this private asylum he found that patients were treated with courtesy and respect, and he enjoyed their discussions on familiar topics from home such as farming and horseracing. Friendly relationships had developed between some patients and the staff. There was a well-stocked library, indoor games, and croquet, bowls and tennis were played in summer. Walks were encouraged, as was regular attendance at church. Selected male and female patients shared afternoon tea. Infrequently, sulphanol or paraldehyde was administered to truculent or aggressive patients, who were put to bed until they had calmed. Nurses suited to the work were asked by the medical superintendent if they had any relatives who might be interested in joining the staff. Although there was no formal training, the head attendant periodically gave instructions to staff. The most proficient nurses were encouraged to submit to the RMPA examination. John read widely, talked to more experienced staff, keenly observed the patients and took copious notes. He passed the examination at Herrison Hospital, the former Dorset County Asylum.

In 1940 the Admiralty placed an advertisement in the *Nursing Mirror* for mental nurses. John applied and was interviewed by senior naval personnel, who wanted men under the age of twenty-eight, in good health, with experience of caring for mentally ill people, and of resilient character to deal with military casualties. As one of twenty-four selected, John went to Skegness, where the recruits underwent a short training to improve their fitness and to be familiarised with weaponry. Eventually they were dispersed in groups of six to naval hospitals at home and abroad. John's group was sent to the Royal Naval Hospital at Chatham. Led by two psychiatrists, their task was to prepare neurosis wards for psychiatric emergencies. The psychiatrists were relieved to have the nurses so that they could dispense with the naval guards, whose heavy-handed approach to restraining distressed patients barely concealed a belief that these men were feigning mental illness to cover their cowardliness. The nurses eschewed the use of padded cells for patients; instead using these for sleeping during air raids.

Shortly after John's arrival the Luftwaffe onslaught began. Meanwhile the German navy was attempting to cut Britain from its vital supplies by sea. Almost every night, numerous casualties, both men and officers, were admitted to Davenport with varying degrees of shellshock. They were mostly sailors, brought in on Robertson stretchers.[15] Some of the victims were distraught; others were conscious, lucid and cooperative. John and colleagues were struck by the vacant gaze of those who appeared to be psychotic, an expression that became known as 'the thousand-yard stare'.[16] Nurses quickly became proficient in arresting bleeding, cleaning wounds and minor surgery. Once patients' physical state had stabilised, psychiatric treatment began; this usually entailed continuous narcosis therapy with close monitoring by nurses.

The medical and nursing staff formed close-knit teams, with a strong spirit of collegiality. Doctor McDonald Critchley, a visiting neurosurgeon, and Desmond Curran, visiting chief psychiatrist, took a keen interest in the work of the mental nurses. Both considered that the care patients received was as important, if not more so, than the treatment they were given. Doctors gave lectures on emergency care and various mental and physical conditions, followed by open discussion. The mental nurses worked alongside the Queen Alexandra Royal Naval Nursing Sisters, whose tutor, specially attached to them, also gave lectures. John married Betty Rickers, who taught anatomy and physiology at the hospital. The nurses were also asked to present aspects of their work so that everyone would appreciate each other's role and skills.

As the war shifted to other parts of the world, the Chatham mental nurses were dispatched to the hospital ship HMS *Vita*. Doctors and nurses worked in confined spaces, conducting physical assessments, intubating patients, preparing intravenous infusions, undertaking minor surgery, and administering medication. Many patients died shortly after being brought on board. Others had injuries that were life-threatening, compounded by heat exhaustion, dehydration, sunburn, poor hygiene and malnutrition. The nurses witnessed the extent of psychological problems in the early stages of adapting to physical deformities, facial disfigurement and multiple disabilities, and gained insights into the long-term *sequelae* that would be endured. The nurses were then posted to the psychiatric hospital in Colombo, where wounded soldiers arrived in a dreadful state: emaciated, flea-ridden, covered in sores and terrified. They seemed like the 'living dead'. Nurses such as John Greene tapped deeply into their personal resources to survive in this adversity. Their experiences would help to change mental nursing for the better.

Cerebral barrage

War did not stop the advance of physical treatments. Insulin coma therapy was curtailed by strict rationing of sugar, although a substitute was found in potatoes, which were crushed to produce a starchy liquid for administration by intravenous injection or stomach tube.[17] However, due to workforce depletion, introduction of this treatment was postponed in many hospitals until after the war.[18] The relatively straightforward convulsive therapy continued, but in a new form. Devised in Italy by Cerletti and Bini, electoconvulsive therapy (ECT) was first administered in Britain in 1939 at the Burden Neurological Institute in Bristol. This clinic for investigation of neuropsychiatric disorders was directed by Frederic Golla, who had run the pathological laboratories at The Maudsley until its closure on the cusp of war. After assembly by W Grey Walter and successful testing at the Burden, the 'shock box' was deployed in nearby mental hospitals.[19]

The electrical method proved technically efficient while gaining better cooperation from patients.[20] Fasting was unnecessary; tea and toast were allowed in the morning before treatment. The temporal region was smeared with contact jelly in preparation for bilateral application of electrodes, dipped in a saline solution for optimal conduction. The greatest advantage of ECT was immediate loss of consciousness, avoiding the terror of the chemical method. On waking, patients had mild and transient symptoms of headache and dizziness, but none of the vomiting or other toxic reactions that arose with Cardiazol. The seizures also appeared less violent, thus reducing musculoskeletal injuries: Hemphill and Walter[21] reported just one fracture in over 200 patients. However, this was possibly due to initial caution with the strength of shock administered, as the fracture rate increased in later reports.

No new theory of action was offered, and the target condition was the same. Acute and chronic schizophrenic patients were treated en masse, three days per week. However, as ECT supplanted Cardiazol, the indication for convulsive therapy was changing. After a year of using ECT in patients with various conditions, Hemphill and Walter concluded that depressive and manic cases fared best, stating that 'the original conception that convulsion therapy had its principal use in the treatment of schizophrenia is now abandoned and early hypotheses on its mode of action cannot be upheld'.[22] However, they suggested that convulsive therapy retained a place in psychosis, adding that 'the possibility of improving the large numbers of old schizophrenics that fill the chronic wards of every large hospital is of special interest'. Although clearly preferable to Cardiazol, introduction of ECT was delayed because many hospitals could not obtain the apparatus.

Meanwhile, the most radical treatment development of the 1930s was beginning to reach British mental hospitals. In 1935 Portuguese neurologist Egas Moniz had announced a new physical procedure that he claimed could relieve the most intractable cases of mental disorder. At this time the frontal lobes of the brain were believed to be the seat of intellectual life, and Moniz was intrigued by reports of experimental removal of the frontal lobes in apes, which had resulted in no loss of function while making the animal more tranquil. There had also been human cases of frontal lobe injury resulting in a calmer, carefree demeanour. Moniz thought that by severing connections to the prefrontal lobes of schizophrenic patients, he could disrupt the neural substrate of their disordered thought patterns.[23] With startling effects on patients with chronic and severe agitation, aggression and paranoia, frontal lobotomy would reach into the darkest corners of the mental hospital, often performed on patients who had failed to respond to shock therapies. By relieving them of their most troubling symptoms, patients could be resocialised, allowing nurses to relinquish the controlling aspects of their work and to engage in nurturing relationships with patients.

In Britain, the first frontal lobotomy (leucotomy) was performed at the Burden Institute in 1940,[24] encouraged by the work of Walter Freeman and James Watts in the USA. Having operated on eighty cases by 1942, Freeman and Watts described their procedure in the textbook *Psychosurgery*.[25] Small holes were bored on both sides of the skull, allowing entry of the leucotome. A blunt edge was protruded from the sheath and rotated to sever the white matter connecting the frontal lobe to the thalamus, although the surgeon could not be sure of cutting only the intended fibres. Frustrated by London County Council medical advisors' restrictions on physical treatments, William Sargant sent patients to St George's Hospital at Hyde

Park, where neurosurgeon Wylie McKissock performed the operation. While posted at the Acute Battle Neurosis Unit in the reception block at Graylingwell Hospital, in anticipation of psychological casualties from the Normandy landings, Sargant selected long-stay mental patients for McKissock's blade. On the year of his arrival, 170 leucotomies were performed, with five deaths. In 1944 Sargant and Maudsley colleague Eliot Slater produced their authoritative *Introduction to Physical Methods of Treatment in Psychiatry*,[26] which cemented the somatic model in mainstream psychiatric practice.

Psychosurgery was embraced by psychiatrists around the world, and as with shock therapy the initial results were promising. However, certified patients were not asked for their consent for an irreversible and potentially fatal operation. In a Board of Control[27] report on 1,000 leucotomies performed from the early to mid-1940s, a heading 'social effects' discreetly recorded an operative mortality rate of 3 per cent, mostly due to damage to vital centres in the brain and intracranial haemorrhage. Another cause of death was post-operative infection, which was partly blamed on lack of aseptic technique by nurses. Yet frontal lobotomy reduced persistently troublesome behaviour, and in the absence of other lasting treatments for severe mental disorder, its adverse consequences were regarded as a lesser evil.

An American nurse in Staffordshire

In April 1943 the 312th Station Hospital and School of Military Neuropsychiatry was established on the Earl of Lichfield's estate near Stafford. Initially intended as a 750-bed hospital for neuropsychiatric rehabilitation, within a short period it had expanded to 1,164 beds with eleven psychiatrists. So high was the demand that the US Command in Europe sent a request to American medical schools to send doctors for a six-week course in military psychiatry in England. One of seventy-five of the US Army Nurse Corps who arrived at the end of 1943 was Hildegard Peplau. Although born in the USA, Peplau had German and Polish ancestry and displayed the typical drive of the immigrant to learn, to be successful, and to make a contribution of which she could feel proud. After enduring the crossing in a military ship on which most of those on board succumbed to influenza and seasickness,[28] she enjoyed a few days in London, having tea at Claridge's and attending afternoon dances with officers at the American embassy at Grosvenor House.

On arriving at Stafford, Peplau found a less hospitable environment. Outside it was damp and foggy, and inside was a traditional hierarchy whereby nurses were mere handmaidens to autocratic doctors. The principal treatment was narcosis, and the sedative of choice was sodium amytal. Patients were given hot soup, followed by six grains of the drug and put to bed. If this did not produce sleep, the dose was increased to as much as eighteen grains. The nurses woke them periodically to help them to the toilet, give them fluids and then administer another dose of the drug. This procedure continued for 72 hours. Anyone who did not recover was given a course of sub-shock insulin therapy, with of daily administrations for at least a week. Patients with hysteria or hallucinations were given intravenous pentothal or sodium amytal until conversion symptoms abated. An advisor to the 312th Military Hospital was William Sargant, who practised a longer form of deep sleep therapy, whereby heavy doses of barbiturate and tranquillisers were administered to keep patients asleep for several weeks to allow the brain to rest. He also administered ECT during narcosis, supposedly to obliterate traumatic memories.[29]

In Peplau's view, such treatments were experimental and of dubious merit, and she saw the potent medication as harmful to distressed soldiers. She courageously challenged senior medical staff in a regimental atmosphere not conducive to critical discussion, and on more than one occasion was reprimanded for her trouble. Her main argument was that patients were not receiving individualised care: nobody took the time to explain narcosis to patients, and to support them in their brief periods of waking. The nursing role was most important when patients regained consciousness and began to talk about their frightening memories. Men told their stories drenched in sweat, agitated, flaccid and disorientated. Many felt that they were failures because they had not withstood the rigours of battle. By acknowledging and soothing anxieties, communicating in a calm and compassionate manner, and serving orange juice, nurses had a remarkable effect. The men came to trust and rely on nurses, who they found more approachable that the military psychiatrists.

Peplau believed that the severe anxiety and exhaustion observed in patients was not a pathological flaw but a rational reaction to the brutality and destruction that they had witnessed. Drawing on her psychology studies and particularly on the work of analytic psychiatrist Harry Stack Sullivan, Peplau instituted individual care plans and group therapy sessions to help restore soldiers' sense of self-worth and dignity. She organised access to the kitchens so that patients could cook meals and cajole each other. Many of her innovations became established routines at the military hospital. On leaving the US Army, she crusaded against the indiscriminate use of lobotomies and ECT, and asserted the primacy of talk in the treatment regime. In addition to being an astute observer, she meticulously recorded her observations, along with her ideas about treatments, and details from the lectures, group discussions and conversations in which she had participated. This material would form the basis of her *magnum opus*, the textbook *Interpersonal Relations in Nursing*.[30]

From eugenics to clinical discipline

British psychiatry was thrown into intellectual turmoil during the war, as assumptions about its role were confronted by the incompatibility of anachronistic institutions with the needs of patients with treatable neuroses, and the influx of analytically minded practitioners from Europe. The eugenics movement, which had been widely supported by mental hospital doctors, was irreparably tarnished by Nazi distortion of the doctrine. On Hitler's authorisation in October 1939, at least 70,000 mentally ill or subnormal patients were exterminated on the basis of *Vernichtung lebensunwerten Lebens* (destruction of life not worth living). Assessments for the National Socialist Euthanasia Programme were conducted by hospital doctors.[31] To dispose of large numbers of patients, some mental institutions such as Sonnenstein used rooms disguised as showers. Carbon monoxide was pumped into the room, in a procedure later modified for the gas chambers of the concentration camps.

> A path that had begun 75 years earlier with Galton's study of the superior traits of the English elite, and had wound its way through the corridors of American science and society, had finally arrived at Auschwitz.[32]

Having been told that they were acting in the best interests of the patients, the country and their profession, nurses played a part in the killings.[33] One nurse who witnessed the euthanasia programme later became a regular speaker at conferences in Britain, where she urged nurses to think critically about the care and treatment of patients, instead of unquestioning compliance with the demands of their superiors.[34] Obedience, traditionally regarded as characteristic to nursing, may be dangerously immoral.

Meanwhile in British mental hospitals the shift from a custodial to medical ethos gathered pace, manifested by the new somatic treatments, but also influenced by general nurses working in mental hospitals wholly or partly taken over for war casualties. All sister tutors in mental hospitals were qualified general nurses who strove to make their environment more like the general hospital. The uniform for female mental nurses more closely resembled that worn by general nurses, and male nurses began to wear white coats to signify the clinical nature of their work. Mental nurse training was increasingly concerned with medication, asepsis, dressings and instruments, and the procedures to aid shock therapy and psychosurgery. The changing focus of mental nursing was epitomised by the book *Modern Mental Treatment: A Handbook for Nurses*[35] by E Cunningham Dax, medical superintendent at Netherne Hospital, which was emerging as an internationally renowned centre of psychosurgery.

Despite the enthusiasm, or indeed hubris, for somatic treatments, psychiatry was far from assimilation with physical medicine. Experience with psychological casualties of the Second World War showed that mental illness cannot be understood by isolating the individual brain or personality, but as a social problem. Highly influential on mental health services after the war was the treatment and rehabilitation of soldiers with battle neurosis at Northfield Military Hospital (the converted Hollymoor Mental Hospital) in Birmingham. In 1942 psychoanalysts Wilfred Bion and John Rickman started a unit at Northfield applying group dynamic theory, but their methods were not appreciated by the military authorities, who terminated the experiment after six weeks. A second experiment began in 1944. The rigid military hierarchy was flattened to open communication channels, promoting social group forces through daily discussion groups and democratic decision-making. As explained by Kurt Lewin's field theory, people respond to social forces at various levels, so it was important to consider the hospital as a whole. No man is an island, and individual behaviour was interpreted as a symptom of the entire social group. Tom Main, one of the 'Tavi brigadiers' who had followed JR Rees, director of the Tavistock Clinic (the centre of psychoanalysis in Britain) to the Army Psychiatric Service, described the approach:

> The Northfield Experiment is an attempt to use a hospital not as an organisation run by doctors in the interests of their technical efficiency, but as a community with the immediate aim of full participation of all of its members in its daily life.[36]

Meanwhile, similar principles were being applied at Mill Hill. Since 1941 Maxwell Jones had been in charge of a 100-bed psychosomatic unit, which received servicemen with similar complaints of pain around the heart, breathlessness, palpitations, giddiness and fatigue – all of which appeared to have psychological rather than physiological origin. Group therapy became the primary treatment for 'soldier's heart', as Maxwell Jones realised the importance of social learning. Formal roles were abandoned and genuine relationships were nurtured as a prerequisite for overcoming defences and resolving conflict.

> By the end of the war we were convinced that people living together in hospital, whether patients or staff, derived great benefit from examining, in daily community meetings, what they were doing and why they were doing it.[37]

Nurses worked alongside doctors at Mill Hill in a democratic and intellectual atmosphere, with regular lectures by eminent Maudsley psychiatrists such as Aubrey Lewis. Mature and intelligent nurses were sought, among whom was Annie Altschul. Having fled her native Vienna in 1939, Altschul had recently qualified in general nursing in Epsom, but it was her experience with mental patients on the observation ward that she found most stimulating. She discovered her flair for caring for 'peculiar' people who tended to be avoided by other nurses, and was struck by the prejudice in the hospital towards gypsies, who were admitted to an annexe where they were treated as if they were mentally and socially disabled.[38] Altschul was one of the first nurses to start training at Mill Hill, arriving in 1943, and she lauded the dynamic atmosphere:

> I found an excitement about the work that I had not encountered before. Everybody was expected to make a contribution. The staff, both doctors and nurses, were very keen to learn and every patient was regarded as interesting and some from whom we could learn a lot.[39]

Most of the nurses at Mill Hill and Northfield were female, and paternalism was evident in the leadership of such units. JR Rees analogised the caring role to mothering, complementing the fatherly nature of the military organisation.[40] An important advance on mental hospital practice was the assignment of each nurse to a group of patients rather than to a set of tasks. For responsibility to be placed in patients, the nursing role became more facilitative, and doctors came to nurses to review clinical and social progress. Mill Hill closed after the war but it made a lasting impression on those who worked there, demonstrating that patients' recovery depended on humanistic methods rather than physical treatment alone. Main developed the Northfield model as the 'therapeutic community' at the Cassel Hospital, a specialist psychotherapy hospital in Surrey. A claim for social therapy was staked in a struggle for the soul of psychiatry.

Return to 'civvy street'

On 8 May 1945, patients and staff at Fishponds gathered in the recreation hall to hear an address to the nation by Winston Churchill. On declaration of victory in Europe (VE Day), joyful celebrations were held, with a bonfire lit next to the nurses' home. A thanksgiving service was held in the chapel, and a plaque was presented in commemoration of the doctors and nurses killed in action. War was not yet over, continuing in the Far East, but the threat of a Nazi sting in the tail had passed. Churchill was a national hero, but now the British public were tired of conflict; they looked forward to better times. On 5 July the Labour Party won a landslide victory in the general election, and the new government led by Clement Attlee promised demobbed soldiers 'a land fit for heroes',[41] with decent housing, employment opportunities, and health and social services for all.

The impact of mental health nurses who had served in the war when they returned to their former hospitals was considerable. Many had volunteered as soldiers while others had joined the medical corps; the former were particularly able to sympathise with patients who had served in the First World War: now they could make sense of the nightly screams as men relived their terror. The returnees encountered nurses who had been recruited in their absence and who had maintained the traditional routines. Some recruits from southern Ireland had been promoted to sister or charge nurse positions;[42] this meant that nurses who had acquired a wealth of experience in the forces had been overtaken in the promotion queue, which inevitably caused resentment.[43]

War broke down the rigid class structure in Britain, and this was evident in mental hospitals where medical superintendents saw the potential of working in partnership with the senior nurses. John Greene returned from the Navy to Herrison in 1946, where he was promoted to assistant chief male nurse. He then applied for a post at Moorhaven near Plymouth, where he was interviewed by medical superintendent Frank Pilkington. Born in Derby of Irish parentage, Pilkington had a fondness for all things Irish, and his experience in the Royal Army Medical Corps (RAMC) and his dislike of the old institutional regime made for a productive 'double act' with John, who he promoted to chief male nurse[44]. Another strong relationship was formed at Warlingham Park in Croydon, where TP Rees, son of a farming family in Carmarthenshire, had been appointed as medical officer back in 1927. After promotion to medical superintendent in 1935, Rees had removed the main gate and begun to unlock doors. Like Rees, chief male nurse Stan Moore spent the war in the RAMC, and they shared a vision for mental health care that would lead to the first community mental health nurses.[45]

Some men, on being demobbed, entered mental nursing for the first time. Those without a job, or not wishing to return to their previous work, were drawn to an institutional environment bearing resemblance to the military organisation, with its uniform, barracks and clear hierarchy.[46] Many were attracted by the excellent sporting amenities. Footballers, cricketers, boxers and athletes, as well as coaches and trainers, were in demand by mental hospitals, as such men were likely to be fit, reliable and good team workers. Tom Richards[47] returned to Tooting Bec Hospital, where he trained on the adjacent common; he went on to win a silver medal in the marathon at the 1948 Olympics in London. When Ronnie Newman, aged twenty-six, went for an interview with the medical superintendent at Roundway Hospital in Wiltshire, the discussion focused on his military and sporting background:

> I was asked what I did in the war and where I had been...He seemed pleased that I played cricket and football in the Army and had been invited to play for a professional team on my discharge. He never mentioned anything about the work, nor what I was expected to do. His last comment before he showed me to the backdoor was: 'Could you start on Monday?'[48]

Strong bonds formed between ex-military personnel, creating an informal hierarchy. Male nurses started daily physical exercise sessions for patients, maintaining the discipline of their wartime experience. However, the many nurses who had left during the war were not easily replaced, and so medical superintendent sent matrons to Ireland for recruitment. Understandably Irish nurses looked to compatriots for support and friendship, but according to Ronnie, they tended to form cliques. Their country having remained neutral in the war, nurses from the Irish Republic lacked the credentials gained by men returning from the armed services.

> The Irish nurses were hard-working, deferential, kind to the patients, but were unable to stand up for patients' rights or contest decisions ... Trained nurses who had vast experience in the Army Medical Corps felt much superior to them in terms of confidence, ability to relate to doctors, patients and senior nurses and they had no hesitation in challenging ideas or practices when it was called for ... Some Irish nurses made reference to the 'military swagger', meant to convey confidence, superiority and seniority. It was voiced on many occasions that serving one's country was a much nobler act than caring for the mentally ill.[49]

While chief male nurses were forging a new kind of relationship with medical superintendents, the female side was also changing. On 4 November 1943 seventy female mental hospital nurses attended a meeting in the aegis of the Royal College of Nursing (RCN) in London. The government had appointed a the Nurses Salary Committee, chaired by Lord Rushcliffe, which had recommended improvements to nurse training and conditions, including a national salary structure. However, mental nurses were not represented on the subsequent RCN negotiating body. Indeed, as the RCN only admitted general nurses, the mental hospital nurses at the meeting were there by virtue of their additional RGN qualification. Disenchantment at the lack of a voice for mental nurses led to the group founding the Society of Mental Nurses. This group met regularly, although it drew opposition from the MHIWU, which feared fragmentation of the workforce. Criticising the RMPA training for conveying an outmoded view of nursing, the Society of Mental Nurses regarded the GNC syllabus as the only thorough preparation for practice, and argued that mental nurses deserved full status on the register. Both wishes would soon be granted.

The Society of Mental Nurses highlighted the stark contrast between the general nursing culture of matrons and sisters, with its middle-class morality, and the male side with its quasi-military discipline and proclivity for team sports. Yet while division of the sexes held firm, some traditional assumptions of the mental hospital culture were beginning to subside. Young women who had experienced a relaxed approach to gender roles in the war were unwilling to accept the petty tyranny of the female side of the mental hospital. The position of female nurses was likely to be strengthened by alignment with the professionalism of general nursing, but also from closer association with unionised male mental nurses. The label 'attendant' was dropped, as staff on both sides identified with the nursing workforce, forging a sense of solidarity that had dissipated since the heyday of the NAWU. Harsh discipline softened in the light of wartime experience, and communication between the three groups of doctors, nurses and patients was gradually opening.

Mental nursing, however, suffered from low status and often dreadful working conditions. Difficulties in recruitment were compounded by a high rate of attrition: young women balked at the unpleasant and extremely heavy work, such as cleaning the doubly incontinent and lumbering barrels of pigswill. Various suggestions were made to attract and retain women in this hostile environment. In 1945 a Ministry of Health and Ministry of Labour subcommittee on mental nursing, chaired by Sir Arthur Hall and Doctor W Rees-Thomas, recommended a four-week introductory period in the training school before the novices went on to the wards, so that their senses would be better prepared.[50] While many in authority acknowledged the need to raise the professional standing of nurses, the priority was quantity rather than quality.

The formal entry requirements of a single school certificate for GNC training was suspended in the war (the RMPA had no academic threshold). Meanwhile, the Nursing Reconstruction Committee established by the RCN in 1941 had recommended a state roll of 'assistant nurses', with a shortened training scheme. This new grade of nurse would add stability to the workforce at a time of acute shortage, and expand regulation of nursing.[51] The Nurses Act 1943 introduced the Roll of Assistant Nurses, but relatively few mental hospital nurses were registered in this way.[52] The report by Hall and Rees-Thomas recommended greater deployment of nursing assistants in routine tasks, thereby freeing trained nurses for patient care and making the work more attractive, but the idea that chronic cases needed basic care but less knowledge was rejected. The MHIWU agreed, fearing that that assistant nurse registration would become the norm in mental nursing.[53] Rees-Thomas pleaded with the Ministry of Health not to limit eligibility by school certificates, explaining that this would hinder the supply of Irish girls.[54]

Bevan delivers

As the nation clambered to its feet after seven years of war, the ideal of the collective good touched every corner of society. Following publication of the Beveridge Report on health and social welfare in 1942, a nationalised health service had been planned. A big question was whether psychiatry and the mental hospitals would be in or out. Initially the Ministry of Health wanted to exclude the mental institutions, but a White Paper of 1944 restated the Macmillan Commission's unifying principle of physical and mental health. In June 1945 a report *The Future Organisation of the Psychiatric Services*, the product of discussion by the RMPA, BMA and the Royal College of Physicians, reinforced the notion that mental hospitals were a health service rather than a remnant of poor relief[55]. Another important influence was a survey by Carlos Blacker,[56] completed in 1944. In the early 1940s it had become apparent that the number of neurotic patients was steadily increasing, not because of the war, but as an emerging trend in use of psychiatric outpatient clinics by general practitioners. As well as substantial expansion of outpatient facilities, Blacker recommended a complete restructuring of mental health services, with each population of 1 million served by a 100-bed psychiatric unit, preferably in a teaching hospital, or otherwise in the general hospital of a large town.

Aneurin Bevan, Minister for Health in Attlee's government, doggedly drove the Bill for a national health service through Parliament, waving aside the BMA's concern for doctors' independence, and the grumbles of Conservative members, who feared an onslaught of socialism. Bevan brought the neglected mental hospitals on board in the National Health Service Act 1946. For the next two years, nurses wondered how the imminent takeover by the health service would affect them. Bryan Johnson, who later became secretary of the West Park Hospital Management Committee, recalled the uncertainties:

> The Act took a good deal of digesting, but this was only the precursor of an avalanche of regulations, circulars and advice, more than a little confused by speculation. The staff, perhaps a little selfishly, applied themselves to a study of new rates of pay, and not least to the new superannuation regulations, compared with which the Asylum Officers' Superannuation Act was like a primary reader in an infants' school.[57]

Anticipating such developments, back in 1941 George Gibson (then president of the TUC) had called for the formation of a trade union covering the whole health service, and on 1 January 1946 the Confederation of Health Service

Employees (COHSE) came into being, with a membership of 40,000.[58] For a brief period before the NHS takeover, some mental institutions run by Labour-controlled councils operated as closed shops, with RCN membership ineligible. In the NHS, however, the RCN would represent the majority of nurses.

The Beveridge Report had presented a triple imperative of tackling poverty, disease and unemployment. In the socialist Utopia none would suffer from want, or from the humiliation of means testing. Experience at Mill Hill and Northfield suggested that all kinds of social problems were amenable to treatment. The scope of psychiatric practice was extended by the opening of the Industrial Neurosis Unit at Belmont Hospital in 1947. Maxwell Jones, having further developed his therapeutic approach with returning British prisoners-of-war, was appointed by the Ministry of Health, Labour and Pensions to this new unit for treatment of social misfits. With their potentially key role in the pursuit of a better society, the mental health services would surely outgrow their narrow remit in isolated institutions.

In a spirit of post-war egalitarianism, not only was the regimental discipline of military service on the male side to soften, but also the authoritarian matriarchy on the female side. If they regressed to their pre-war subservience, nurses would be unable to reproduce the revelatory social *milieu* of wartime psychiatry. As a craft, nursing needed practitioners who could fulfil its human and social potential. From quasi-Poor Law attendants to a health service profession, mental nurses were beginning a new era.

Notes

1 Taylor R (2001): Death of neurasthenia and its psychological reincarnation: a study of neurasthenia at the National Hospital for the Relief and Cure of the Paralysed and Epileptic, Queen Square, London, 1870–1932. *British Journal of Psychiatry*.
2 Winter J (2006): *Remembering War*.
3 Barham P (2007): *Forgotten Lunatics of the Great War*.
4 Hunter R, Macalpine I (1974).
5 Johnson BCT (1969). 16.
6 Pearce D (2011).
7 Sargant W (1967).
8 Personal communication (NM, 2014).
9 Early DF (2003). 60.
10 Sargant W (1967).
11 Hunter R, Macalpine I (1974).
12 Pearce D (2011).
13 Trimingham A (2008): *Out of the Shadows: a History of Mental Health Care in Sussex*. Lewes: 101.
14 Personal communication (PN, 1995).
15 Designed for removing the injured from spaces where access was too restricted for use of regular stretchers.
16 A phrase coined by American artist and war correspondent Tom Lea.
17 Sargant W (1967).
18 For example, insulin coma therapy started at Brentwood in 1946. Nightingale GS (1990): *Warley Hospital Brentwood: the First Hundred Years 1853–1953* incorporating *Into the Second Century*.

19 Cooper R, Bird J (1989): *The Burden: Fifty Years of Clinical and Experimental Neuroscience at the Burden Neurological Institute.*

20 Fleming GWTH, Golla FL, Grey Walter W (1939): Electric-convulsion therapy of schizophrenia. *Lancet.*

21 Hemphill RE, Walter WG (1941): The treatment of mental disorders by electrically induced convulsions. *Journal of Mental Science.*

22 Hemphill RE, Walter WG (1941).

23 Partridge M (1950): *Pre-frontal Leucotomy.*

24 Hutton EL, Fleming GWTH, Fox FE (1941): Early results of prefrontal leucotomy. *Lancet.*

25 Freeman W, Watts J (1942): *Psychosurgery: Intelligence, Emotion and Social Behavior following Prefrontal Leucotomy for Mental Disorders.*

26 Sargant W, Slater E (1944): *Introduction to Physical Methods of Treatment in Psychiatry.*

27 Board of Control for England and Wales (1947): *Report on Prefrontal Leucotomy in 1,000 Cases.*

28 Callaway BJ (2000): *Hildegard Peplau: Psychiatric Nurse of the Century.*

29 Shephard B (2003): *A War of Nerves: Soldiers and Psychiatrists in the Twentieth Century.*

30 Peplau H (1952). *Interpersonal Relations in Nursing.* See more on Peplau in Chapter 6. In the 1990s she was voted 'Psychiatric Nurse of the Century' by colleagues who recognised her courage and impact as the mother of psychiatric nursing.

31 Lifton RJ (1988): *The Nazi Doctors: Medical Killing and the Psychology of Genocide.*

32 Whitaker R (2002): *Mad in America: Bad Science, Bad Medicine, and the Enduring Mistreatment of the Mentally Ill.* 66.

33 Schulz M (2012): Mental health services in Germany. In *Mental Health Services in Europe* (eds N Brimblecombe, P Nolan).

34 Steppe H (1992): Nursing in Nazi Germany. *Western Journal of Nursing Research.*

35 Dax EC (1947): *Modern Mental Treatment: a Handbook for Nurses.*

36 Main TF (1946): The hospital as a therapeutic institution. *Bulletin of the Menninger Clinic.*

37 Jones M (1968): *Social Psychiatry in Practice: the Idea of the Therapeutic Community.* 17.

38 Nolan P (1999): Annie Altschul's legacy to 20th century British mental nursing. *Journal of Psychiatric and Mental Health Nursing.*

39 Quoted in Nolan P (1993). 101.

40 Rees JR (1945): *The Shaping of Psychiatry by War.*

41 Kynaston D (2007): *Austerity Britain 1946–51.*

42 Bingham S (1979): *Ministering Angels.*

43 John Greene (personal communication with PN, 1995).

44 Ardern P (2001): John Greene (obituary). *Guardian.*

45 Nolan P (2005).

46 Nolan P (1987): Jack's Story. *History of Nursing Group at the Royal College of Nursing.*

47 Richards was still working at Tooting Bec in the 1960s, when co-author PN started training there.

48 Personal communication (PN, 1995).

49 Ronnie Newman (personal communication with P Nolan, 1995).

50 Ministry of Health and Ministry of Labour: Nursing Services Interdepartmental Committee (1945): *Report of the Subcommittee on Mental Nursing and the Nursing of the Mentally Handicapped.*

51 Department of Health and Social Security (1971): *The State Enrolled Nurse: a Report by the Sub-Committee of the Standing Nursing Advisory Committee.*

52 By 1949 there were 318 SENs in the mental nursing workforce, and by the end of the 1950s they had almost disappeared. Glenister DA (2008): *Matrons, Mental Nurses and Madness: a Sociological Historiography of Mental Nursing from the Nurses Act 1943 to the Nurses Act 1969, Critically Adopting Some Sensitising Aspects of Giddens' Structuration Theory.*

53 Glenister DA (2008).

54 Ministry of Health and Ministry of Labour: Nursing Services Interdepartmental Committee (1945).
55 Jones K (1993).
56 Blacker CP (1946): *Neurosis and the Mental Health Services*. Blacker was director of the Eugenics Society, and eugenic assumptions probably influenced his idea of separate services for neurotic patients, leaving the mental institutions to chronic psychotic cases.
57 Johnson BCT (1969). 19.
58 Glenister DA (2008).

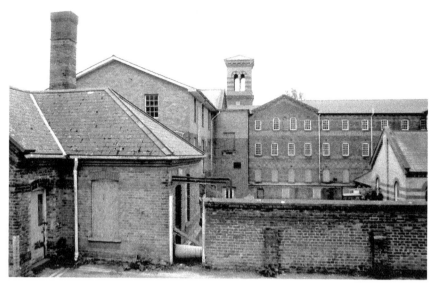

Plate 1 Built to last: Sussex Asylum, Hayward's Heath

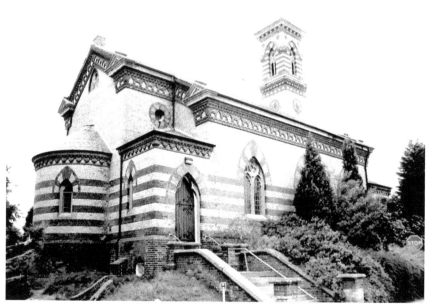

Plate 2 Chapel, Sussex Asylum

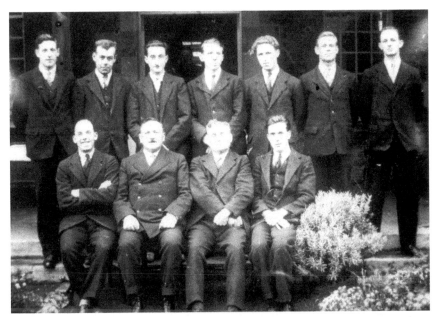

Plate 3 Attendants at Littlemore Mental Hospital (1930s)

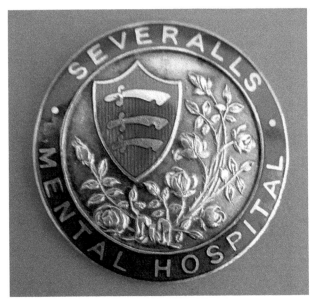

Plate 4 Nurse's badge, Severalls (1930s) (reproduced with the kind permission of Peter Malecek: petersnursingcollectables.com)

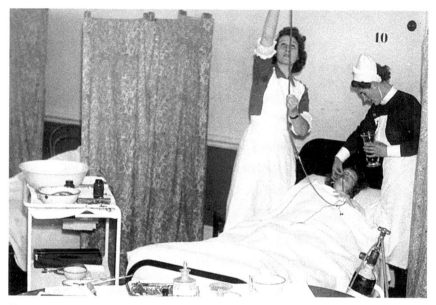

Plate 5 Insulin coma therapy at Graylingwell (1950s) (reproduced with the kind permission of Barone Hopper)

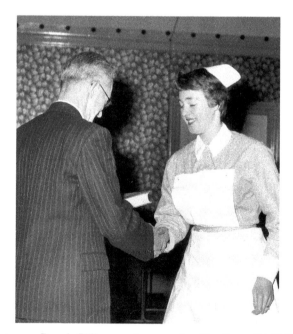

Plate 6 Student nurse Brenda Billings receives award at Graylingwell (c1960) (reproduced with the kind permission of Brenda Billings)

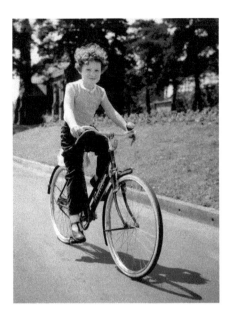

Plate 7 An institutional childhood: psychiatrist's daughter (and future nurse) Fiona Couper at Digby Hospital, Exeter (1960) (reproduced with the kind permission of Fiona Couper)

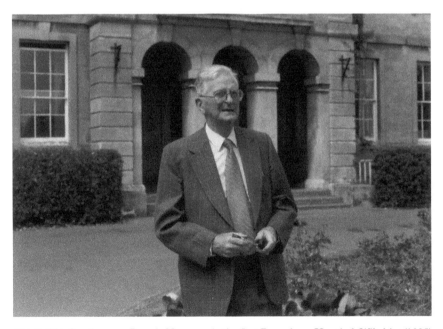

Plate 8 Chief male nurse Ronnie Newman (retired) at Roundway Hospital, Wiltshire (1995)

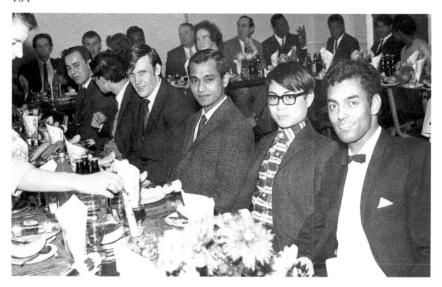

Plate 9 Tom Chan (second from right) at Christmas meal for single foreign nurses, Park Prewett (1967) (reproduced with the kind permission of Tom Chan)

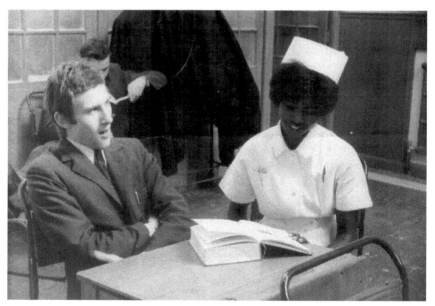

Plate 10 Peter Robinson, student nurse at Cane Hill (1967) (reproduced with the kind permission of Peter Robinson)

135

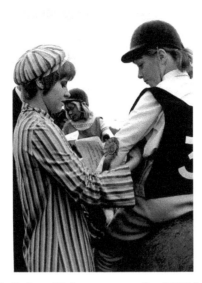

Plate 11 Actress Prunella Scales at Netherne summer fête (1967) (reproduced with the kind permission of Ann Bagheea)

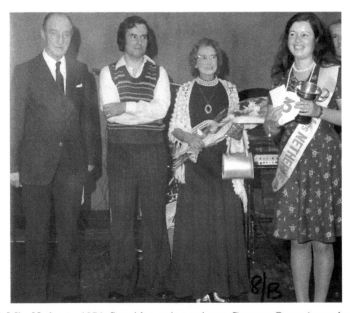

Plate 12 Miss Netherne 1974: Spanish nursing assistant Carmen Otega (reproduced with the kind permission of Ann Bagheea)

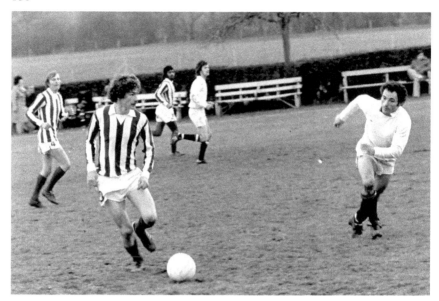

Plate 13 London mental hospitals football league match at Netherne (1970s) (reproduced with the kind permission of Ann Bagheea)

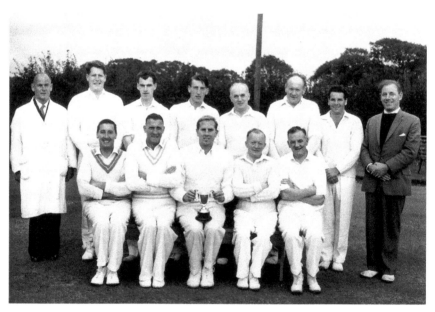

Plate 14 Graylingwell cricket team (1980s): nurse John Pay holding trophy (reproduced with the kind permission of John Pay)

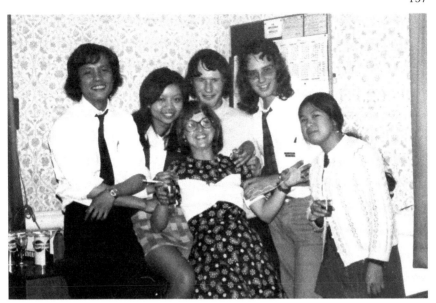

Plate 15 Ian Norman (second from right) and colleagues at Phoenix House, Long Grove (1974) (reproduced with the kind permission of Ian Norman)

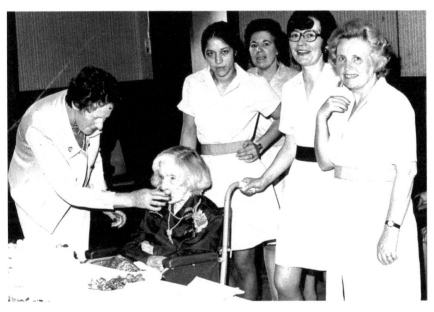

Plate 16 Senior nursing officer and nurses celebrating patient's 104th birthday party at Netherne (1970s) (reproduced with the kind permission of Ann Bagheea)

5   A new dawn

On the appointed day on 5 July 1948, all county and borough mental hospitals were transferred to the National Health Service. Hospital management committees were formed, with medical and lay members. On their baptism in the NHS, several mental hospitals were sanctified. The Brighton Borough Mental Hospital at Haywards Heath became St Francis' Hospital; Winson Green in Birmingham became All Saints. Such renaming evoked the caring tradition of religious orders, but the principle was to make mental institutions indistinguishable by name, thereby reducing stigma. In Cornwall, for example, instead of being sent to the institution still fearfully known as Bodmin Asylum, patients were admitted to the newly christened St Lawrence's.

However, the NHS did not suddenly transform life in the mental hospitals. For nurses in these isolated institutions the routine continued as before, with the same patients in the same wards, the same airing courts, the same counting of cutlery and locking and unlocking of doors. Indeed, overcrowding was getting worse, while staffing on the female side was dangerously low. In 1947, sixty-seven of the nation's 140 mental hospitals housed more than 1,000 patients; some had grown to over 3,000. After the stringencies of war, many buildings were in structural decay.

An interesting perspective on British mental hospitals was from a tour by the National Mental Health Foundation, a US government body, in August 1947. The visitors drew contrasts with the state institutions on their side of the Atlantic. American psychiatry had been scandalised by novelist Mary Jane Ward, whose best-selling book *The Snake Pit* (1946) described her experience of treatment for a schizophrenic breakdown at Rockwell State Hospital in New York. Dramatised in an Oscar-winning film in 1948, starring Olivia de Havilland, *The Snake Pit* raised concern in American society for the mentally ill. Alongside excessive use of sedation and ECT, unfeeling nurses were a prominent feature in Ward's account. Meanwhile Albert Deutsch's book *The Shame of the States* (1948) exposed dreadful conditions at Byberry Hospital, known as the Bedlam of Philadelphia, where hundreds of incontinent men spent each day naked, winter and summer. Bybery had 6,100 beds at the time Deutsch visited, and was hopelessly understaffed, but it was relatively small compared to the awesome, multi-storey monolith of the

Pilgrim State Hospital at Brentwood, New York State. With 10,000 beds, this was surely the largest asylum in the world.

For Dallas Pratt and his National Mental Health Foundation colleagues, everything seemed smaller in England, including the sixteen mental hospitals that they visited (the average public mental hospital population in 1945 was 1,261 in England compared to 2,658 in USA). They graded the hospitals from 'progressive' to 'backward', but generally observed relatively high standards. Then in their final year of local authority control, the English hospitals were criticised for 'red tape', old-fashioned furniture and inadequate clinical facilities, but a homely atmosphere was found in most wards, with enclosed gardens lacked by the American multi-storey blocks. Over half of admissions were voluntary. Unlike the almost total reliance on unqualified attendants in the USA (where a senior graduate nurse oversaw several wards), the English nurses were mostly trained or in training. The ratio of physician to patients was similar, at about 1:250, but it was noted that doctors performed little psychiatric treatment, merely dealing with physical maladies. However, the refractory wards in England were calmer, which was attributed to 'intelligent and humane nursing care, the frequent use of occupation and recreation, the absence of physical restraint and other violent methods, and active physical treatment including shock therapy and prolonged narcosis'.[1]

The major difference between the USA and Britain was the mixed public, private and military veterans' services in the former, and the uniform institutional provision in the latter. However, as urged by CP Blacker's influential report, separate hospital services for acute and chronic cases were beginning to appear. In Lancashire, where several former Poor Law institutions became general hospitals in the NHS, the old observation wards were relabelled as psychiatric units. On its return by the Royal Navy in 1947, Barrow Hospital in Bristol issued an admissions policy excluding 'mental defectives, chronic psychotics, chronic epileptics, senile and infective cases', stating that these categories 'will be admitted directly to Fishponds'.[2] The modern facilities of Barrow would be reserved for new and recoverable cases, a decision that appeared to condemn Fishponds as a dumping ground. Such division would cause increasing concern in the British mental health system: professionally rewarding work with treatable cases would attract the best doctors and nurses away from stultifying Victorian institutions.

The dawn of the NHS coincided with the growth of physical treatments. Insulin coma therapy units became standard, although there were long delays in some hospitals due to limited resources. According to Morah Geall[3], insulin treatment started at Hellingly as late as 1951. She attended the first session in the admission hospital. Nurses were not told much about the procedure, except their responsibilities to measure vital signs and to record the period of coma. A dozen patients were treated, in darkness; none went into coma in the first session, as the insulin dose was to be gradually titrated. Once psychiatrists and their teams of nurses learned from their experience, the mortality rate declined. However, around one patient in a hundred did not survive the course. Patients were not out of danger once they returned to their wards, as a former Prestwich nurse recalled:[4]

At night time they'd slip into a coma again; there'd be only one nurse on duty for about sixty patients so it happened that sometimes people would go into a coma and never come out of it.

Insulin come therapy had gained ascendancy over convulsive treatment for schizophrenia, but ECT was widely used for acute cases, and long-stay patients were periodically subjected to refresher courses. In 1950 a study of 'regressive electroplexy' on eighteen schizophrenic patients at Mapperley Hospital in Nottingham reported complete failure of a regime of seven shocks per day, which induced 'a state of complete confusion and utter apathy, mute, incontinent and unable to take food without assistance'.[5] ECT proved particularly effective with acute psychotic depression, with a recovery rate of up to 80 per cent in involutional melancholia.[6] Convulsive therapy was made safer and more acceptable by use of a muscle relaxant, preceded by injection of a small dose of anaesthesia. The violent motor seizures, which caused a litany of musculoskeletal injuries, could now be avoided without diminishing the success of the treatment. However, some psychiatrists continued to believe that an unadulterated fit was necessary in resistant cases. In nurse training at Graylingwell in the 1950s, John Pay[7] met a patient who had not responded to the modified treatment, but who made a remarkable recovery on receiving 'straight' ECT.

Meanwhile, operating theatres were installed in mental hospitals throughout the land. At Haywards Heath the admission villa Hurstwood Park, opened in 1938, reopened as a neurosurgical unit in 1946. Doctor McCartan, the medical superintendent, engaged the services of a neurologist and envisaged the unit as a centre for leucotomy operations.[8] In 1946 Thomas Tennent at St Andrew's Hospital in Northampton organised a systematic study of frontal lobotomy, with 300 patients from various public and private mental hospitals brought to the operating table under the steady hands of surgeon Wylie McKissock, the most prolific lobotomist in Britain. Whereas most researchers had only studied short-term outcomes of the operation, the St Andrew's project examined patients at six months, twelve months and two years. There were nineteen deaths related to the operation (4 per cent), and other *sequelae* such as epilepsy and incontinence were carefully recorded. The outcome of most interest to psychiatrists was personality change, and the St Andrew's study produced clear evidence of loss of inhibition, lack of spontaneity and motor retardation. Some lobotomised patients found great difficulty in getting up in the morning. Social disinhibition was illustrated by some patients undressing or urinating in public, without embarrassment. However, the operation appeared to reduce agitation and obsessional behaviour.

One sees a patient who has been insidiously ill for 8 years, with an increasing deterioration which culminates in the eating of faeces while in the padded cells, and sees him, a year after operation, physically robust, and singing excellently in a well-known choir, having taken the bus from his home to get there.[9]

Forty years later, co-author NM worked with a patient who had been lobotomised in the 1950s. A well-spoken man from the affluent Surrey 'stockbroker belt', Malcolm[10] was normally pleasant but would sometimes erupt in explosive rage on being prompted by care workers to wash and dress. He was barred from several local shops for making enquiries of a sexual nature to staff and customers. NM asked him about his psychosurgery:

> *Why did you have this operation?*
> I couldn't talk to people very clearly.
> *Was that the only reason?*
> I used to get angry with my mother for nagging at me, or my colleagues at work ticking me off for things I'd done wrong – I'd tell them to shut up and leave me alone.
> *What did you do when you became angry?*
> I would hit my mother.
> *How did you feel about the leucotomy?*
> I wasn't very happy about it, I'm afraid.

After three admissions to Brookwood Hospital, Malcolm was unable to keep his job in the City. His father consulted William Sargant, who referred him for unilateral leucotomy by surgeon Harvey Jackson at Queen's Square. On the next day he was transferred to Belmont Hospital, where he did a course in printing, but sadly he failed to recover and went to Netherne. A few years later he received another leucotomy, on the other side.

According to a ministerial report,[11] 12,000 leucotomies had been performed in Britain by 1954. About half the patients were discharged after the operation, although many were readmitted. A disproportionately high number of women were selected for psychosurgery. There was no specific diagnostic indication: some patients with persistent anxiety or obsessional states were brought in from home; at the other end of the spectrum were persistently troublesome schizophrenics in the back wards, who had not responded to shock therapy. As the current 'Red Book' predated the physical treatments, nursing students learned procedures from American mental nursing manuals, or British textbooks on neurosurgical nursing. During her nurse training at Graylingwell in the late 1950s, Brenda Billings[12] asked to observe a leucotomy being performed. She was surprised by the apparently mundane procedure: visiting surgeon Wylie McKissock[13] bored a hole in the skull and the whole operation took half an hour. Brenda never saw any patient improve as a result.

Undoubtedly there were improvements to mental hospitals in the early years of the NHS. The proportion of patients admitted under the Lunacy Act steadily declined. At Moorhaven in Plymouth, for example, certification accounted for 23 per cent of the admissions in 1948, falling to 8 per cent in 1950. Modest refurbishment programmes began, though typically limited to repainting. At Denbigh Hospital, for example, the corridors were stripped of the oppressive thick brown paint by blowtorch, making way for lighter colours.[14] The degrading communal bathing ceased, providing a vacant space for other uses. At West Park, the general bathroom was converted to a hospital shop and locker room for staff sports. Yet for all the enthusiasm generated by new treatments and the NHS, overcrowding and impoverishment was worsening.

Although younger patients with a first admission were discharged as soon as possible, the mental hospitals were steadily becoming geriatric institutions by default. Noting the high prevalence of social causes in older patients, Aubrey Lewis at The Maudsley presciently warned that within thirty years the majority of the resident population would be elderly.[15] Medical superintendents argued that their hospitals should not be the sole repository of senile dementia. A Ministry of Health circular of 1950 proposed observation units and long-stay annexes within the geriatric department of a comprehensive general hospital. However, such provision failed to materialise, and it was left to mental hospital management committees to plan for a multitude of older people who needed medical and social care, but not necessarily psychiatric intervention.[16] Reporting an increase in proportion of elderly patients from 18 per cent in 1938 to 24 per cent in 1948, Bexley doctors Cook, Dax and Maclay[17] commented:

> We do not want to advocate that the mental health service should shelve any of its proper responsibilities, but we think the care and treatment of patients exhibiting simple cerebral deterioration due to age should be shared by the general hospitals.

The population of the female side of mental hospitals had grown disproportionately, yet this was not always reflected in resources. Figures from the adjacent hospitals of Rubery Hill and Hollymoor in Birmingham show a failure to respond to the gender imbalance (see Table 5.1)

At Rubery Hill almost two-thirds of the patients were female, with a 36 per cent excess on official capacity. One factor was longevity and the incidence of

Table 5.1 Male and female population at Rubery Hill and Hollymoor, 1954[18]

| | Rubery Hill | | | |
	Male	Female	Female proportion	Total
Authorised accommodation	353	439	55%	792
Number in residence, 21 June 1954	337	598	64%	935

| | Hollymoor | | | |
	Male	Female	Female proportion	Total
Authorised accommodation	327	307	48%	634
Number in residence, 21 June 1954	329	384	54%	713

dementia: 31 per cent of women were aged over sixty-five years, but merely 19 per cent of the men. A higher proportion of women were certified. In 1953, of 253 female admissions to Rubery Hill, 127 were compulsorily detained, compared to fifty-one of the 151 male admissions. More female nurses were urgently needed, but in areas such as Birmingham, once known as 'Workshop of the Empire', young people had a wide range of career options.

> Recruitment of student nurses is most difficult, especially in the Midlands, where the ratio of employment in industry is very high. The nursing staff is about 35% below its proper establishment, and much use has to be made of married women who may only work part of their time.[19]

The marriage bar was lifted after the war, but recruitment problems worsened. Open days, exhibitions and costly advertising campaigns proved futile.

Old habits die hard

A 1950s booklet by the hospital management committee at Long Grove promoted mental nursing as a stimulating and rewarding career:[20]

> Patients suffering from mental disorders are ordinary people like the rest of us, whose way of thinking and behaviour has become unusual owing to illness. Most can be restored to health and enabled to live, work and enjoy themselves in a perfectly normal way. A few remain too seriously handicapped to live without the help and shelter of a hospital, but much can be done to make their lives happier and more useful. The methods of treatment used in a progressive hospital like Long Grove are most varied. They include the use of drugs, electrical treatment, and the technique of influencing the minds of patients towards healthy behaviour, known as psychotherapy. The mental nurse has a vital part to play in relation to all these methods. In addition to the interesting technical work of nursing there is the fascination of learning to handle patients in the way that will best fit them once more for normal life, and in a few cases to make the most of their remaining capacities. If you decided to adopt this career, you will find it to be an absorbing study that holds your interest and appeals to your imagination.

This optimistic marketing, however, contrasted with the reality of mental nursing, as recruits discovered on their first ward. Typically they were placed on a ward for frail elderly patients, and this was like being thrown into the pool at the deep end. These wards housed upwards of ninety patients, mostly bed-bound, with barely sufficient space to clamber between the beds. Some patients were in the tertiary stage of syphilis; as their flesh sloughed away from their bones, they expired in misery and pain.

Despite the positive spin of recruitment campaigns, mental nursing was the 'Cinderella' of the nursing profession. A government working party chaired by Sir Robert Wood on recruitment, training and retention of nurses, noted:

> There can be little doubt that discontent and apathy amongst nursing staff are deeper and more widespread in the mental hospitals.[21]

The Whitley Nursing & Midwifery Council, established in 1948 following the Rushcliffe Committee, agreed to issue mental nurses a £20 lead over general nurses in their annual salary. This was a pragmatic response to staff shortage, although it came to be misconceived as 'danger money'. The Nurses Act 1949 amalgamated the male nurses' section with the general part of the register, but male nurses and mental nurses were ineligible for full RCN membership until 1960.[22] Illustrating the difference in culture, 65 per cent of mental nurses were members of a trade union (mostly COHSE), compared to merely 6 per cent of general nurses.[23] Disparaging attitudes to mental nursing persisted, with the middle-class snobbery of the senior ranks of general nursing barely concealed, as David Glenister described:

> Incorporation of mental nurses within the nursing statutory framework and occupational culture presented several problems for the professionalisation of nursing. Mental nurses came from a lower social class than general nurses, were apparently intellectually less able, undertook work which, unlike general nursing, lacked positive public regard, and allegedly adopted industrial rather than professional approaches to advancement.[24]

Notwithstanding advances in clinical treatment, most mental hospitals would have been instantly recognisable to a Victorian time traveller. ruled by moralistic matrons, and by military disciplinarians on the male side. Obedience to superiors was more important than respect for patients. Nurses were not told patients' diagnoses, and had no access to medical records. The cursory notes made by an exhausted nurse at the end of a long shift featured stock phrases such as 'settled' or 'restless', with no attempt to present the patient's perspective. Such individual attention was quite impossible due to the sheer workload. A *Nursing Times* article described a ward at Menston Hospital near Leeds containing 103 patients; on each evening mattresses were laid on the floor between beds.[25] This was certainly not the largest or most overcrowded ward in the country, but it illustrated the deprivation. In many hospitals it was necessary to convert day-rooms to dormitories, and to use the corridors for similar purpose. As described by Joyce Archer, a nurse at All Saints in Birmingham, there was insufficient hot water, soap and towels for bathing, and patients wore the same grimy clothes for weeks.[26]

With their insurmountable workload, nurses tended to reduce care to a production line.[27] Contempt was openly expressed, as in the term 'wet and dirty' for those past caring for the toilet. Perhaps nurses thought that patients would not understand. Paul Warr was a newspaper reporter who decided to start a career in mental nursing, recording his experiences in his account *Brother Lunatic*. Warr recalled being told by senior nursing staff at Shenley that the chronic patients, and especially those suffering from epilepsy, 'must be watched because they are crafty and murderous'.[28] Nurses told the medical superintendent what he wanted to know, while behind the scenes there was much rough handling in the showers, teasing and intimidation. Nurses protected each other, and if a patient had been bruised for his trouble, the unwritten rule was: 'Don't tell the Super'.

Ronnie Newman,[29] a nurse at Roundway Hospital in Wiltshire, described the paucity of drug treatment in the post-war years. The medicines cupboard, to which only the charge nurse had the key, contained three large Winchester bottles labelled 'white mixture', 'brown mixture' and 'paraldehyde'; these were refilled every Friday afternoon and liberally dispensed without prescription. The white solution was a purgative; the 'brown mixture', composed of laudanum and treacle, was used as a sedative. The medical superintendent came to each ward in the morning, and a junior doctor in the evening, but according to Ronnie they merely spoke to the nurse in charge, and rarely spent time with patients.

Use of paraldehyde was ubiquitous in the more turbulent wards. Bridget Dickson-Wilde[30] recalled an incident during her training at Netherne in 1952. As the only nurse on night duty in the female disturbed ward, she was sitting by the open fire believing all the patients to be asleep. The six side-rooms, used for the most challenging patients, were normally locked by the sister prior to her departure. Bridget had inadvertently drifted to sleep when she woke to find a patient drinking the contents of a bottle of paraldehyde, taken from Bridget's pocket. The patient's side-room had not been locked. Luckily Bridget was not caught napping by the night superintendent, who visited each ward three times per night. Presumably the patient had a good sleep. Although patients were addicted to paraldehyde, nurses hated the odour, which clung to their clothes and hair. Morah Geall told of cycling from Hellingly to the cinema in Hailsham, worrying that she smelled of the mental hospital.[31]

Olive Slattery[32] recalls a tragedy with medication at Gartnavel in Glasgow in the mid-1950s. A nurse had come to Olive's ward seeking medicine to calm a disturbed patient for the night, and as there was none of the clear draught available, she took some of the cloudy mixture (paraldehyde). Nurses were warned never to combine the two types of medicine, as this could be lethal. At 2 a.m., Olive learned that a patient on the ward to which the nurse had returned had collapsed and died. The duty doctor arrived some time later and pronounced the patient dead from a 'heart attack', and although he asked the ward nurse about the medication given, he made no record of the likely cause of death. The doctor covered up the nurse's fatal error.

Meanwhile ECT was used liberally and indiscriminately, sometimes as a behavioural rather than curative intervention. In an autobiographical account of a life spent in psychiatric institutions,[33] Jimmy Laing was given raw ECT among other punitive responses to his persistent absconding. Laing had been sent to Gartloch from remand at Barlinnie Prison in Glasgow, on a criminal section of the Lunacy Act. After taking unauthorised leave, he was told he would be given a new treatment:

> They put me on a dreaded drug which was later taken off the list – Sulphonal. The effects were unbelievable. Within three days I lost the power of my voice, I was speaking as if I was gaga. I couldn't walk, to such an extent that the nurses had to lift me on to a commode if I wanted to go to the toilet. All this time the dreadful thing was that my brain was functioning normally but I couldn't tell anyone because I couldn't speak. I lay in bed for three months and during that time they brought a speech therapist to teach me how to speak again. They stopped the treatment after three months and, fortunately, they stopped using the drug at all not long after that. It took months to get my voice back. Some of the other patients were given increased doses of Sulphonal. They turned into virtual zombies, drooling at the mouth, and, like me, unable to walk; men, whom I'd seen in the past out playing football and being full of life, now shadows of their former selves.[34]

A highly toxic drug, sulphonal was supposedly a last resort for severe agitation, but as Laing illustrated, it was also used to control the irascible patient. After several more escapades, a course of ECT was prescribed. In the ante-room Laing laid waiting alongside three others, all in their surgical gowns:

> I heard this blood-curdling scream. It scared the living daylights out of me. I leapt up and ran along the corridor as fast as I could and out of the first door that I could with all the nurses chasing after me. Eventually they caught me on the football pitch. I was screaming when they brought me back. I don't think I have ever been so afraid in my life. They put me on a trolley and covered me with a sheet … Then there is one almighty flash.[35]

Laing received a course of twelve shocks, each time without pre-medication, and after hearing the screams of patients who preceded him.

> I found out later that the way the nursing staff gauged whether or not the blast had penetrated was by one watching your feet. If your toes turned in they would say, 'that was a good one, that was a beauty'.[36]

School days

Having agreed to relinquish nurse training after the war, the RMPA held its last examinations in 1951, but it did not abandon its involvement. Psychiatrists such as Ian Skottowe at St John's in Buckinghamshire, Rolf Strom-Olsen at Runwell and TP Rees at Warlingham Park were engaged by the GNC Mental Nurses Committee in syllabus design. Meanwhile the long-awaited revision of the 'Red Book' appeared in 1954. Expanded to 476 pages, the manual no longer attempted to cover the whole scope of nursing: sections on physical diseases and wound care were omitted. In their place were detailed chapters on the various mental disorders. On page 283 was a chapter on mental nursing, which described general duties of the nurse including basic care, with an emphasis on maintaining safety. Exercise and recreation were given prominence, with an example of an activity schedule. While acknowledging that the number of trained occupational therapists was small, the textbook asserted that engaging patients in work and recreational activity was fundamental to the nursing role. For example:[37]

> Dancing is usually a favourite form of recreation among patients, of which full use should be made. Dances are held frequently in hospitals in the winter months, and all patients who can should be encouraged to attend them and to take special care over their appearance on such occasions, for dances introduce an element of normality which, despite all efforts, is too often lacking in mental hospital life. In addition to ballroom dancing, country dancing has of recent years become an established form of recreation in many hospitals. It is remarkable how greatly this is enjoyed even by many deteriorated patients, who take pleasure in the simple rhythms and in the co-operative nature of the performance. Many patients are able to work off both aggression and surplus energy in this pursuit which often arouses interest and a willingness to participate where other methods have failed.

The eighth edition of the 'Red Book' maintained a low level of abstraction, with no theoretical framework for mental nursing. In the section on treatment, social methods were promoted, with reference to wartime success in group work. It was recommended that wards be divided into groups of four to eight patients, but limited guidance was given on the principles and practice of social therapy. The authors steered clear of prescribing any particular social treatment, and the term 'therapeutic community' was absent. Perhaps this could have given nurses ideas above their station. The role of the nurse as a therapeutic agent was limited to general guidance, suggesting reluctance of the authors to undermine medical authority

The 1954 text belatedly brought student nurses up-to-date with physical treatments. Shock therapies were described in detail, with particular attention to the nurses' procedures in preparing patients, assisting the doctor with administration, and observation and support in the recovery stage. Insulin coma therapy was presented as the most effective treatment for schizophrenia, particularly in apathetic or self-absorbed cases. The typical course was a daily administration for three months, and the manual briefly mentioned modified sub-coma treatment for neurotic illness. Acute schizophrenia and depressive disorder were the indications for ECT, although it was noted that some doctors preferred the chemical method for maintenance treatment. Prolonged narcosis was stated to have declined in use due to the effectiveness of insulin and ECT. The chapter on psychosurgery acknowledged undesirable personality changes resulting from the operation but emphasised the beneficial effects on cases unresponsive to other methods. A chapter on sedation promoted hydrotherapy, despite this being abandoned in most mental hospitals. Drugs were presented as a second-line treatment for agitation or excitement, normally barbiturates such as sodium amytal, while extreme cases could be calmed by paraldehyde or hyoscine. The revised text was unfortunately timed, as psychiatry was about to undergo a drug revolution; until the next edition in the 1960s, student nurses read of treatments that had been long discarded.

Students now spent whole days in the nursing school, in blocks of one or two weeks. Full uniform was worn at all times, and apart from the hours in the classroom, there was no exemption from duties on the wards. In Morah Geall's training at Hellingly,[38] students went to their ward as usual at 7*a.m.* to get the patients up; they returned at four o'clock and finished at 7.30 p.m. On one occasion in her training at Graylingwell, Brenda Billings[39] made the mistake of arriving on duty wearing lipstick. 'Get here, my girl', exclaimed the ward sister, who marched Brenda to a basin where she washed off the offending adornment. Brenda accepted this as a lesson in professionalism.

From open wards to the open hospital

Many medical superintendents endeavoured to change what they saw as an oppressive if not brutal institutional system. At Dingleton Hospital in the rural Scottish borderland, George Bell began to unlock the wards in 1946 and by 1949 the whole hospital was open. This was not the first time this had been achieved: Barony Parochial Asylum near Glasgow had opened the doors back in 1881, and similarly Saxty Good at Littlemore in the 1920s, but in both of these institutions wards reverted to lock and key. With reports of successful outcomes at Dingleton, a momentum began to develop. In 1952 Duncan Macmillan declared all wards open at Mapperley in Nottingham, only the outer hospital doors being closed at night. At Warlingham Park TP Rees had unlocked all but two wards by 1954. Moorhaven in Devon and Central Hospital in Warwickshire were fully open by 1956, and Fulbourn by 1958.

At Dingleton, Bell believed that had he consulted the nurses, they would have rejected the idea outright. In a report in *The Lancet*, ES Stern[40] stated that no ward was unlocked at Central Hospital until the charge nurses were ready. Perhaps progressive medical superintendents had seen the pitfalls of imposing radical change to the running of the hospital without the support of those responsible for its implementation: resistance could lead to sabotage. As Liam Clarke[41] explained, the nurses had genuine fears about escape, and sexual liaisons, violence or suicide; they knew of colleagues fined or dismissed for lapses in care and security. As nurses saw that their worst fears were not realised by the open door, they became more enthusiastic. Stern reported a dramatic change in the *milieu*:

> The whole staff–patient relationship is transformed. Nurses are no longer regarded as turnkeys.[42]

In 1953 JAR Bickford was appointed as deputy medical superintendent at De La Pole Hospital in Hull, then a typically gloomy mental institution of traditional order. Bickford focused his attention on the most disabled patients on the male side. He divided the forty men in a long-stay villa into groups of ten, each with designated nurses who supervised a schedule of work and recreational activities. The average age was thirty-two, but all of these patients had been destined for a lifetime in the institution. The groups worked on a rota to construct a bowling green, and they also went potato-picking on neighbouring farms, earning some pocket-money. The men derived much benefit from working: the physical activity, fresh air and rapport with fellows in a shared endeavour. Educational discussions were held by a nurse, who planned the topics in advance, including 'how to run a smallholding, chrysanthemum growing, dairy farming, the Liberal point of view, local government, the job of a cricket captain, care of a motor-cycle, prospects for the Derby, and how to run a seaside boarding house'. Impressive results were reported by Bickford in a *Lancet* article on 'the forgotten patient':

> One young man who for eighteen years had been smiling and grimacing to himself, wildly gesticulating, and constantly talking or shouting out to himself, often striding up and down and never saying a sensible word, is now a neat hardworking, quiet, pleasant man.[43]

Bickford acknowledged that none of this would have been possible without the enthusiasm of chief male nurse Peter Archer. Several other hospitals around the country were boasting of their liberal advances, but Bickford cautioned that opening of doors was not treatment by itself. Most chronic schizophrenic patients showed no desire to leave the hospital; in the absence of social activation, freedom was a fallacy.

> One sees the open ward containing fifty voluntary patients who never leave it except on their visit to hospital entertainments, and then well-escorted, or the open ward where ten or more patients are always to be found in bed because otherwise they would run away. There are open wards whose patients are by day turned out into an airing-court with a high iron railing. If the patients want to reach the grounds on the other side of the rails they have to go up an iron staircase from it to reach another ward.[44]

In 1953 televisions arrived on the wards, a remarkable development spurred by live broadcast of the Coronation. However, for a meaningful sense of liberty, patients needed real contact with the outside world. At Moorhaven Hospital in Devon, medical superintendent Francis Pilkington and chief male nurse John Greene espoused a policy whereby not only were patients allowed out, but the local community were invited in. Pilkington greatly increased the number of patients on 'daily pass' (a term he substituted for the penal-associated 'parole'),[45] giving them freedom to wander in the hospital grounds or visit the nearby village. Social skills training was initiated and an industrial therapy unit was built. Lecturers were invited from nearby Dartington Hall to provide art, drama and music therapy. While patients were encouraged to practise their religious beliefs, attendance at Sunday service was no longer compulsory. Years later, Greene assimilated his working relationship with Pilkington to the historic partnership between Philippe Pinel and head attendant Jean Baptiste Pussin in Paris.[46]

Following Joshua Bierer's innovation in Hampstead in 1946, one of the first day hospitals developed in the conventional mental health system was in Bristol, where a large house accommodating long-stay female patients from Fishponds was converted in 1951. Alongside a doctor and occupational therapists, the day hospital was staffed by full-time nurses.[47] A more ambitious deployment of mental nurses in the community was planned by TP Rees at Warlingham Park Hospital. Observing the tendency for patients who had spent years in hospital to relapse on discharge, Rees worked closely with ward sister Lena Peat to establish a nursing service to support discharged patients, and the innovation was highly successful. Credited as the first community psychiatric nurse,[48] Peat was initially deployed on a six-month stint, but she made the job her own for twenty-three years. She was followed by Arthur Groves, a charge nurse on the male side.

Despite the solidity of the traditional institutional regime, social approaches were making inroads.

A pioneer was David Clark, who was appointed as medical superintendent at Fulbourn Hospital in 1953, at the relatively young age of thirty-two. In his training under David Henderson at the Royal Edinburgh Hospital, Clark had learned the importance of the social aspects of mental illness. However, perhaps the most poignant influence was his wartime experience as a paratrooper, and his horror at the Nazi concentration camps. Seeing the plight of patients on the back wards of Fulbourn as a slow death sentence, Clark pledged to liberate them from institutional oppression.

> Grey, big courts, paved with tarmac surrounded by a wall 12 foot high and a hundred men milling around. A few of them walking, some running, others standing on one leg, posturing, the urine running out of their trouser legs. A couple of bored young male nurses standing on 'points duty', looking at them ready to hit anybody who got out of line, but otherwise not doing anything. A scene of human degradation.[49]

Inspired by the work of Maxwell Jones at Belmont, Clark introduced a 'Work for All' programme in 1954. He then selected the female disturbed ward to apply his emerging model of social therapy.[50] F5 had occupied a separate building furnished with merely long tables and wooden benches, where the patients spent most of the day unoccupied and having little interaction with the nurses. Moving F5 into a freshly renovated ward in the main building, Clark unlocked the door, abandoned the padded room, brought in occupational therapists, and allowed visitors to come to the ward instead of seeing their relatives in a central hall. Impressed by sociological analyses of mental institutions in the USA, Clark invited a researcher to study the social mechanisms of change. Improvements were modest: the custodial hierarchy persisted, and the officially open door was repeatedly locked by nurses. Yet by unlocking the whole of Fulbourn's wards by 1958, Clark reached a milestone, marking five years of battles fought and won:

> Opposition groups were reasoned with, cajoled, but if necessary overruled. Much staff enthusiasm was liberated, and from being custodial and rather dreary, the hospital became lively and optimistic.[51]

A remarkable experiment in a refractory ward at Gartnavel Mental Hospital was reported in *The Lancet* in 1955. Psychiatrists John Cameron and Ronnie Laing and psychologist Andrew McGhie selected twelve of the most disabled schizophrenic patients for an intensive nursing environment, which they labelled the 'Rumpus Room'. Here, two nurses spent each day with the patients in a brightly decorated, well-furnished room with gramophone, material for drawing, sewing and knitting, and cooking facilities. Instead of reacting to violence by injecting patients with paraldehyde, nurses were encouraged to stay calm and to understand why the patient was acting in this way. The patients showed dramatic improvement, resulting in their discharge. The authors argued that by developing genuine relationships with patients, nurses became the primary therapeutic agent.

> We conclude that the physical material in the environment, while useful, was not the most important factor in producing the change. It was the nurses. And the most important thing about the nurses, and other people in the environment, is how they feel towards their patients. Our experiment has shown that the barrier between patients is not erected solely by the patients but is a mutual construction. Removal of this barrier is a mutual activity.[52]

The summit – at last

Ironically, while some progressive medical superintendents were transforming mental hospitals, their position was threatened. As mental health services began to grow out of institutional isolation, the medical overlord was challenged in clinical practice by the autonomy of consultant psychiatrists, and in administrative authority by the increasingly centralised NHS bureaucracy. In 1954 a review, *Internal Administration of Hospitals*, by a committee chaired by Lord Bradbeer recommended a management triumvirate for hospitals comprising a lay administrator, a doctor and the matron. A partnership of equals was intended, although in most mental hospitals the medical superintendent remained in post well into the next decade. Whether charismatic or autocratic in style, they did not readily let go of the reins.

After decades of relentless rise, the mental hospital census finally reached its peak in the 1950s. The high-water mark in England and Wales was in 1954 and three years later in Scotland. Although we can see the tide turning in retrospect, at the time there was little sense of relief in the mental hospitals. Moreover, while the end-of-year head count was beginning to fall, the rate of admissions was soaring. The threshold for admission had lowered: people with common neurotic disorders such as depression and anxiety were being sent by general practitioners. Apart from cities with observation units, or the few general hospitals with psychiatric wards, there was nowhere else to go for treatment. At St Francis' Hospital in Sussex, for example, there were 160 admissions per month in 1957, compared to annual totals averaging 250 in the 1930s. The symmetry here was typical: in this hospital of 900 beds, 900 entered and 900 left over the year. Such throughput could be misleading, as the back wards had little flux: for chronic patients the horizon stretched no further than the airing court.[53]

In 1954 long-overdue reform of the Lunacy Act was begun by the Royal Commission on Mental Illness and Mental Deficiency. Chaired by Lord Percy, who had sat on the Macmillan Commission in the 1920s, the eleven members included TP Rees, alongside three other doctors, two lawyers, and mental nurse Claude Bartlett (president of COHSE).[54] Mental nursing was afforded little attention by the Percy Commission, which did not dwell on the detail of care but instead focused on re-orientating a traditional mental health system towards the community. Seventy per cent of the resident population of mental hospitals in 1955 was confined,[55] and the requirement for voluntary patients to sign for their willingness to accept treatment was seen as an unnecessary distinction from physical health care.[56] Urging abolition of the frightfully outmoded terminology of lunacy, the Percy Commission regarded admission as a purely medical decision.

Wonder drugs

In 1953 Joel Elkes, professor of experimental psychiatry at the University of Birmingham, and a pioneer of research on potential uses of lysergic acid diethylamide (LSD), tested a new drug on chronic schizophrenic patients at All Saints Hospital.[57] Since first reports in 1952, chlorpromazine had produced startling results in acute psychosis, but Elkes found that patients who might have been described as hopeless cases also made dramatic improvement. Men who had been embroiled in delusions and hallucinations were stabilised, some engaging in social and occupational activity for the first time, only to relapse when the pills were replaced by placebo.[58] The drug revolution – the most poignant moment in the development of modern psychiatry – had begun.

Chlorpromazine, like many medical advances, arose through serendipity. Henri Laborit, a French naval surgeon in colonial Tunisia, was seeking a solution to the problem of surgical shock. Laborit believed that the lowering of blood pressure was caused by secretion of histamine, a substance known to be involved in allergic reactions. As an antihistamine, promethazine was tried by Laborit in a cocktail of anaesthesia given to patients prior to surgery. The experiment confirmed promethazine as the most effective agent; patients were so calmed that post-operative morphine was unnecessary. In 1951 Laborit moved to the Val-de-Grâce military hospital in Paris, where he received a new antihistamine compound (coded 4560TP) synthesised by pharmaceutical company Rhône-Poulenc. It reduced pre-operative anxiety to the extent that some patients became indifferent to their situation. Laborit saw the implications for psychiatry, and he persuaded doctors to test the drug on a manic patient, who showed remarkable improvement within two weeks of treatment. Hearing of this experiment, in 1952 Jean Delay and Pierre Deniker conducted the first clinical trial of this drug on manic patients, and their results confirmed the effectiveness of the drug, which was named chlorpromazine. Soon the wards of Parisian mental hospitals were transformed. After Delay and Deniker presented their results at a conference, American company Smith, Kline & French gained a licence to market, the drug as Thorazine in the USA. In Europe it was sold by Rhône-Poulenc as Largactil (inferring 'large action'), and in 1954 it was introduced in Britain by May & Baker. As with shock therapy and leucotomy, there was neither a known mechanism nor a specific diagnostic indication for chlorpromazine: it appeared particularly beneficial in schizophrenia and mania, but also in agitated depression and other neurotic states.[59]

After a positive report on fifty patients at Warley Hospital, published in 1954,[60] a large evaluation was reported by Leslie Cook and colleagues[61] at Bexley Hospital. Their study included 200 consecutive cases on the female wards, plus forty-eight women with mental and motor disturbance who were randomised to either the drug or placebo. In the sequential series, sixty-two of the 103 patients with chronic schizophrenia improved, as did fifty-two of the ninety-seven with affective or other states. In the case-control experiment, sixteen of the twenty-four women taking the drug improved, compared to just five of those taking placebo. The Bexley doctors concluded:

> Generally speaking chlorpromazine controlled psychomotor excitement and agitation, aggressiveness and tension, and allowed better rapport, enabling the patients to become occupied and resocialised. On the other hand, the basic schizophrenic symptoms – thought disturbance, delusions and hallucinations – appeared to be much less influenced, and continued, though frequently reduced in intensity.[62]

From the outset, Cook and colleagues did not regard chlorpromazine as a miracle cure – far from it. They noted that it diminished excitatory states while exacerbating inhibitory symptoms. They observed complications in 22 per cent of cases, with instances of collapse, pyrexia and skin rashes, although they found that most side effects declined after three weeks of administration. Emaciated patients who had suffered from persecution by voices and persistent restlessness gained weight. The wards were quieter, with less shouting, screaming and lashing out, creating an environment conducive to socialisation and enabling some patients to go on leave. Nonetheless, the Bexley report concluded:

> Chlorpromazine is a valuable though limited addition to the therapeutic armamentarium.[63]

Pharmaceutical companies developed various other drugs of the phenothiazine class in the late 1950s, but none was found superior to chlorpromazine in clinical action or tolerance.[64] Reserpine, after much promise, was withdrawn due to excessive sedation. Sober analysis did not temper enthusiasm for this instantly effective and convenient treatment: Largactil required no elaborate, time-consuming procedures (unlike insulin coma), it apparently caused no irreversible change to the personality (unlike psychosurgery), and it could be used for as long as necessary (unlike ECT).

Within a few years of the introduction of chlorpromazine, most insulin treatment units were abandoned. Research had already cast doubt on the benefits of insulin coma. In 1953 an influential article in *The Lancet* on 'the insulin myth' attributed positive results to flawed evaluation.[65] The death knell was sounded in 1957 by a randomised, controlled trial of insulin versus barbiturate-induced coma, by Brian Ackner and colleagues at the Bethlem Hospital, which debunked any specific action of insulin.[66] Meanwhile a large trial in the USA showed no difference in outcomes between insulin coma and chlorpromazine, and while such results justified continuing use of the former treatment by some psychiatrists for many years to come, the prevailing view was that patients need not be subjected to a laborious and dangerous procedure when the same outcome could be achieved with pills and syrups administered by nurses.[67]

Another casualty of the drug revolution was psychosurgery. Some psychiatrists expressed regret for their involvement in a treatment of such dubious merit. Ivor Browne, a trainee psychiatrist at Grangegorman Mental Hospital in Dublin in the 1950s, assisted with lobotomies on Saturday mornings, and was distressed by the nonchalance of the visiting neurosurgeon, who whistled while he cut.

> I feel shame and regret. But it is senseless, in retrospect, to react with such emotions of guilt, nor does it make sense to blame the surgeon, for neither of us knew any better. This was an accepted procedure at the time, recommended by supposed experts and the senior psychiatrists who were in charge of the hospital.[68]

Henry Marsh, author of an acclaimed book on his experiences as a leading neurosurgeon found little clinical justification for the operation in the medical records of lobotomised men at a large mental hospital, where he briefly worked as a nursing assistant in the 1970s.

> The lobectomized men were, it seemed to me, some of the worst affected of the patients – dull and apathetic and zombie-like. I was shocked to find, when surreptitiously looking at their notes, that there was no evidence of any kind of follow-up or post-operative assessment. In all the patients who had been lobectomised there would be a brief note stating 'Suitable for lobectomy. For transfer to AMH'. The next entry would read 'Returned from AMH. For removal of black silk sutures in nine days', and that was it.[69]

The number of psychosurgery operations was declining in Britain before the introduction of Largactil, partly because so many long-stay schizophrenic patients had already been leucotomised, but also because the modest benefits were perceived as a price too high to pay for the irreversible changes to personality, and the high mortality. Furthermore, the operation was doing little to reduce the mental hospital population. According to JAR Bickford, 'a past prefrontal leucotomy may be the only thing that makes a patient's recovery impossible'.

Meanwhile, troubling effects of prolonged use of Largactil and other phenothiazine drugs were emerging. Although drowsiness tended to reduce once the optimal dose was set, lasting neurological impairments were suspected. Tardive dyskinesia became noticeable in about a quarter of patients after three years of taking neuroleptic drugs. Involuntary, repetitive movements of the lips and tongue gradually worsened, leading to grotesque facial mannerisms and impaired speech. As most patients were taking the drugs *ad infinitum*, the incidence was steadily increasing. The wonder drugs were thus a double-edged sword, calming psychotic disturbance but producing embarrassing effects that hindered socialisation.[70] Often used excessively, they were dubbed the 'chemical cosh'.

The mission, in a word

In 1955 a sociological study of the causes and prevention of aggression began on the disturbed wards of Netherne Hospital in Surrey.[71] Under medical superintendent RK Freudenberg, Netherne was changing its focus from leucotomy and other physical treatments to social methods. By this time the hospital housed 1,909 patients, a small but significant reduction from the peak of 2,062 in 1946. Four of the forty-one wards and villas had been unlocked in 1936, but despite steady progress fifteen wards remained locked. With the advent of tranquillising drugs, further liberalisation was planned. The number of leucotomies had fallen to nineteen in 1955, but physical treatments were used extensively: 1,216 patients received ECT and ninety-five insulin coma therapy. Occupational activity was increasing, and 985 patients had some form of parole, but patients in the disturbed wards had little liberty.

MS Folkard (previously a mental nurse) conducted the research on Ward F11A and M5. The fifty patients on the female disturbed ward were mostly schizophrenic, with a few epileptic, psychopathic and manic-depressive cases. They were placed there due to aggressive or antisocial behaviour, and ineffectiveness of ECT or leucotomy. Frequent aggression was attributed to the authoritarian regime, overcrowding, patients being held in a state of irresponsibility, and punitive staff response to incidents (e.g. use of the padded room or heavy sedation). Freudenberg, who supervised Folkard's study, was striving to relieve patients from chemical, electrical and social restraint. Paraldehyde was withdrawn. Folkard found that whereas the doctors saw the priorities of the nurses' role in understanding patients and keeping them occupied, the five senior nurses responsible for F11A emphasised cleanliness and order, and keeping patients safe from harm or escape. In Freudenberg's view, the perceived need to control patients was a self-fulfilling prophecy.

Contrasting the two wards, Folkard observed considerable differences in aggression between male and female patients. M5 had half the number of patients as the female ward, but in two ten-week periods in 1955 and 1956, the number of incidents on F11A was 547, compared to just sixty-three on M5. Nurses were assaulted five times on M5, but 101 times on the female ward. Folkard suggested childhood experiences of female patients as a factor, particularly in the relationship with their mothers, but he also commented on the gendered response to aggression: women with violent tendencies were usually diagnosed as mentally ill, while men were more liable to imprisonment. Also, there were staffing differences: F11A was run by a sister with three students or nursing assistants, while the male ward had more staff nurses and therefore less turnover.

F11A was unlocked in 1956. Many of the women spent most of the day off the ward, either in occupational therapy or on parole. Yet nurses were apprehensive about the change. Folkard's comparison of ten weeks before and after unlocking of the ward showed a reduction from 249 to 193 aggressive incidents, and from four to three patients absconding. Over the three years of Folkard's study, ten more wards were unlocked, although as Folkard acknowledged, this was only one factor in reducing aggression. Perhaps more destructive was nurses' failure to engage with patients:

> The ways in which the staff avoid or ignore the patients, for fear of some disturbance in their routine, tends to provoke the very reaction which they are trying to forestall. Nurses in the hospital can be seen, when they are alone, moving swiftly away from a patient, which provokes the patient into pursuit. Similarly a group of nurses, seeing a patient get agitated with one of their colleagues, will close in around the disturbed and frightened patient who will then thresh out in terror.[72]

Meanwhile a trial of reserpine on F11A showed little difference in aggressive incidents between cases and controls. Chlorpromazine was highly effective in controlling psychotic symptoms, but neither tablets nor the liberalised but orderly regime were sufficient as treatment. Surveys in the 1950s indicated that large numbers of patients did not need skilled medical and nursing care, but the chronic schizophrenic would be prone to relapse in the community. Medication was no use if lost or poured down the sink. To survive in the community, patients needed better preparation than simply complying with the routine on 'dead end' wards. Long-stay patients needed a social, occupational and recreational push. In a word: rehabilitation.

With its numerous villas, Netherne was an ideal setting for a graded programme of rehabilitative work. The resettlement unit, started in 1958, enabled intensive resocialisation of patients prior to their return to the community. However, while the ultimate goal was discharge, rehabilitation was a principle applied throughout the mental hospital to improve patients' functioning. Group living was emphasised, and depersonalising routines were abandoned. Instead of dining at long benches in the main dining hall, patients had meals in the wards, in a dining area with tables for four or six. For TP Rees,[73] rehabilitation was merely a rewording of the moral treatment regrettably neglected since the early idealism of the asylum. Work, so prominent in the nineteenth-century institution, returned to prominence. Instead of merely performing ward chores, patients needed occupational training, preparing them for the realities of modern industrial society. Whereas the inmates of yore toiled in the fields, patients would now be primed for the production line. The Vale workshop opened at Netherne in 1956, with industrial subcontracts for simple assembly tasks; three years later another workshop was created specifically for severely disabled patients.

A pioneer of industrial therapy was Donal Early at Glenside (formerly Fishponds). In 1957 John Turley, managing director of the Tallon Pen Company, was introduced to Early by a general practitioner in Bristol. Turley was invited to Glenside and agreed to a trial of ballpoint pen assembly. A disused section of the night nurses' accommodation was used as a small factory. Seven carefully selected patients were paid at the attractive rate of 2s 6d per gross of completed 'Wagtail' pens – the same rate paid to Turley's outworkers. Soon one-third of the hospital population was employed in an expanding industrial therapy department. However, once this bonanza became known to National Insurance officers, the earning limit for hospital patients was imposed. The workshop at Glenside was supervised by Louis Walker, a senior charge nurse. Walker was receiving treatment for hypertension, and needed relief from his responsibilities on a 115-bed ward. It was typical for a trusted old hand to be given such a position: a nurse who knew the patients well, and who could motivate them without pushing them too far.

A major development in integration with the community was led by Joshua Carse, medical superintendent at Graylingwell. With admissions higher than ever, Carse sought a substitute for hospital admission, and he gained Medical Research Council funding to launch the Worthing Experiment. From 1957 onwards, admissions from the Worthing district were avoided wherever possible, with most psychiatric referrals receiving outpatient treatment, domiciliary visits or day hospital care at The Acre, a large house previously used for convalescent female patients. Graylingwell admissions reduced dramatically from 1,038 in 1957 to 764 in 1958. Evaluated by leading research psychiatrist Peter Sainsbury, the Worthing Experiment was a catalyst for the development of services elsewhere. The day hospital movement gained momentum, as evidence indicated the role of such facilities in the welcome reduction in hospital admissions in the late 1950s.[74]

The Worthing Experiment showed that a high proportion of psychiatric patients could avoid admission to the mental institution, but those with severe and enduring psychotic illness needed more support than could be provided in the community. The longer the period of treatment, the harder it was for the patient to return home. Rehabilitation helped patients who would otherwise have stagnated in long-stay wards, but they would not necessarily be welcomed back by their families and neighbours. For many long-stay patients, links with their community had been lost long ago. Partly due to the remoteness of mental hospitals, such patients were cast adrift, their social world confined to fellow patients and nurses. Enid Mills conducted a survey of patients admitted to Long Grove Hospital in 1956 and

1957 from Bethnal Green. This borough had a dark history of treatment for the mentally unwell, from the infamous Warburton's madhouse of the last century, to the common knowledge of people sent to a distant asylum, never to be seen again. Relatives from this poor district found great difficulty in visiting their loved ones.

> The journey to Long Grove by public transport will take at least 1½ hours. It can mean a bus ride, a journey on the tube with an awkward change at Bank Station (elderly relatives unable to manoeuvre the spiral iron staircase between the Central and Northern lines were forced to travel by bus), followed by a train journey and another bus trip of 20 minutes' walk. Some people prefer to find their way by the Green Line coach route to Epsom. But there is no simple and direct route to the hospital, and it is practically impossible to make the journey for less than 7s.[75]

Rehabilitation would be incomplete without involving the patient's family, but some relatives were unable or unwilling to support a discharged patient. In 1959 Elly Jansen, a Dutch theology student, was so concerned about such difficulties that she invited a few patients from Long Grove to live with her in a large house in Surrey. Jansen founded the Richmond Fellowship, and this was followed by other voluntary schemes to help those afflicted with mental illness and social exclusion. Mental illness remained a taboo in society, but an enlightening series of programmes by the BBC helped to confront fear and prejudice. *The Hurt Mind*, presented by Christopher Mayhew,[76] examined the rationale and practice of psychiatry, and life inside the mental hospital from the perspectives of patients and staff. Meanwhile the popular periodical *Picture Post* presented damning images of the poor conditions in which patients were being held. The question began to be asked about whether people with mental health problems should be removed from society to mental institutions.

New horizons

When a pigeon landed on the window ledge of Ward 1B at Denbigh Hospital, Bill warned the nurses to watch out. Since reading a newspaper article on a Nazi experiment in espionage, Bill had a paranoid delusion that he was being watched by winged spies, and he became agitated if nobody took him seriously. So the nurses would enter his fantasy world, and offer a counter-explanation. The pigeon was once a German agent, but it had defected to our side. Such an approach would not be found in the 'Red Book' or in medical instruction, but with caring intent the staff pacified Bill, and helped him to cope with his distressing aversion. As Andrew McCrae[77] recalled, there was thus no need to call the doctor, or an extra dose of tranquillising medication. In this caring spirit, nurses kept the torturing demons of schizophrenia at bay.

Denbigh was one of the hospitals involved in an innovative scheme with De la Pole, where JAR Bickford had initiated holiday exchanges. Every summer, a ward was ferried en bloc by coach to Hull, with a similar group taking their place in

North Wales. Bickford and HJB Miller, physician superintendent at Ailsa Hospital in Ayrshire, described the 'therapeutic holiday' for their long-stay schizophrenic patients:

> On a morning in May a motor coach left each of our hospitals with 20 patients and 5 nurses. At the midway point they stopped for lunch, exchanged passengers, and returned to their starting-point. The result was that the nurses and patients spent a little over two weeks in a strange hospital with a culture and a countryside differing considerably from their own.[78]

The Ailsa patients visited the maritime museums of Hull, the fish docks, brewery, ice cream factory, monasteries and the theatre. However, the Yorkshire patients felt that they had a better deal in the pleasant Ayrshire setting; as well as country walks they visited the American air force base at Prestwick, and had day trips to Loch Lomond and Edinburgh. For the accompanying nurses, the holidays were seen as a skive, particularly as any unstable or troublesome patients were left behind. They had a free sightseeing trip and relief from the arduous routine, but the exchange also exposed them to the culture of another hospital, perhaps giving them ideas for improvement on their return. Andrew McCrae remembered patients and nurses returning to Denbigh in high spirits. Bickford's travel agency would not have been possible without the drug revolution, but it also depended on nurses relinquishing control.

As the importance of interpersonal relationships to patients' recovery was appreciated, mental nurse training was under the spotlight. Staffing levels improved in the mental hospitals in the 1950s, but most of the increase was in nursing assistants, who doubled in number over the decade, while full-time qualified nurses increased modestly from 11,056 in 1949 to 11,415 ten years later.[79] The level of qualification on the male side was double that on the female side, where merely a third of nurses were qualified by the mid-1950s. In response to high attrition of nursing staff, a study was commissioned by Manchester Regional Hospitals Board[80] on the role of the mental nurse. Finding that nurses were excessively engaged in routine administrative tasks, while less than 5 per cent of their shifts was spent in conversation with patients, the Manchester report concluded that training was failing to prepare nurses for therapeutic practice.

In 1957 the GNC introduced an experimental syllabus, removing mental nursing students from the foundation year in knowledge and skills for physical nursing, so that their entire training would be in the psychiatric field. For nurses to be effective therapeutic agents, they would need more preparation in psychosocial treatment. A book *Chronic Schizophrenia* by psychiatrist and psychotherapist Thomas Freeman, written with Gartnavel colleagues Cameron and McGhie, urged a reorientation of nurse training to psychoanalytic principles.[81] Recruitment for mental nurse training began to change direction, as head tutors or senior nurses sought candidates with personal qualities best suited to the work and most likely to engage with patients, instead of someone who would simply follow ward routines.[82] However, psychologically minded nurses were not easy to find: understaffed hospitals continued to accept almost anyone who applied: as always, ideals were trumped by reality.

Ten years in the NHS

Long dormitories with a sea of beds inches apart: after a decade in the NHS the wards of the old institutional block looked much the same as before. Doors were unlocked and airing courts dismantled, but the mental hospital system remained stigmatised and oppressive, with scarce individualised care and nurses whose main concern was to maintain order. Yet major changes were happening. The overall population was slowly but steadily falling. This was a trend that began before the introduction of chlorpromazine, but the drug revolution had radically changed the atmosphere in the mental hospitals, and raised therapeutic optimism. Psychiatry had become dualistic, with both physical and social interventions to the fore. Indeed, whereas in the past occupational and recreational activity had been regarded as adjuncts to medical treatment, in progressive hospitals social methods had primacy. Psychiatrists of humanistic orientation saw tranquillising drugs as a mere accessory to patients' socialisation and reintegration to the community. Legislative changes were imminent, confirming progress in attitudes to mental illness, and in redefining the hospital from a place of incarceration to part of a broader service rooted in the community. Liberalisation of the institutional regime benefited nurses as well as their patients, but as we shall see, it would also threaten the very existence of the mental hospital.

Notes

1 Pratt D (1948): *Public Mental Hospitals in England: a Survey.*
2 Quoted in Early DF (2003). 82.
3 Personal communication (NM, 2014).
4 Hopton J (1999).
5 Weil Pl (1950): 'Regressive' electroplexy in schizophrenia. *Journal of Mental Science.*
6 Stafford Clark D (1963) *Psychiatry Today* (2nd edition).
7 Personal communication (NM, 2015).
8 Gardner J (1999).
9 Partridge M (1950). 473.
10 Personal communication: pseudonym (NM, 1995).
11 Tooth GC, Newton MP (1961): *Leucotomy in England and Wales 1942–1954.*
12 Personal communication (NM, 2015).
13 McKissock performed over 3,000 of these operations in England and Wales. In an obituary, he was described as 'a leucotomist of extraordinary surgical speed'. Bell BA (1996): Wylie McKissock – reminiscences of a commanding figure in British neurosurgery. *British Journal of Neurosurgery.*
14 Michael P (2003).
15 Lewis A (1946): Ageing and senility: a major problem of psychiatry. *Journal of Mental Science.*
16 Hilton, C. (2005). The origins of old age psychiatry in Britain in the 1940s. *History of Psychiatry.*
17 Cook LC, Dax EC, Maclay WS (1952): The geriatric problem in mental hospitals. *Lancet.*

18 Rubery Hill and Hollymoor Hospitals (1954): *Visit of the French Delegation – Monday 5th July 1954.*

19 Rubery Hill and Hollymoor Hospitals (1954). 9.

20 Quoted by Day T (1993): *More like Home: the Story of Long Grove Hospital and How it was Closed to Improve Mental Health Services.* 33–34.

21 Ministry of Health (1947) *Report on the Recruitment and Training of Nurses.*

22 Arton M (1998).

23 Ramon S (1985).

24 Glenister DA (2008). 140.

25 *Nursing Times* (28 November 1953): Friends of Menston Hospital.

26 Personal communication (PN, 1996).

27 Chatterton C (2004): Caught in the middle? Mental nurse training in England 1919–1951. *Journal of Psychiatric and Mental Health Nursing.*

28 Warr P (1957): *Brother Lunatic.* 42. The author's name was a pseudonym.

29 Personal communication (PN, 1995).

30 Personal communication (NM, 1997).

31 Personal communication (NM, 2014).

32 Personal communication (PN, 2014).

33 Laing J, McQuarrie D (1992): *50 Years in the System.*

34 Laing J, McQuarrie D (1992). 73–74.

35 Laing J, McQuarrie D (1992). 76–77.

36 Laing J, McQuarrie D (1992). 78. After his next escape, Laing was sent to the Criminal Lunatic Department in Perth, and later to Carstairs State Hospital (the Scottish equivalent of Broadmoor).

37 Royal Medico-Psychological Association (1954). 305.

38 Personal communication (NM, 2014).

39 Personal communication (NM, 2015).

40 Stern ES (1957): 'Operation Sesame'. *Lancet.*

41 Clarke L (1993): The opening of doors in British mental hospitals in the 1930s. *History of Psychiatry.*

42 Stern ES (1957).

43 Bickford JAR (1955): The forgotten patient. *Lancet.*

44 Bickford JAR (1958): Shadow and substance: some changes in the mental hospital. *Lancet.*

45 Pilkington F (1958).

46 Personal communication (PN, 1995).

47 Early DF (2003).

48 Nolan P (2005).

49 David Clark in conversation with Brian Barraclough (1986). *Bulletin of the Royal College of Psychiatrists.*

50 Clark DH (1958): Administrative therapy: its clinical importance in the mental hospital. *Lancet.* Having drawn much attention from American psychiatrists, Clark conducted a lecture tour in the USA.

51 Clark DH (1965). 76.

52 Cameron JL, Laing RD, McGhie A (1955): Patient and nurse: effects of environmental changes in the care of chronic schizophrenics. *Lancet.*

53 Gardner J (1999).

54 Bartlett was appointed as president of the NAWU in 1927 and was re-elected every year (as the MHIWU and later COHSE) until he retired in 1962. In 1960 he became president of the TUC.

55 Royal Commission on the Law Relating to Mental Illness and Mental Deficiency (1957): *Report on the Royal Commission on the Law Relating to Mental Illness and Mental Deficiency.*

56 Busfield J (1986): *Managing Madness: Changing Ideas and Practice.*

57 Le Fanu J (2011): *The Rise and Fall of Modern Medicine* (2nd edition).
58 Elkes J, Elkes C (1954): Effect of chlorpromazine on the behaviour of chronically overactive psychotic patients. *British Medical Journal.*
59 The mechanism was unknown until 1963, when the drug's action on dopamine, a chemical neurotransmitter, was discovered.
60 Anton-Stephens D (1954): Preliminary observations of the psychiatric uses of chlorpromazine (Largactil). *Journal of Mental Science.*
61 Vaughan GF, Leiberman DM, Cook LC (1955): Chlorpromazine in psychiatry. *Lancet.*
62 Vaughan GF, Leiberman DM, Cook LC (1955).
63 Vaughan GF, Leiberman DM, Cook LC (1955).
64 In the 1960s thioridazine (Melleril) was introduced as a substitute for Largactil, having fewer side effects. A more potent tranquilliser, haloperidol, was also widely used.
65 Bourn H (1953): The insulin myth. *Lancet.*
66 Ackner B, Harris A, Oldham AJ (1957): Insulin treatment of schizophrenia. *Lancet.*
67 McCrae N (2009): Nonelectrical convulsive therapies. In *Electroconvulsive and Neuromodulation Therapies* (ed. CM Swartz). 17–44.
68 Browne I (2013): *The Writings of Ivor Browne: Steps Along the Road – The Evolution of a Slow Learner.* 136.
69 Marsh H (2014): *First Do No Harm: Stories of Life, Death and Brain Surgery.* 115. AMH is Atkinson Morley's Hospital, where Wylie McKissock reigned.
70 Scull A (1995): Psychiatrists and historical 'facts'. Part one: the historiography of somatic treatments. *History of Psychiatry.*
71 Folkard MS (1957): *A Sociological Contribution to the Understanding of Aggression and its Treatment.*
72 Mills E (1962): *Living with Mental Illness: a Study in East London.* 52.
73 Rees TP (1957): Back to moral treatment and community care. *Journal of Mental Science.*
74 Farndale WAJ (1961): *The Day Hospital Movement in Great Britain.*
75 Mills E (1962). 38.
76 BBC (1957): *The Hurt Mind: an Enquiry into Some of the Effects of Five Television Broadcasts about Mental Illness and its Treatment: Audience Research Report.*
77 Personal communication (co-author NM's father, 2012). Pseudonym used for the patient.
78 Bickford JAR, Miller HJB (1959): Exchange of patients by mental hospitals.
79 Glenister DA (2008).
80 Joint Committee of the Manchester Regional Hospital Board and the University of Manchester (1955): *The Work of the Mental Nurse.*
81 Freeman T, Cameron JL, McGhie A (1958): *Chronic Schizophrenia.*
82 Gallaher EB, Levinson, DJ, Erlich, (1957) *The Patient and the Mental Hospital.*

6   Time is called

The Victorian legal framework for insanity was finally abolished when the Lunacy Act 1890 was repealed by the liberalising Mental Health Act 1959. A similar statute removed the last vestiges of the Lunacy Act (Scotland) 1857. Parliament had accepted the premises of the Percy Commission that mental illness should be treated like physical illness, and that services should be developed in the community. Although these two aims dovetailed, they required very different professional and administrative effort. Changing the pattern of provision within the NHS would prove easier than persuading social services to provide for highly dependent people who had spent much of their lives in the mental institution.

As well as making admission a decision for doctors rather than lawyers, the Mental Health Act shortened the periods of detention: 72 hours in Section 29 (for emergency), 28 days in Section 25 (for observation), and one year in Section 26 (treatment order, renewable with six-monthly reviews). More importantly, compulsory admission was to be a last resort, with rights of appeal established. The legal duties of the medical superintendent were delegated to a 'responsible mental officer' for each patient, giving consultant psychiatrists the same clinical autonomy as in other fields of medicine. Hospitals were required to provide outpatient care on discharge, but there was no statutory obligation on local authorities. Mental welfare officers replaced the duly authorised officers, although the role was basically similar and no qualification was required; often this was simply the same workers relabelled. The Board of Control disbanded, its function transferred to the regional hospital boards.

On the appointed day of 1 November 1960, a major administrative exercise began in reclassifying each 'certified lunatic', a process of formal discharge and readmission that took months to complete. Within a few years only a tenth of the mental hospital population was formally detained, and typically only one locked ward was retained on male and female sides. Yet the legions of long-stay patients did not march to the gate. The hospital remained their home, as it did for the majority of nurses. Better the devil you know …

A bolt of lightning

In March 1961 Minister for Health Enoch Powell addressed the National Association for Mental Health conference in London. [1] Without prior consultation or warning, he announced the beginning of the end for the mental hospitals.

These bold words … imply nothing less than the elimination of by far the greater part of this country's mental hospitals as they exist today. This is a colossal undertaking, not so much in the new physical provision which it involves, as in the sheer inertia of mind and matter which it requires to be overcome.

An astute minister of the Harold Macmillan's cabinet, Powell acknowledged the Herculean task ahead.

There they stand, isolated, majestic, imperious, brooded over by the gigantic water-tower and chimney combined, rising unmistakable and daunting out of the countryside – the asylums which our forefathers built with such immense solidity. Do not for a moment their power of resistance to our assault … Hundreds of men and women, professional or voluntary, have given years, even lifetimes, to the service of a mental hospital or a group of mental hospitals. They have laboured devotedly, through years of scarcity and neglect, to render the conditions in them more tolerable, and of late they have seized with delight upon the new possibilities opening up, and the new resources available, for these old but somehow cherished institutions. From such bodies it demands no mean moral effort to recognise that the institutions themselves are doomed. It would be more than flesh and blood to expect them to take the initiative in planning their own abolition, to be the first to set the torch to the funeral pyre.

Soon after Powell's speech, a Ministry of Health survey supported the case for closure: Tooth and Brooke[2] predicted that the ratio of mental hospital beds would fall from 3.1 per 1,000 in 1959 to 1.8 by the mid-1970s. The small but significant drop in the mental hospital population from 1954 to 1959 was attributed to better treatment of acute cases, outpatient clinics and rehabilitation of long-stay patients, and it was envisaged that advances in pharmacological and social treatment would hasten the arrival of a 'Brave New World' of mental health care.

In 1962 the *Hospital Plan for England and Wales*[3] signposted psychiatry away from its asylum origins. The district general hospital would replace all the smaller specialist, maternity and cottage hospitals; long-stay institutions for mental illness and mental subnormality would continue to exist but would eventually become redundant[4]. Containing thirty to sixty beds, the general hospital psychiatric units were a stark contrast to the remote and daunting mental institution. Evidence from such units opened in Manchester Region in the 1950s showed that the stream of admissions to mental hospitals slowed to a trickle: a consultant psychiatrist covering the Blackburn area stated that 95 per cent of the caseload in a population of 250,000 was treated without recourse to Lancaster Moor.[5] The *Hospital Plan* predicted a decrease of 40 per cent in psychiatric beds by 1975, with the number of institutions of over 1,000 beds to fall from sixty-nine to twenty-six. The trend was already visible: by 1963, the mental hospitals in England and Wales housed 20,000 fewer patients than in the peak of the mid-1950s.

The Worthing Experiment produced the best evidence to date that patients could be successfully treated in the community. Peter Sainsbury's evaluation contrasted a district served by a mental health centre based in a residential street, with a traditional hospital system in Salisbury. Although the amount of referrals by general practitioners was substantially higher in Worthing, the proportion of admissions to Graylingwell was half that at Old Manor Hospital in Salisbury (excluding elderly patients, who were admitted in similar numbers). The community-based service was reaching hitherto untreated sufferers in society, yet fewer beds were needed.[6]

Meanwhile day hospitals were spreading rapidly: there were 153 in England and Wales by 1962, although few had opened in Scotland.[7] It was administratively convenient and less costly to use a converted ward in the old mental hospital, but this was less accessible for patients and perpetuated institutional conformity. A more favourable option was a large villa in town, where an informal, homely setting could be created, while providing a link between the hospital and community[8]. In Plymouth a comprehensive community mental health centre opened in 1963, comprising offices for social workers, day hospital facilities and rooms for psychotherapy. The day hospital was staffed by three mental nurses and two trainees. This was one of the earliest instances of psychiatric and social services staff working together on the same premises.[9] Yet such schemes were exceptional, relying on the determination of psychiatrists, local authority officers and family doctors to overcome the bureaucratic obstacles. The Plymouth centre, despite funding by the Nuffield Trust, took six years to fully open.

In most cases, an acute episode was followed by discharge as an outpatient or day hospital attendee. Admission to the remote mental institution was avoided wherever possible. In London, the observation units at Fulham, Bow, St Pancras, Battersea, Tooting and Dulwich were established buffers for mental hospital admission, and these were gradually replaced by psychiatric units in general hospitals. At St Clement's, the former City of London poorhouse in Bow, 350 people were admitted annually to the emergency psychiatric unit, of which just 10 per cent were transferred for longer-term care at Long Grove.[10] By 1959 the population of the distant Epsom hospital had already fallen by 500 from the peak of 2,320 four years earlier.[11] The easiest way to reduce a mental hospital population was simply to stop sending patients there.

Psychiatry was dividing into a first and second class. Unlike the medical superintendent, younger doctors had little emotional attachment to the mental hospital, and their clinical environment was very different to that of assistant medical officers in past decades. Sectorisation was introduced, with each consultant covering a catchment area and spending increasing amounts of time away from the mental hospital, perhaps only visiting for two or three sessions per week. Psychiatrists openly referred to mental hospitals as 'bins'. The future was outside the institution, as a fully fledged medical specialty in a modern hospital. In 1963 the RMPA renamed its journal *British Journal of Psychiatry*, its pages increasingly filled with psychopharmacological studies sandwiched between glossy advertisements for the latest hubristic remedies. For nurses, the drug trolley was brimming over with new tablets and syrups: the expanding range of antipsychotic drugs and an array of anti-Parkinsonian drugs for their side effects, monoamine oxidase inhibitors for depression, and benzodiazepines for anxiety or a sleeping draught.

As sister on an acute psychiatric ward at St Thomas' Hospital in London, Felicity Stockwell worked with controversial psychiatrist William Sargant. Believing that mental illnesses were caused by difficulties in forming social relationships, Sargant wanted to create a therapeutic milieu whereby nurses were continually engaging with patients, in an environment that could pass for a posh hotel. He disparaged the industrial, occupational and recreational therapies provided in the mental hospitals, and rejected all forms of psychotherapy. Furthermore, he had no time for mental nurses, accepting only general nurses on his wards (Felicity was doubly qualified). The fact that the majority of the staff comprised general nursing students, who spent only six weeks on the wards, did not concern him. He just wanted smartly uniformed women who were bright, cheerful and socially competent. As little time as possible was spent in the office because Sargant believed that nurses should be visible at all times. Felicity recalled:

> There was a great mix of patients with different conditions and from different backgrounds. The amazing thing was that they all got on well together and helped each other.[12]

For a large number of patients, however, the mental hospital was their destiny. The validity of government projections was disputed by some psychiatrists: it was relatively straightforward to release patients with less severe illness who would comply with a medication regime at home, but this was 'skimming off the cream'. While the phenothiazines were effective in treating acute psychosis, the underlying illness remained, and social withdrawal resulted in a downward spiral in mental and physical well-being.[13] A 'revolving door' syndrome emerged, as patients who relapsed at home accounted for an increasing proportion of psychiatric admissions. Psychiatrists urged caution in discharging the more disabled patients, for whom prospects of independent living were poor. Highlighting the lack of investment in hostels and other community resources to replace institutional care, critics suspected underlying economic motives for the policy.

Much-needed investment in the fabric of mental hospitals was at risk, as the Ministry of Health did not want money wasted on upgrading outmoded buildings. Old hands became disillusioned: what was the point of improving the mental hospitals, only for the government to run them down? Yet there were tangible improvements as dormitories became less crowded. Defunct insulin coma therapy units became industrial therapy workshops, and the admission blocks of the 1930s were ideal for a rehabilitation unit. The medical superintendent's house was split into flats for junior medical staff. For the first time, in the 1960s the size of the asylum estate went into reverse. The hospital farm was neither economically viable nor an appropriate occupational preparation for patients, and land was sold for private housing, bringing the mental hospital into the suburban fringe.

Perhaps the most poignant change was the precipitous demise of the iconic water tower.[14] Always a target for lightning, some of these steeples of Victorian lunacy were erased from the skyline.

Humanising the institution

At noon the deputy chief male nurse inspected the dining hall to ensure that the long tables were correctly set, before ringing a bell sounding in Wards 6 to 10. The doors of these male wards were unlocked and the patients were counted out by nurses and trooped along the corridor. After they had eaten and all cutlery was checked, the patients were escorted back to their wards before the next sitting. This was Hartwood Hospital in 1968, where Charlie Russell embarked on his career in psychiatric nursing.[15] The old order lingered here: the physician superintendent's reign, pronounced gender segregation, and a barely adequate nursing staff responsible for 2,000 souls. Routines were followed unthinkingly and inflexibly, with little time or inclination for individualised care.

Hartwood would have had much in common with a large mental institution across the Atlantic. Through several months of observation at St Elizabeth's in Washington, sociologist Erving Goffman conceptualised the 'total institution', run for the convenience of administrators and staff. Nurses kept social distance from their stigmatised patients, who occupied the bottom rung of a social hierarchy. Hostility between these two groups was readily apparent, yet both depended on each other. Although the ward was the patients' home, nurses perceived it as their property. Goffman's book *Asylums* was highly influential in Britain but more so in the USA, adding a devastating critique to previous studies by Belknap, and Stanton and Schwarz. Following a report *Action for Mental Health* by the National Institute for Mental Health in 1961, two years later President Kennedy launched a major federal investment in community mental health centres. Most nurses in British mental hospitals would have been blissfully ignorant of the American programme of deinstitutionalisation, although this blazed a trail for policy-makers and community-orientated psychiatrists in the UK.

From an organisational perspective, the regime at hospitals such as Hartwood was efficient. Younger nurses may have been aware of shortcomings in patient care, but they were soon inculcated to the institutional culture, and the tried and tested ways of managing large numbers of mentally ill patients. Great credit is due to a few enlightened psychiatrists who coaxed nurses from their custodial function to a more dynamic and rewarding role. One of the most notable in this respect was Russell Barton, who was appointed as the third (and last) medical superintendent at Severalls in 1960. Instead of following tradition by appointing the deputy medical superintendent, the regional hospital board sought a leader with vision and drive to reform an inward-looking institution. As Diana Gittins[16] explained, they got more than they bargained for.

Barton had made his name with his book on 'institutional neurosis',[17] a syndrome superimposed on chronic schizophrenia, featuring apathy, lack of initiative and spontaneity, blunting of emotional response, submissiveness and an abnormal posture or gait. It was attributed to loss of contact with the outside world, enforced idleness and dependence, lack of personal space and possessions, an authoritarian regime with bossy nurses, and the iatrogenic effect of medical treatment (Barton blamed excessive use of tranquillising drugs, but another factor may have been that many schizophrenic patients had been leucotomised). Barton did not pull punches: the system was making patients worse.

The cause and effects of 'institutionalism' were illuminated by a seminal paper by psychiatrist John Wing and sociologist George Brown of the Medical Research Council Social Psychiatry Unit.[18] In a study of three mental hospitals, Wing and Brown compared long-stay female patients on a range of variables including symptoms, personal possessions, occupational activity, medication and attitudes to discharge. Two of the hospitals chosen, Mapperley and Netherne, had a reputation for social therapy. The other hospital was Severalls, where a regressive regime was yet to be overhauled by Russell Barton, who was appointed just before fieldwork began. The hospitals ranged in population from 940 at Mapperley to 1,860 at Netherne, with 1,590 at Severalls.[19] The results showed that the patients at Severalls were the most socially withdrawn: they spent an average of 5 hours and 39 minutes doing nothing, compared to 2 hours and 48 minutes at Netherne. Almost half of the Essex women had no personal possessions; 70 per cent were indifferent about the future or preferred to stay in the hospital, compared to 54 per cent at Netherne; nurses at Severalls were less optimistic about patients' occupational ability and prospects for discharge. Wing and Brown concluded that an impoverished social environment exacerbated the negative symptoms of schizophrenia. Importantly, Wing and Brown found no evidence that changes to drug treatment accounted for clinical improvement. For psychiatrists to rely on mediation alone would be 'like fighting with one hand behind one's back'.[20]

It was said that there were no chronic patients in mental hospitals, only neglected ones.[21] Wing and Brown described Longfield Villa at Netherne as an exemplar of social treatment for chronic schizophrenia. For many years at Netherne clinical energy had been channelled to the long-stay wards; elsewhere, as consultant psychiatrist Douglas Bennett reflected, 'psychiatry was upside-down, with the least ill and least disabled patients treated by the most able and qualified staff'.[22] Since 1956 Longfield had been used for resocialising severely withdrawn patients. Habit training was abandoned, as it was thought to reinforce passive dependence on staff. Workshops and therapeutic groups were shared with a neighbouring villa of similar purpose for male patients. Doors were open from the outset, and male and female patients mixed freely, some being allowed to leave the grounds together. Each patient had a locker, there were mirrors in all dormitories and the kitchen was always accessible; at mealtimes, milk and sugar were placed on dining tables. Taken for granted by most people, these were luxuries for long-stay mental patients. On returning in afternoons from the occupational therapy workshop, patients attended a small group meeting with their assigned nurse. Many Longfield patients showed sufficient improvement for transfer to the resettlement ward, or discharge.

Within a year at Severalls, Barton had dismantled all airing court railings, removed restrictions to visiting times, ensured patients had personal clothing instead of the ill-fitting communal garments, began a programme of domesticating the wards, and established an industrial therapy unit for men. He faced considerable resistance. The matron fought him tooth and nail over his reforms, and much resentment was caused in the male ranks after the deputy chief male nurse retired and was replaced by an outsider. To change outmoded practices, Barton introduced refresher courses and symposia for the nursing staff. Meanwhile, as hundreds of patients were discharged, senior nurses and administrators were concerned that their salaries would be cut, due to the pointage system related to the size of the hospital (a perverse incentive that led to the official number of beds in mental hospitals consistently exceeding the number of patients).

Further investigation by Wing and Brown in 1964 showed significant improvements in the Severalls cohort. A major factor was the industrial therapy pushed by Barton. Traditional gender roles were apparent in the work offered: at Severalls there was a household management unit with cookers and ironing boards, while men had a carpentry workshop. Sewing pink bows on to lingerie for Marks & Spencer was a job for women, but men assembled wooden doll's houses.[23] The mental hospital, however, was not a normal work environment. Building on achievements at Glenside in Bristol, in 1960 the Industrial Therapy Organisation was founded as a non-profitmaking company, providing work for people with physical or mental health problems. Minibuses of patients from Glenside and Barrow Hospitals went daily to the factory, and similar ventures followed elsewhere in the country. Nurses working in these units added to a small but increasing number based outside a hospital.

Meanwhile a more radical change to mental hospital practice was waiting in the wings. At the social therapy unit at Belmont, an American anthropologist Richard Rapoport[24] described four tenets of the therapeutic community model:

1 Democratisation: sharing of responsibility and decision-making in a flattened hierarchy.
2 Permissiveness: experiential learning from trial and error.
3 Communalism: nurturing a strong group identity with free communication.
4 Reality confrontation: analysing incidents to understand cause and effect, thereby enabling people to learn about their effect on others.

A friend of Maxwell Jones, David Clark had proceeded tentatively in introducing the therapeutic community at Fulbourn, acknowledging that nurses would struggle to cope without the certainties of rules and routine. In 1958 a female convalescent villa became the testing ground. Community meetings were introduced and the patients were made responsible for all housework, and nurses were instructed to step back from their customary function. Hospital managers were horrified by the mess, and on one occasion the fire brigade were called to a fire. A rumour circulated that the hospital renovation programme was postponed due to the frequent and costly repairs needed on this villa. Despite Clark's support, the doctor in charge of the villa and the nurses felt ostracised by other staff in the hospital; the sister stopped taking her meals in the canteen.[25] Junior doctors found the ward demoralising. Yet in 1960 Clark courageously extended the model to a disturbed ward. Initially, the daily ward meetings were chaotic.

> Women shouted at their hallucinations, or surge across the room to assault someone. Fights were common, and on some occasions the meeting had to be abandoned. Window-breaking increased, and a crisis was reached when the most disturbed patient pushed the Ward Sister down the stairs so that she broke her ankle.[26]

Clark and the nurses persevered and eventually the meeting became calmer, allowing issues to be explored. With more open communication between patients and staff, improvements in behaviour and psychiatric symptoms were observed and some refractory patients progressed to rehabilitation and discharge. The therapeutic community was thus a challenging but ultimately rewarding enterprise.

Psychiatry undermined

Radical politics came to the fore in the 1960s. As Marxist agitators, sociologists and students challenged the structure of society and its institutions, psychiatry was interpreted as an oppressive device of the Establishment. Criticism, however, started within the system. In 1961 Thomas Szasz, a Hungarian psychiatrist in New York, launched a sustained attack on his profession. In *The Myth of Mental Illness* Szasz argued that psychiatric diagnoses were a bogus medicalisation of 'problems in living'; mental illness was a category error as distress is of mind, not body. Psychiatry was portrayed by Szasz as no less a tyrannical social control than the communism that the Americans were opposing in the 'Cold War'. In tune with the rebellious 'beat poets', Ken Kesey's *One Flew over the Cuckoo's Nest* added fuel to the fire of an anti-psychiatry movement. While Kesey promoted recreational drugs, he demonised psychiatric drugs and ECT as an assault on humanity. In his eloquent historical treatise *Madness and Civilisation,* French philosopher Michel Foucault[27] described how the concept of insanity evolved with the contemporary values of society; labelling of deviant behaviour as madness thus tells us more about prevailing social attitudes than about mental illness.

Undoubtedly the most influential critic of psychiatry in Britain was RD Laing, who had moved from Glasgow to the Tavistock Clinic. For Laing, all behaviour of the person labelled mentally ill was intelligible and indeed a justifiable response to a hostile family or hospital staff. Instead of helping the person to cope with stress and social adversity, psychiatrists were colluding with the family to project deviance on a convenient target. His book *The Divided Self* had an impact far beyond the intellectual spheres of psychiatry and psychoanalysis. In the counter-culture of the 1960s, Laing rose to *guru* status, worshipped by followers around the world. In 1962 South African psychiatrist David Cooper, an accomplice of Laing, began 'an experiment in anti-psychiatry'[28] in the defunct insulin unit at Shenley Hospital. Patients with first or second psychotic breakdown were admitted for interpersonal therapy at Villa 21, where use of tranquillisers was minimised. Young nurses without engrained institutional attitudes were selected. Patients were allowed to get up when they liked, and they were encouraged but not forced to attend daily meetings; only by taking responsibility for themselves could they make progress, as this bizarre incident was meant to convey:

> At one time all the occupants of a six-bed dormitory rebelled against the community meeting by staying in bed until after eleven o'clock. Frank, one of the charge nurses, went upstairs to see what was going on. One of the patients left to go to the toilet and Frank seized the opportunity to take off his white coat and climb into the vacant bed. The patient, on his return, appreciating the irony of the situation, had little option but to take the vacated staff role, put on the white coat, and get the others out of bed.[29]

Cooper rejected the prevailing notion that patients must be kept busy all day. A paper in 1971 stated that 'eighteen thousand mental hospital patients still staple, stick, pack and hammer away' in workshops on or off site, but attitudes to industrial therapy were changing.[30] Imposition of the National Insurance limit to patients' earnings, set at 39 shillings, removed the incentive to boost workers' performance. Meanwhile trade unionists were concerned about cheap labour. Quality control was inevitably a problem, and as contracts became more elusive, the factories became less dynamic and more dependent on benevolent companies. This was not a real job for real pay. Arguably, dozens of passive patients sitting on benches sorting piles of plastic parts into packets was akin to the exploitative labour of the past.

The rehabilitation honeymoon was ending. Impressive progress recorded by Wing and Brown in Netherne and Mapperley patients was not sustained, with some reversal by the time of their last assessments in 1968. Social therapy had proven value in the mental hospitals, but it relied on energy and enthusiasm of staff. Without constant encouragement, patients defaulted to idleness and apathy. Nurses told Wing and Brown of their difficulty in socialising withdrawn schizophrenic patients:

> On a ward like this there is not much chance to draw them out – we've not enough staff.[31]

Ageing patients in aged buildings

In 1964 journalist Gerda Cohen wrote an account of her tour of NHS hospitals for the Penguin *What's Wrong with ...* series. Visiting a former LCC asylum, she was impressed by the relatively recent admission villa, but in the main block conditions progressively deteriorated as she passed from the convalescent wards at the front to the chronic wards at the rear.

> Along the corridors, sunk in apathy, sat putty-face men in clothing from a common wardrobe. Here, no money had been spent on the floribunda wall-

paper which rampaged over the 'front blocks'. Everything was an indecisive beige, from the sick lino to the meat pie.[32]

In an effort to humanise the environment, ward numbers were dropped in favour of names. At Deva Hospital in Cheshire, the theme was local villages; for example, M6 became Frith Ward.[33] Elsewhere literary figures and founders of psychiatry were common. Cohen found that forty-two numbered wards had recently been named after trees on the male side, and flowers on the female side, but this did not mask the degrading conditions:

> The incongruity had pathos. 'Willow' and 'Crocus' denoted a dim caserne for the senile. 'Daffodil' was like a bad joke outside a labyrinth reeking of stale urine.[34]

Although their population was in steady decline, it was obvious that the mental hospitals would survive for longer than government policy predicted. With the ravages of wear and tear in buildings 100 years old, the cost of maintenance was a drain on NHS resources. Hospital managers struggled to fulfil expectations of a modern health service: lack of comfort was regrettable, but poor hygiene was a fundamental failing. At St Francis' Hospital in Sussex, for example, hospital management committee visitors noted in one long-stay ward a single bath for ninety-six patients.[35] For elderly residents, many of whom were constipated or incontinent, the paucity of toilets was particularly galling. Cohen found little privacy afforded to patients.

> 'They don't notice', the charge nurse crisply reminds a visitor upset by the spectacle of five mute men being undressed and swiftly bundled into five grubby bath-tubs alongside each other. Here, every door is lockable except the lavatory. 'Greyhound traps, we call 'em,' the charge nurse laughed. 'Open top and bottom for a good view; otherwise they'd sit here for hours.'[36]

Sometimes the authorities were forced to invest. On the night of 24 February 1968 a tragedy at Shelton Hospital in Shropshire led to an overhaul of safety procedures in mental hospitals throughout Britain.[37] Twenty-four patients died and eleven were seriously injured in a fire at Beech Ward, a locked ward housing forty-three women, whose escape was impeded by top-to-tail beds in an overcrowded dormitory. Sedated and bed-ridden patients were carried to the fire escape by nurses as the blaze spread. Most of the deaths were caused by asphyxiation. Patients in the row of single rooms survived due to the heavy wooden doors, and because they slept on mattresses on the floor for their safety. The fire had started in the day room, where an open fire remained in use, although the cause was believed to be a smouldering cigarette. Following this incident fire doors were fitted in every hospital, and emergency signage proliferated.

Wards were gradually renovated, to a hybrid social and medical design. Walls were repainted in brighter colours, and space between beds was demarcated by plywood or curtain screens. Fluorescent lighting was installed; bare floorboards were covered by linoleum, a non-slip surface easier to clean. Standard issue NHS wheeled beds were procured, enamelled and glass equipment such as urine bottles and syringes were replaced by plastic, and sanitary facilities at the end of Nightingale dormitories were extended and modernised.

The mental hospital populace was already ageing due to greater longevity, but the opening of admission units in general hospitals exacerbated this by diverting younger acute cases. Wards accommodating older residents remained severely overcrowded. Vacant beds were rapidly filled by frail patients who had nowhere else to go. As shown in Table 6.1, in hospitals with a high frequency of elderly admissions as much as a third of the turnover was due to mortality. In the Epsom Cluster fewer older people were being sent from the distant catchment areas, but a high number of patients died at Tooting Bec, which received patients with dementia from across the metropolitan area.

With minimal support from the Ministry of Health, some psychiatrists introduced dedicated care for older patients. Patients admitted in old age were very different to the chronic schizophrenics who had lived in the hospital for thirty or forty years, but they quickly became institutionalised. The ideal was brief treatment in hospital followed by support in the community, and this required active medical and nursing input. Following a similar innovation at Crichton Royal three years earlier, in 1961 Russell Barton created a psychogeriatric unit

Table 6.1 Admissions, discharges and deaths in 1966 at selected mental hospitals[38]

Hospital	Residents (31 December 1966)	Admissions	Discharges	Deaths	Admissions aged >65
Long Grove, Surrey	1,550	1,379	1,265	148	12%
Banstead, Surrey	1,392	1,332	1,274	113	14%
Deva and annexes, Cheshire	2,058	3,198	2,938	241	14%
Horton, Surrey	1,550	1,541	1,361	205	15%
Central, Warwick	1,359	1,855	1,659	226	15%
St Bernard's, London	2,208	2,163	1,832	284	19%
High Royds, Yorkshire	2,020	2,099	1,849	246	21%
Park Prewett, Hampshire	1,570	1,307	1,119	233	24%
Brookwood, Surrey	1,476	1,437	1,220	297	25%
Exe Vale, Devon	1,682	2,379	2,104	274	30%
Highcroft, Birmingham	1,034	1,750	1,507	219	31%
Tooting Bec, London	1,757	1,499	999	520	35%

at Severalls, comprising four male and six female wards (with 145 and 229 beds respectively).[39] This unit provided not only inpatient care but also a day hospital, a 'month-in / month-out' scheme, boarding-out for long-stay patients, and emergency domiciliary visits. Sadly such attention to older people was missing in most mental hospitals, where the most vulnerable patients occupied the worst wards, in the care of a few devoted nurses alongside colleagues deemed incompetent in other wards.

Wards with elderly patients gave novices an opportunity to practise basic nursing care, although the learning environment left much to be desired. Starting nurse training in 1968 at Park Prewett in Hampshire, Tom Chan[40] was first posted at Ward M1, where dozens of older men, mostly with dementia, slept in a vast dormitory. The few side-rooms were given to patients with privileges (the 'trusties'). Dressing and toileting was a laborious task for nurses, with little concession to patients' dignity. Bedside lockers were provided, but no personal clothing was worn. Dentures were supposed to be washed separately and soaked in a cup overnight, but some older nurses put them in a single bowl of water. Patients queued naked for their weekly unscreened bath. Charlie Russell recalled the sister of a female psychogeriatric ward at Cane Hill who deprived patients of tea because it made them incontinent, and the diet was restricted so that they did not get too heavy for nurses to lift.[41]

On starting her training at Netherne in 1965, Carmel Piris[42] was placed at Highfield Villa, which had previously served as an isolation ward for tuberculosis (hence its verandahs). It housed elderly women, under the strict rule of a sister who Carmel likened to a mother superior at a nunnery. Twice a week, patients were given an enema. Thick red rubber sheets were placed on each bed. A pint and a half of the green soapy substance was slowly poured through a funnel into a rubber anal tube, which had a mark to indicate correct insertion. Some patients were restrained for the period of five minutes needed for the treatment to work. Then the patient was led to the toilet, and the nurse estimated the amount of faecal matter passed in the 'bowels book'. According to Carmel, the sister led this twice-weekly procedure with warped vigour.

Mental nursing revised

Two months after his 'water tower' speech, Enoch Powell opened a mental nursing school at Littlemore Hospital in Oxford, where he urged nurses to play a leading part in creating a new system of mental health care. Unlike psychiatrists, who were increasingly active in the general hospital and community, records of the Association of Chief Male Nurses suggest that nurses had not been persuaded that their future lay outside the mental hospitals.[43] Nominally professional, mental nursing remained inward-looking, attracting a particular type of person who wanted the certainties of a job for life. The need for change was emphasised by a study of four Scottish hospitals by Audrey John, whose thesis at University of Edinburgh was subsequently published in 1961. A general nurse, John's recommendation for a 'comprehensive basic training'[44] arose from her observation of limited proficiency in physical care among mental nurses, but she also highlighted the paucity of psychological knowledge and skills. She saw little distinction between the work of a nursing assistant and a staff nurse, as if there was only one grade. The term 'nurse', John argued, should be respected and not used by hospital managers to include unqualified workers. Although indispensable in running the wards, nurses were not regarded as part of the treatment team. Deriving comfort from routine, nurses told John that domestic duties helped them to avoid thinking. Such behaviour blatantly illustrated the dehumanising process found in a general hospital study by Tavistock psychoanalyst Isobel Menzies,[45] who described how nurses exhibit unconscious defence mechanisms to reduce anxiety.

There were many obstacles in shifting mental nursing from a household management role to one of active engagement in human relationships with patients. When Doctor MC Moss and psychiatric social worker Peter Hunter at Moorhaven Hospital in Devon asserted that patients instead of nurses should clean the ward, allowing nurses to play a more active role in therapy, both the patients and the nurses reacted negatively:[46]

> This change in role for the nurses and loss of function as a near-domestic was a very hard one to accept, symbolising the laying aside of collective defence mechanisms acquired over the years, against the stress of working with disturbed patients in an environment where they had no support except for each other, and where no attempt was made to achieve an understanding through discussion.

In some hospitals the wards had two charge nurses, with separate teams, and difficulties arose when one tried to liberalise the regime without support of the other. In 1965 Bryn Davis[47] was appointed as charge nurse on Lister II, a male refractory ward at Holloway Sanatorium. This ward had been run on traditional lines, with sparse furnishing and security dominating all procedures and activities. While Bryn strove to personalise the ward, his counterpart maintained custodial control. Rearranging the chairs in the day-room to create small social circles, on the next day Bryn found that the opposite shift had pushed them back against the walls.

Maxwell Jones,[48] appointed as physician superintendent at Dingleton Hospital in 1962, built on the work of his predecessor George Bell to apply the therapeutic community to an entire hospital for the first time. However, the model required commitment that nurses were not necessarily keen to give, as Dennis Martin found:

> The male nurse tends to settle down in hospital, marry and build a home. Any apparent threat to his promotion prospects therefore strikes economically at the roots of his security and his home life. For this reason alone, he has a much stronger resistance to change if he feels it runs contrary to the approve policy of senior nursing staff on whom his promotion depends.[49]

According to JKW Morrice, psychiatrist at Dingleton, a transitional period was required to support nurses in abandoning a 'relatively simple and structured relationship for a complex, vaguely defined one'.[50] Nurses trained in the 1950s or earlier had not been equipped for understanding individual mental processes or group dynamics. Progressive psychiatrists such as Russell Barton and David Clark appreciated the need for close medical supervision of nurses in developing a therapeutic role; otherwise they would surely flounder in emotional strain.

Despite pressure from the GNC to raise entrance standards, there remained no compulsory educational criteria for enrolment at a mental hospital school of nursing. Trainees were students in name only, the needs of the hospital taking precedence over learning. Meanwhile, as recruitment problems persisted, a lower tier of nursing qualification was established. In 1961 the title of the assistant nurse created by the Nurses Act 1943 was changed to State Enrolled Nurse (SEN). Assistant nurses had been consistently opposed by COHSE, who feared dilution of mental nursing, compounding difficulties in recruiting nursing students and consequently the number of qualified nurses. However, unqualified nurses in psychiatric hospitals were allowed to apply for enrolment in 1964; in the first year, nearly 4,000 nursing assistants (including part-timers) were granted SEN status.[51] A training syllabus was introduced in the same year, with 'pupil nurses' qualifying on completion of a two-year course (later reduced to eighteen months), and eventually SEN awards were restricted to the examination route. No school certificates were necessary for pupil nurses. Students failing the final RMN examination at the third attempt were registered instead as SENs. Debate ensued on the scope of the SEN role and responsibilities such as administering medication, but in reality most hospitals were too short of staff to impose restrictions. In another bid to boost recruitment, a cadet scheme was introduced, whereby school-leavers too young for nurse training could start work at the age of sixteen. They were given experience of various wards and ancillary departments, while receiving further education for two days per week in English, arithmetic and practical skills. Meanwhile the entry threshold for general nursing of two 'O' levels was belatedly applied to mental nurse training in 1966.

The Committee on Higher Education,[52] which reported in 1963, excluded nurse training from its enquiry into expanding tertiary education. Chairman Lord Robbins espoused the liberal notion of knowledge as an end in itself, and nursing, as a practical vocation, was not considered as an academic pursuit. Wary of the threats to the professional status of nursing should educational standards fall behind other disciplines, in 1964 the Royal College of Nursing[53] established a committee on nurse education, chaired by Sir Harry Platt. Mental nursing was represented by John Greene from Moorhaven and Annie Altschul of the Bethlem and Maudsley Hospitals.

Despite (or perhaps because of) her lack of experience in conventional mental hospitals, Altschul was a guiding light for mental nurse education in Britain. Since sister tutors were appointed in the 1930s, there had been no requirement for teaching qualifications. The first course for nurse tutors began at Battersea College in 1932, although this was not endorsed by the GNC. The few sisters from mental hospitals who attended this one-year course did so at their own expense, but in 1947 Altschul's training was funded by The Maudsley Hospital. While developing the nurse training school at The Maudsley, she completed a degree in psychology at Birkbeck College, graduating in 1951.[54] With her psychological insights Altschul presciently saw the significance of Hildegard Peplau's book *Interpersonal Relations in Nursing*,[55] which introduced psychodynamic principles to the nurse–patient relationship. Inspired by Peplau, in 1957 she wrote a textbook on psychiatric nursing.[56] In 1958 Altschul was awarded a Commonwealth Scholarship to study nurse training in the USA, where she was impressed by the focus on therapeutic relationships and the regular supervision sessions for trainees. Revised in 1964 and 1969, her textbook presented a distinctly social model of nursing, guiding trainees in group dynamics.[57] On the RCN committee, Altschul expressed her frustration at the omission of nursing by the Robbins Committee, fearing the loss of bright recruits so vital for the development of mental nursing.[58] AR May of the Ministry of Health shared her concern:

> Concepts of dynamic psychiatry are difficult to communicate to nurses with limited intellectual ability, and such nurses are often unable to fulfil the role expected of them in a therapeutic community. In fact, many of them are relegated to the chronic wards, where often the emotional strain placed upon them is greater even that in acute short-stay wards, and where a lack of active clinical interest may isolate them still further in a quasi-custodial role.[59]

Altchul's book was followed by several other training manuals written by nurse tutors in the mental hospitals; for example, by Bird and Bray at Tone Vale in Somerset.[60] However, their use was restricted by the continuing dominance of the 'Red Book', which would remain the standard text for many years to come. In 1964 a new edition appeared, edited by psychiatrist Brian Ackner.[61] As David Glenister[62] commented, the revised text emphasised the shift from a moral concept of 'duties' to a sociological concept of 'role'. Yet physical care continued to dominate the content of the first half of the course, and the questions in the intermediate examination. Barry Hopper,[63] who started RMN training at Graylingwell in 1967, found the 'Red Book' informative but bland, and devoid of sociological and philosophical critique of psychiatry. In many mental hospital nurse training schools the RMPA manual was used well into the 1970s.[64] Meanwhile the perceived inadequacy of RMN training was underlined by the routine secondment of newly qualified nurses to a general hospital to gain the SRN certificate. Co-author PN, for example, on qualifying at Tooting Bec in 1965, went to May Day Hospital in Croydon for eighteen months, on his staff nurse salary.

Tutors had leeway to recruit candidates able to think more theoretically about their role, but the gap between the ethos of nurse education and the institutional culture was wide. While tutors were preparing the nurses of the future, ward staff asserted that the real training was 'on the job'. Harsh or tyrannical attitudes to patients were becoming less socially acceptable, but the priorities of security and discipline were impressed on students. Most hospitals retained at least one padded room, a tangible reminder of the lurking dangers of the job. At Netherne this was on the male side, on K Ward. Known as 'The Slammer', it had leather walls and a bed fixed to the floor, a high ceiling and a tiny window beyond reach, an inner door with an observation slit and a thick outer door, and a lingering odour of paraldehyde. Patients were sometimes confined here for several hours, while awaiting a psychiatrist's assessment.[65] Some young recruits, such as Peter Robinson,[66] perceived restraint and seclusion as punitive; in 1967 he left nurse training for art school:

> I was there approximately ten months – not very long, but long enough to get a glimpse of goings-on in such places. It opened my eyes in many ways, but overall I found the atmosphere somehow oppressive … Years later I saw the film *One Flew over the Cuckoo's Nest* and I think that captured the totality that was Cane Hill.

Older nurses may have been behind the times, but their methods were often vindicated when nursing students brought idealistic principles without the benefit of experience. Wards were orderly most of the time, but there was an underlying volatility, and some patients would test the reactions of a newcomer. On her first ward at Warlingham Park, Janet Herd[67] recalls a female patient striding towards her with a chamber pot over her head, with faeces dripping down her face; fortunately the sister came to Janet's rescue. Beryl Hepworth,[68] a general nurse who started a conversion course at St Bernard's in 1969, disliked the female locked ward, where she thought that tight restrictions worsened patients' behaviour. One woman was kept in her room all day except for short periods accompanied by two nurses. Beryl asked the ward sister if she could let this patient out of her room for a while to sit in the verandah. The sister agreed, probably to teach Beryl a lesson: a wave of destructive energy was unleashed as the patient swept all the crockery off the tables and threatened further violence, before being swiftly returned to her room.

As AR May[69] argued, it was wrong to describe everything negative in a mental hospital as 'custodial' and everything good as 'permissive'. Nurses needed an active therapeutic approach to replace the traditional regime. When Clark returned from a sabbatical year in California in 1963, he reorganised the Fulbourn wards to create an intensive nursing unit, comprising the five male and female disturbed wards. Clark realised that whereas principles of social treatment could be applied to a whole hospital, the therapeutic community needed a concentrated effort, staffed by workers with the desired attitudes. There was more fertile soil for nurse training after appointment of head tutor Reg Salisbury, who was liberally minded and popular with trainees,[70] but the pace of change to the nursing culture was slow. Clark deployed social science graduates as nursing assistants, but as he later described to John Adams, these bright young workers were not always accepted by the qualified staff:

> Of course there were tensions. There was one stage when the staff group at Hereward House was completely split between 'them as went to college' and

'them as didn't'. And I and the doctors were seen as being on the same side as these nursing assistants, whereas the trained nurses felt they were being put down with long words.[71]

As well as overcoming the institutional practices of older staff, Clark was troubled by recruits drawn to mental health by the ideology of RD Laing.

> The only pity is that his books are mainly read by people who know nothing of the pain and suffering of mental disorder and the real problems of living with it. They are liable to accept the whole conspirational picture and leap to naïve simplistic conclusions (such as that all episodes of mental disorder are entirely caused by evil and vicious parents, aided and abetted by purblind doctors and nurses). Those who, inspired by Laing, come to help in the work of institutions give fine service – but have a long and bitter time discovering that the human truth is far more complex than the black-and-white pictures of the poets ever tell.[72]

Many nurses were perturbed by what was happening at Fulbourn, particularly when the therapeutic community model was extended to admission wards. It was certainly not a laissez-faire approach, despite the perceptions of its critics. Nurses were expected to take risks, but the contingencies of coercion remained: seclusion and injection of tranquillisers were sometimes forced upon patients, many of whom were admitted under the Mental Health Act. Yet in this relatively free environment many patients recovered, replicating the past achievements of The Retreat.

In 1965 Clark was appointed to chair a Ministry of Health committee to examine the role of the psychiatric nurse (the term 'mental' was now eschewed). Apart from Duncan Macmillan and JAR Bickford, all other members were nurses, including Fulbourn matron Queenie Brock. The report *Psychiatric Nursing: Today and Tomorrow*, published in 1968, promoted a therapeutic remit. As Altschul had described, the essence of nursing was in interpersonal relationships; psychiatric nursing, in particular, was primarily for human *beings* rather than human *bodies*. Although the GNC's experimental syllabus had become the standard for mental nurse training in 1964, physical care could not be wiped off the menu. However, Clarks' report opposed the learning of anatomy and physiology by rote, and the recent initiative of seconding trainees for three months in a general hospital. Prioritising of technical knowledge and tasks over interpersonal skills perpetuated a tendency for emotional detachment:

> When you keep your distance from patients and regard them as irrational objects, their fate is not too important. If you get to know them as people and enter their lives, you may appreciate the terror of schizophrenic hallucinations or the deep despair of recurring melancholia. If things go awry and someone you have worked with closely kills herself, the pain and grief may be very heavy.[73]

For all that nursing in mental hospitals was stuck in the past, it would be unfair to portray an 'old guard' lacking in therapeutic interest. Nurses knew the patients best: their foibles, and their breaking points. Often nursing skill calmed a violent situation, preventing its escalation. Barry Hopper[74] was impressed by the handling of an incident at Graylingwell. Urgently summoned from the canteen to Amberley 1 Ward, he met staff nurse Tom at the doorway to the day room. Alan, a manic male patient was standing on the billiard table, a ball in each hand, having already hurled several balls across the room at random. Another patient was enraged at being struck by one of these missiles, and charge nurse Bob's arm had been cut by a smashed mirror. After Barry had ushered patients to safety, Bob calmly stepped forward and stated in a reassuring rather than reprimanding tone: 'It's okay, Alan – it's all over now.' Instead of the expected confrontation, Alan was disarmed by this humane response, and the balls simply dropped from his hands. Alan came down from the table, mumbled 'Sorry, nurse' and walked away. The nurses picked up the balls and the shards of glass, and all was well.

Demise of the old hierarchy

Until the 1960s most matrons and chief male nurses and their deputies had worked in the same hospital since their training. Living on site, they were totally immersed in the institutional culture, which they stamped upon junior staff. Discipline and respect for superiors was unstintingly imposed, as Mary and Sophie Slevin[75] found at All Saints. Matron ruled the roost; when she entered a ward, each nurse would instantly stop what she was doing and stand to attention with her hands behind her back. While inspecting the nurses' appearance and the precision of their bed-making, this imperious madam paid little attention to the patients.

For the many ward sisters who were unmarried, their world was the mental hospital. As recalled by Carmel Piris,[76] five of the older ward sisters at Netherne shared a house in the grounds, and apart from the two Barrett siblings, they all disliked each other and rarely interacted. In the morning Sister O'Hara was always first out, followed in single file by two of the other sisters, at a certain distance from each other. When Sister O'Hara retired, Carmel knocked on the door for contributions to a leaving gift, but the other sisters said that they did not really know this woman. According to Carmel, sisters guarded stock as if it were personal property: for example, on Sister Norton's ward underwear was hidden under a piano lid, and night nurses counted draw-sheets every morning. While some sisters were fastidious, they were protective of patients, typically referring to them as 'my girls'.

Although medical superintendents such as Clark and Barton deserve their accolades, some senior nurses were the linchpins in the transforming the mental institution from an authoritarian to a humanistic culture. Following his National Service in the Royal Air Force, Andrew McCrae[77] was dismayed by the much stricter regime in his nurse training at Denbigh Hospital. His father urged him to stay, to gain a qualification. Thankfully, a new chief male nurse was appointed by the hospital management committee, who did not believe that reform was possible through internal promotion. Sidney Badland had a testy reception, but he gradually persuaded charge nurses to think beyond petty rules and routines, and to take more therapeutic interest in patients. He introduced social therapy, with nurses assigned to small groups of patients, who they would accompany to the workshop, art therapy and dining room. This had remarkable results: Andrew remembers a statuesque character who became a keen painter. While the head tutor simply read out scripted lectures, expecting students to write copious notes, an assistant tutor appointed by Badland encouraged discussion and debate.

In 1963 the government appointed a committee chaired by Brian Salmon to consider a new structure for senior nursing. In mental hospitals, promotion to deputy or chief male nurse/matron was like 'Buggins' turn', in a hierarchy built as much on nepotism as managerial competence. Senior nursing was insular, detached from wider health service organisation and of the community served by the hospital. The report presented data showing that many sisters and charge nurses had occupied the same level for twenty years or more. There were more charge nurses than staff nurses, and many female wards were run by SENs, who could never be promoted to the level of matron or deputy (see Table 6.2).

The Salmon Report, implemented in 1968,[79] had major impact on mental hospitals. The division of male and female sides was officially abandoned. Out went the chief male nurse and matron as the nursing hierarchy was unified with a single leader. Atop the pyramid was the principal nursing officer; senior nursing officers managed an 'area' (e.g. acute, psychogeriatric); and nursing officers led a 'unit' of perhaps three or four wards. Two charge nurses (the 'sister' title remained in use but was optional in the new structure) ran each ward; night charge nurses covered a whole unit. The report recommended that nursing staff divisions match

Table 6.2 Staff nurses and charge nurses in mental hospitals (30 September 1964).[78]

Rank	England and Wales			
	Male	*Female*	*Total*	*Total(WTE*)*
Staff nurse	3,385	1,197	5,302	4,702
Charge nurse	3,383	3,400	6,783	6,693
Total RMN	6,768	4,597	12,085	11,395

Rank	Scotland			
	Male	*Female*	*Total*	*Total (WTE)*
Staff nurse	775	543	1,318	1,258
Charge nurse	409	404	813	808
Total RMN	1,184	947	2,131	2,066

* Whole-time equivalent

the geographical sectors of consultant psychiatrists, with rotation of nurses to include stints in long-stay wards and the general hospital psychiatric unit. Cleaning was to be taken over by a domestic staff, enabling nurses to concentrate on patient care.

In 1972 a DHSS report[80] stated that the Salmon structure was working well in psychiatric hospitals. However, not everybody liked it. The new structure gave management an opportunity to appoint people with fresh ideas, but this broke the unwritten contract of internal promotion. More often than not a man was appointed to the lead nursing post, as many a matron was deposed from her erstwhile matriarchy. Senior nursing officers took their place alongside psychiatrists and administrators in tripartite management but their influence was relatively weak. Moreover, some of the most talented nurses were detached from clinical practice. A common criticism from informants for this book was the emergence of an officer class that sat in smoke-filled rooms in the administration block, visiting wards only to speak to the charge nurse behind a closed door. There were more chiefs than Indians.

As the management structure was overhauled, cracks appeared in the rusting hull of the institutional culture. Society was changing, and the mental hospital was not immune. Youth of the 1960s had grown up free from the rationing and respect for discipline of the post-war years. The 'Angry Young Men' playwrights and rock 'n' roll music led to the 'counter-culture' of the 1960s with its revolutionary ideology, provocative fashion and recreational drugs, challenging the assumptions of the relatively stable post-war society. Nurses began to free themselves from the shackles of a regimental hierarchy and medical hegemony. Unlike their older colleagues, recruits to mental nursing would not slavishly defer to their superiors: there would be no more doffing the cap to the lord of the manor.

Although the medical superintendent position was officially withdrawn by the 1959 Mental Health Act, which confirmed clinical responsibility for each consultant psychiatrist, in most mental hospitals the incumbent retained his title.[81] Until they retired, these men retained their oak-panelled office above the main entrance, while enjoying the privileges of a grand house with domestic service. Many consultant psychiatrists saw this role as an anachronism, and not all medical superintendents had the liberal ideology and social dynamism of the likes of Bickford or Barton. Indeed, a few stood against progress. Consultant psychiatrist Richard Crocket, who established a therapeutic community in an acute annexe of Warley Hospital at a general hospital in Romford, scathingly described 'little frightened men in big jobs'.[82] Symbolising their defensive mentality, some had covered walkways erected from their residence to the main building. Powers that had previously rested with medical superintendents were shifting to medical advisory committees, in which consultants at the mental hospital met to discuss treatment and professional matters. Gradually, these committees expanded to include psychiatrists from other hospitals in the locality, eventually becoming area and regional groups. While they had no authority to formulate policies, their recommendations had considerable influence. Some medical superintendents refused to serve on the committees, while castigating those who did. Norman

Imlah at All Saints returned from leave to find that the consultants had formed a medical advisory committee without his consent. He immediately ordered that the group be disbanded and declared himself in sole charge of clinical policy and practice in the hospital. Imlah's reluctance to relinquish power was a source of friction until his retirement many years later.[83]

By the late 1960s, most nurses were working for consultant psychiatrists' 'firms', and needed to adapt to their new medical leader's philosophy of care and treatment. Consultants jealously guarded their wards and nurses as their personal domain, but while some exercised autocratic control, others nurtured a democratic, liberal ethos. Most psychiatrists were eclectic, complementing drug treatment with psychosocial interventions, while affording nurses some say in patients' care. However, flattening of the hierarchy was a rude awakening for some psychiatrists, who could be undermined by the collective strength of the nursing staff. Tom Harrison,[84] during his medical training at Hollymoor, was told by Peter Hall of his experience as one of the first consultants. On entering a ward, Hall was given two documents to sign by the charge nurse: one for a bulk prescription and the other for cleaning materials. When he asked to see the patients, the charge nurse told him in no uncertain terms that it was not a convenient time, ushering the bewildered consultant to the door. Charge nurses were more experienced if less educated than younger doctors, and for the first time they began to openly challenge medical decisions. Nurses were beginning to claim territory in their field of practice, as in this nurse's experience on being appointed in charge of a ward at Fulbourn, where the consultant psychiatrist was determined to instil order:[85]

> He grabbed my arm as I walked across the grass and said, 'Now, I shall tell you how I want *my* charge nurse to behave'. And I said, 'Well, let's get one thing straight, I am not *your* charge nurse, I have a profession in my own right … If you want to run the ward – you go and do three years of nurse training'. 'Oh – I'm going to have problems with you then.'

Consultant psychiatrists established their position as clinical leaders, clubbing together in hospital medical advisory committees to determine treatment policies. Yet nurses, managing wards around the clock, had a major influence on patient's treatment, in practice if not by prescription. On a disturbed ward at Long Grove, Ian Norman[86] was impressed by a charismatic charge nurse who boldly did things his way. This tall Welshman with a shock of white hair was also the COHSE shop steward, a position that made him less susceptible to managerial control. When a manic patient booked himself a holiday in Spain, the charge nurse allowed him to go, on the condition that he come back to see him on his return. The young doctor Tom Burns, who later became a prominent psychiatrist, did not overturn this illicit and risky decision, respecting the nurse's experience and stature.

Boys and girls come out to play

The sexual revolution was late in reaching a bastion of puritan Victorian values. The female nurses' home remained out of bounds for men, its door locked by the matron in the late evening. Yet forbidden fruit was frequently taken. Sophie and Mary Slevin spoke of the 'affairs' that flourished on night duty at All Saints. Nurses on duty would sometimes disappear for up to two hours, senior male nurses regularly visited the female wards despite having no responsibility for that side of the hospital, and doctors also appeared at night on the female wards for contrived reasons. As well as consensual relationships, there was also a malevolent aspect to nocturnal liaisons; a notoriously sleazy male tutor frequently made unannounced visits to the female nurses' home at night. [87]

At Parkside in the mid-1960s, Yvonne Beaumont[88] recalls that while most colleagues spent their evenings in the sitting room of the female nurses' home, she went to the staff canteen, where a light supper was served at 9 p.m. for nurses finishing a late shift. Often she chatted to an older male charge nurse with literary interests, who recommended classic and modern novels. Yvonne also got to know some younger male nurses. On one occasion, she and a friend were cavorting with two men, who climbed through a window of the nurses' home. This was reported and all involved were summoned to a disciplinary meeting with the matron and chief male nurse. Yvonne and colleagues were severely reprimanded. The hospital, they were told, had a responsibility for the welfare of its staff. Indeed, managers were acting in *loco parentis* for young female recruits. Judy Lunny[89] recalls that while the female nurses' home at Graylingwell was locked at night by the home warden, nurses above the 'age of majority' (twenty-one in England until 1970) had a key. Ruth Valentine's history of Horton Hospital included this quote from a storeman who was surprised by the strict staff segregation when he arrived in 1967. He and colleagues were lured by an underground passage to female company:

> We found the ducts that led to the nurses' home, so one evening we crawled along them. We came up inside there, right next to the phone. There was a young lady on the phone, and suddenly there were these men coming up through the floor. We said 'good evening', but she dropped the phone and ran off.[90]

Fired by 'Dutch courage', female nurses at Lancaster Moor sometimes ventured into the tunnels at night, taking the long passage to the male nurses' home at the edge of the grounds. This 'tunnel of love' was dimly lit and infested with cockroaches, but romantic pursuits were undeterred, until the authorities padlocked the underground entrances.[91] Introduction of the contraceptive pill was a factor in relaxation of the rules, but officially the hospital frowned upon sexual liberty on its premises. An informant for this book[92] was enjoying a 'foursome' with three others in the nurses' home in the early hours of the morning, when there was a knock on the door. Naked, he tentatively opened the door to a tall man in jacket and tie – the night nursing officer! He instinctively slammed the door shut, got dressed and opened the door again. Someone had complained about the noise. The nursing officer offered a few words of advice, but did not take the matter further.

A starkly visible sign of reform at Fulbourn was the decision to allow nurses to come out of uniform. In most mental hospitals, female nurses wore a white or pale-coloured dress with belt, buckle and cap; the dress had gradually shortened over the decades. By the 1950s the men's blue suit and cap had been replaced by a grey suit, more akin to a civil servant than a prison officer. Male apparel also included a white coat for physical nursing duties, and colours on the epaulettes and women's dress differentiated RMN (blue) from SEN (green), and trainees accordingly. Stripes denoted the rank: one for students and two for staff nurses, three for charge nurses, although sisters were more readily identified by their blue dress. Neil Chell, an interviewee in John Adams' study of Fulbourn, described the correct alignment of insignia on the jacket at St Edward's in Staffordshire, where he was trained:

> Your State-Registered badge had to be on the top, your hospital badge had to be second, and your trade union badge was third. And you were reported to the Nursing Office if your badges were in the wrong order or one was missing.[93]

On moving to the Cambridge hospital, Chell was shocked to see nurses in their own clothing. The *mufti* policy befitted the therapeutic community ideal of breaking down the barriers between staff and patients, but the lack of obvious difference from first-year student to charge nurse caused confusion. Disparaging remarks were made by staff elsewhere in the hospital: nurses in therapeutic community wards were indistinguishable from the patients, and not only in attire – an intended slur that was water off a duck's back to Clark and his acolytes. A more widespread change was the use of first names by nurses, although some senior colleagues denied such familiarity. When Judy Lunny was promoted to sister at Graylingwell, an older sister said that she could now address her simply as 'Ryan'.[94]

Working hours, shortened from forty-eight to forty-four per week in the late 1950s, went down to forty-two a few years later. Managers accepted that nurses on a series of long days were too jaded to provide optimal care, as highlighted by Audrey John's study. The shift pattern changed to a combination of long and short shifts. At Denbigh, Andrew McCrae[95] worked a four-day sequence of a late shift from 1.30 p.m. to 9 p.m., followed by two long days and ending with an early shift from 7 a.m. to 2 p.m. The traditional shifts were preferred by nurses, partly because it gave them more days off and made childcare easier for married couples; in some hospitals the unions opposed this change[96]. Meanwhile pay was improving. After ten years of voluntary wage constraint to curtail inflation, in 1959 the government awarded nurses a 12 per cent rise; this was followed by a 14 per cent increase in 1962, and 5 per cent in 1963.

In many ways these were 'salad days' for mental hospital nurses, who now had more money and more time to spend it. While many filled the gaps in their week with overtime, others took advantage of the amenities on site. The social club was the hub of the staff community, frequented by all ranks. In the late 1960s, regular discotheques began, where young mini-skirted women gyrated 'freestyle' to the latest pop records. Meanwhile, staff dances in the main hall remained major events, as at Tooting Bec, where co-author PN started his nursing career in 1962; leading jazz musicians such as Humphrey Lytttleton, Chris Barber and the Ambrose Band were hired.

Institutional entertainments, however, were unfashionable. In the late 1960s and early 1970s mental hospitals were infiltrated by 'hippie' culture, a Californian youth movement espousing harmony with nature, communal living, experimental art and recreational drugs. Unlike the the regimental 'short back and sides' of older peers, many young male nurses sported long hair and beards. As well as marijuana and LSD, there was a ready supply of psychoactive drugs in the hospital. According to Imelda Bures[97] at Netherne, theft of Mandrax and Valium (sedatives of the addictive benzodiazepine class) were so frequent that tablets had to be checked after each handover. Mental nursing was attracting people with a rebellious streak, but a minority had underlying psychological problems. Carmel Piris[98] told of a student nurse at Netherne who overindulged at the Christmas party in 1966. In the morning after a senior male nurse locked the intoxicated student in the padded cell to keep him out of sight. When they opened the door, the student went berserk. He had stripped himself in the cell, and ran out of the hospital naked. The next day he was found on the downs, still naked and badly cut. He did not continue his training.

The 'Berlin Wall' dividing the two sides of the institution was breached by patients as well as nurses. Sometimes close friendships developed between patients of opposite sex, and there was no formal guidance on when and how nurses should intervene. A couple holding hands in the grounds was tolerated, but any sexual activity was definitely out of bounds. Some female patients were known to prostitute themselves for a cigarette ('a fag for a shag', as co-author recalls the unwritten contract). Some women had an intra-uterine coil inserted, while a few predatory men were prescribed testosterone suppressants.[99] Occasionally there were unplanned pregnancies; after the Abortion Act 1968 patients could be taken for a termination at the general hospital, on the basis that birth would be detrimental to mother and child. Recent writers such as Diana Gittins suggest that gender segregation benefited female patients, some of whom felt uncomfortable with men around,[100] but in the spirit of sexual emancipation it was perceived as a remnant of Victorian repression. Normalising the environment was vital for rehabilitation, and for long-stay patients interaction with the opposite sex was as much a right as a privilege. Nurses found that the presence of female patients moderated men's behaviour, and vice versa; sexual interest was reinterpreted as a sign of recovery.

The Salmon Report made male and female nurses fully interchangeable. Female nurses and domestic staff worked on male wards, and in some cases men took charge of female wards. Although this was anathema to nurses accustomed to segregation, in the 1960s mixed-sex wards began to appear.[101] The majority of wards remained single-sex; for example, wards for most categories of patient (acute admissions, long-stay, senile and infirm) at Graylingwell remained so when Barry Hopper completed his training in 1971.[102] Many hospitals were not readily amenable to this innovation, having mostly large dormitories with a few side rooms. Co-author PN remembers senior nurses at Tooting Bec Hospital opposing the idea, believing that patients needed protection from themselves and the temptations of others.[103] The hospital management was cautious about male and female patients visiting each other's wards; notices appeared forbidding their association in bedrooms. If a female patient were impregnated the hospital could be sued; venereal disease could spread; or a patient might develop an uncontrollable sexual appetite! However, such restriction was swimming against the tide: patients met in the bushes, behind sheds or in disused buildings. They had not committed themselves to a life of celibacy. Gerda Cohen was told by a doctor of the secret rendezvous in the tunnel connecting the two sides of the hospital, known as 'the snoggery'. Policing of illicit sexual contact between patients was replaced by disparaging humour:

> 'He's got a crush on that psychopath in Twelve', reported a nurse at the weekly case conference. 'She won't do him any good, a right tart.' A stifled titter came from the junior houseman. 'She's a nymph, isn't she?'[104]

Scandal and solidarity

On 10 November 1965 a letter was published in *The Times* alleging widespread neglect of elderly patients in mental hospitals, and inaction by the Ministry of Health in response to relatives' concerns. The floodgates opened to a wave of public anger, repeatedly expressed in the correspondence pages of newspapers. The authors of the original letter were of various backgrounds including scholar Brian Abel-Smith,[105] and campaigner Barbara Robb, who collected the subsequent material in a book *Sans Everything: a Case to Answer*,[106] published in 1967. The foreword was written by outspoken psychiatrist Russell Barton, who described a self-serving institutional culture of oppressive rules, misplaced loyalties, personality conflict and victimisation of anyone who failed to toe the line.

Kenneth Robinson, Minister of Health in the Labour government, was angry with Barton. Like many politicians in the early decades of the 'welfare state', Robinson idealised the NHS and doubted claims of desertion of duty or deliberate harm. He feared electoral consequences for the government and also a loss of confidence in the cherished NHS, and his instincts were to defend the system.[107] Although Robinson promised that nurses who made complaints would not face reprisals, the nursing bulletins warned of scapegoating. Hospitals were anonymised throughout *Sans Everything*, but their identities were requested by the Ministry of Health, which ordered regional hospital boards to investigate. The report[108] amounted to little more than whitewashing: most of the allegations were discredited as inaccurate or exaggerated, while those upheld were portrayed as isolated incidents. Nonetheless, *Sans Everything* was a catalyst for exposure of the hidden evils in hospitals for mental illness and mental handicap.

In summer 1967 a nursing assistant wrote to the *News of the World* newspaper describing a series of specific instances of maltreatment and theft at Ely Hospital, a former Poor Law institution in Cardiff. The hospital mostly housed mentally subnormal patients, with some psychogeriatric wards. A regional hospital board enquiry was led by the Conservative politician and lawyer Geoffrey Howe, who refused to amend or abridge the report for publication, insisting that all 83,000 words be released. Nurses were named and shamed, but the most damning criticism was of the nursing management, who had attempted to quash dissent.

> Members of the nursing staff who were genuinely concerned about conditions at Ely must have come to feel that it was almost more than their life was worth for them to voice any feelings of concern.[109]

Conditions described at Ely should not have surprised mental hospital nurses. In his ministerial office at Whitehall, Richard Crossman was aware that Ely was not exceptional, and that a 'can of worms' could be opened in most if not all of the large mental institutions. His published diary reflected on his first visit to a mental hospital:[110]

> God, I remember Littlemore. I went there once when I was a councillor. It was a Dickensian nightmare of huge great shadowy halls, with about 150 people in each. As you came in they crowded around you, women with their grey hair in disorder and long nails. It was a kind of nightmare madhouse.

While the NHS was by design a national and equitable system, it had not standardised the quality of care. Stark differences were observed by itinerant nurses, who might find a friendly and caring atmosphere in one hospital, and an oppressive regime in another. Yvonne Beaumont, for example, moved from Parkside in Macclesfield to Lancaster Moor Hospital in 1968 and found the latter 'very behind the times'.[111] Extreme variation in staffing, maintenance and hygiene between mental hospitals had shocked WAL Bowen, physician superintendent at Naburn and Bootham Park Hospitals in York, on conducting a survey in one region. Speaking at a symposium on psychiatric hospital care in 1964, Bowen warned of much wider disparities across the country: 'Even the cursory perambulation around those hospitals which feel secure enough to receive the various meetings of the Royal Medico-Psychological Association confirm this fact.'[112] Bowen recommended an inspectorate of three psychiatrists to highlight deficiencies and promote good practice. However, his peers were wary of reviving the 'punitive fault-finding authority' of the past.[113]

In the aftermath of *Sans Everything* the *Sunday Times* sent reporter DAN Jones around Britain to examine the state of mental hospitals, the article featuring on the cover of the magazine supplement in September 1968. Jones and photographer

Lord Snowdon were welcomed at Severalls, where Barton's progressive leadership was apparent. Images contrasted the admission block and long-stay wards, the former represented by a young woman with fashionable hairstyle choosing an album in the music room, and the latter by an older schizophrenic lady 'who spends most of her day slowly knitting, then unravelling, a skein of wool'. The article described hospitals where older patients were clean and comfortable, and others where the wards had a pervading stench of urine. Jones suspected that he had not seen the worst:[114]

> Hatton in Warwickshire persistently refused to let us in; they had suffered too much 'bad publicity'. But I am reliably informed that this 112-year-old hospital contains 1365 patients where there should be no more than a thousand; that beds are jammed tight together in every available corner; that wards meant for 50 people contain 86; that there are 85 male nurses when the establishment is for 145. An official visitor assures me that there are members of the Regional Hospital Board who have never been inside this place.

Lord Shaftesbury would have turned in his grave at conditions that Jones partly blamed on the lack of a national inspectorate – that great achievement of the nineteenth century reformers. Clearly there was a need for rigorous monitoring and an effective complaints procedure. John Martin, in his book on the hospital scandals, considered as part of the problem a complacent optimism in the 1960s, inspired by the drug revolution, the Mental Health Act 1959 and investment in the NHS:[115]

> Prevention of abuse had not been a major issue in the modern era, although of course it had been of great importance in earlier times. It was a reasonable assumption that hospitals existed to do good to their patients, or at least provide civilised care; their staff were dedicated and the reduction of abuse was seen as a natural by-product of improving standards as a whole. The beneficent role of the hospital was almost taken for granted.

In 1969 Crossman chaired a Post-Ely Working Party, which included Geoffrey Howe, Professor Peter Townsend (who had studied the plight of the elderly in institutions), and Eileen Skellern (nursing superintendent at Bethlem and Maudsley Hospitals). The group met fortnightly and made influential recommendations on the problems of communication, clarification of responsibilities and quality of care. The recently renamed Department of Health and Social Security established a new inspection body on 1 November 1969. The Hospital Advisory Service, chaired by psychiatrist Alex Baker, comprised practitioners seconded from NHS clinical posts.[116] Visits began in February 1970, lasting about a week at each hospital, culminating in a final meeting with managers and staff. Reports were sent to the Secretary of State but not published; instead, an annual report presented overall findings from HAS visits.

Meanwhile another scandal erupted. In summer 1969 two senior members of staff wrote directly to the Secretary of State about improprieties and suppression of complaints at Whittingham Hospital in Lancashire. In July 1967, forty-five nursing students had attended a meeting with the principal nurse tutor to discuss various allegations including mistreatment of patients and fraud. Psychologist Patricia Bunn and assistant psychiatrist AB Masters identified with the dissidents' cause. The chief male nurse demanded that the normal channels of communication be used for any complaints, including the students' supervisors and trade union representatives. He put up a poster mocking 'Bunn and the Bunnies', but when Mrs Bunn and others demanded an apology, the chairman of the hospital management committee told them that 'they could leave the hospital as far as he was concerned'.[117] In response, Bunn and Masters wrote their letter to Whitehall. Consequently, an auditor was sent to the hospital and police were informed.

Hearing rumours from Whittingham, the *Lancashire Evening Post* opened a 'press desk' at the pub in the nearby village of Goosnargh. Editor Barry Askew asserted the principle of public interest, and with lubrication by beer, information was gleaned from insiders. Reports of cruelty featured prominently in the newspaper edition of 7 February 1970. This drew a vociferous defence from hospital staff and COHSE, but in June the police produced evidence of maladministration and victimisation. Soon after the police had completed their enquiry, a male nurse assaulted two patients, one of whom died. Charged with murder, the nurse was convicted of manslaughter.

In August 1970 Askew went to London to urge Sir Keith Joseph, the new Secretary of State, to order a public enquiry.[118] In fact this was already planned but could not commence during the murder investigation. Eventually a committee of enquiry was appointed on 15 February 1971,[119] including WAL Bowen, whose views on the shortcomings of mental hospitals were known. On arrival at Whittingham the committee members were struck by the expanse of the hospital, much of it comprising three-storey blocks built in the 1870s, surrounded by pleasant but deserted grounds. While some facilities were modern, many older wards had eighty beds or more. The hospital population had fallen by a third from its peak in the mid-1950s, but 2,000 mostly long-stay patients remained.

Facing a culture of denial, the committee compelled witnesses to public hearings, applying a clause of the National Health Service Act. While noting that care at Whittingham was mostly satisfactory, the report in February 1972 found persuasive evidence of abuse on four wards, the worst run by a sister who had worked there continuously for 47 years. Barbaric practices included 'wet towel treatment', which entailed twisting a towel around a patient's neck until he lost consciousness. Although strenuously denied by the nurses, a student nurse who had left the hospital claimed that this method was frequently used to control violent patients on Ward 3. Sadistic abuse was alleged in an instance of a nurse pouring and igniting methylated spirits in the breast pocket of a blind man's dressing gown, the patient shrieking as he was engulfed in a large flame; allegedly the nurse laughed aloud while dousing the flame with a towel.

A major revelation at Whittingham was the extent of theft. In the financial year 1968–1969 the takings of the hospital shop were £42,000, yet £91,000 had been issued by the hospital bank to patients, for the majority of whom the shop was their only retail outlet. Therefore, £49,000 had disappeared. Furthermore, goods bought at the shop did not necessarily reach patients. Much of the money dispensed by the treasurer went into the hospital shop tills via nurses, who supposedly purchased items such as cigarettes, confectionery and clothing on patients' behalf. Records of such spending were not maintained, but it was apparent to the auditor that cigarettes were bought collectively for the ward, including contributions from patients who did not smoke. Furthermore, cigarettes were sold singly to patients at a profit.

According to many informants for this book, petty pilfering was rife in mental hospitals. There was casual acceptance on some wards that nurses took a share of patients' food and cigarettes. Carmel Piris asked the sister on a ward for the frail elderly at Netherne why some women only received half a banana in their evening meal; she was told that these patients did not want any more, but clearly a portion of the food supplied by the central kitchen was being withheld for staff consumption.[120] Such misappropriation was at the minor end of the scale, but there was also more serious theft, as witnessed by Philip Barton-Wright.[121] Years before he started nursing, Philip worked as an electrician at High Royds in Yorkshire. One Saturday he was working in a room above the rear entrance to the kitchen, and saw several members of staff arriving and leaving with boxes of food and crates of beer (which was sometimes prescribed for debilitated patients). He recognised them as porters and nurses. Philip raised this with a colleague, who warned him to keep his mouth shut.

Organised embezzlement of NHS and patients' property was probably rare, but every hospital had weak spots that could be exploited by crooked staff. At Whittingham, irregularities found by the auditor led to two male nurses being convicted for stealing suits. The management group secretary recited what he had been told by these two nurses:

> Everyone at the hospital is in the racket. Just everyone. You don't need me to tell you who these people are. All you need to do is to take a look around and see which of the staff change their cars every year, and which of the staff go abroad for holidays every year and who take their wives out two or three times a week and who have built bungalows recently.[122]

Following the Whittingham scandal, administration of patients' money was taken over by the hospital bank. According to Dermot Hennessy,[123] this was not appreciated by Banstead Hospital charge nurses, many of whom had taken an illicit source of income for granted. As Dermot recalled, Banstead was staffed by nurses who had failed their examinations or run into disciplinary trouble at other hospitals. It was a closed community, but Dermot was accepted after scoring six goals on his debut for the hospital football team. The charge nurses worked every Tuesday for the weekly distribution of patients' money; some came in on their days off. Patients were brought to the office to sign for their 10 shilling allowance, which many did not receive. 'They were all at it,' recalled Dermot. One patient regularly threw his weekly money in the toilet; the charge nurse fished it out and allegedly kept it for himself.

Whittingham was the classic 'corruption of care'.[124] A contributory factor was the devalued role of the hospital, which since the Hospital Plan had been reduced to care of ageing, long-stay patients (in 1969, 86 per cent had been there for over two years[125]). The five consultant psychiatrists had commitments elsewhere and they were not sufficiently present to know what was happening on the wards; indeed, only one full-time equivalent was devoted to the long-stay blocks. The Manchester Regional Hospital Board, so progressive in opening psychiatric units in general hospitals around the county, had neglected its former asylums:

> Their plan is no more than half a policy when the problem which it entails of running down and closing out of date hospitals has not been fully thought out. Without adequate recognition of the continuing need for elderly long-stay patients, an old hospital can never close. Appreciation of this fact had led to a frank disbelief and dichotomy of aim between the Board and the Whittingham Hospital management. Worse, there is a danger that it could lead to a two-tier system of psychiatry – well staffed 'acute' units and 'long-stay dumps'.[126]

From his observations as HAS chairman, Baker stated that while neglect was sadly common in the mental hospitals, abuse was a rarity.[127] Indeed, a nurse who bullied patients was likely to be ostracised. Tim Mosses,[128] who was at Bexley from 1971 to 1979, once witnessed a nursing student on a male geriatric ward slap a patient who had wet himself. The charge nurse grabbed the student by the scruff of the neck and dispatched him to the corridor, telling him he must never return to that ward; the shamed student withdrew from his training. According to Tim, nurses were aware of scandals elsewhere but did not believe that abuse would be tolerated at Bexley. However, several informants for this book were aware of sadistic behaviour in the darker recesses of their hospital. Tom Chan[129] told of an instance at Park Prewett when a doctor observed redness and bruising on both sides of a patient's head; there were no witnesses, but the injury could only be explained by the patient being picked up by the ears. Reflecting on his experiences as a nursing student at Cane Hill, Peter Robinson wishes that he had acted on cruelty that he witnessed on Zachary Ward:

> One old man who was blind, deaf and dumb, epileptic and schizophrenic, was regularly slapped around the face by a very stupid and nasty staff nurse. Alfie would start screaming and the staff nurse thought it was hilarious. There was another old man, John, who constantly wrote letters and underlined every word, and when he argued with this same nurse the latter threw him out of his chair on to the floor, filled a hypodermic syringe with Largactil, splayed out the needle point on a nearby cast-iron pipe, and stabbed this instrument of torture into the poor patient's backside, pumping the drug in so fast that a swelling the size of a golf ball appeared. It must have been agonisingly painful. I'll never forget that and the fact that I did nothing about it.[130]

In the past a medical superintendent could summarily dismiss a nurse suspected of abuse, but doctors in the 1960s lacked such licence, as illustrated by a case at St John's in Buckinghamshire:[131]

A doctor had to interview a woman who had been an in-patient for a long time to tell her that her husband had decided to divorce her because she seemed to be incurable. When she came into the office he noticed that she had two severe black eyes, but she was unwilling to talk about them. Neither the daily nor nightly nursing reports made any mention of them, or any accident or fight, and there was nothing in the accident-report book. The ward sister looked uncomfortable but was unwilling or unable to explain, and the lack of any mention of the black eyes was itself a misdemeanour. The Medical Director took the matter up with vigour. He held private interviews with a number of nurses and with other patients in the ward. It emerged that the night nurse had struck the patient, and indeed was known in some circles as a rough woman. The Director thereupon suspended her from duty, and reported her to the HMC with the suggestion that she was unsuitable to nurse psychiatric patients and should be dismissed. The Committee were upset in two ways. In the first place the Director was *ultra vires*: he was not in charge of the nurses and had no authority to suspend or dismiss staff. Secondly, a nursing union was already making threatening noises on behalf of the nurse … None of the nurses who had spoken to Dr Watt in private were willing to come forward and give evidence in public. The Chairman therefore closed the matter and ordered the night nurse to be reinstated.

The reputation of an entire hospital could be tarnished by a few miscreants. Yet the cases coming to light may have been merely the 'tip of an iceberg'. In the third edition of *Institutional Neurosis*, Russell Barton[132] belatedly realised why some patients walked past nurses in a cowed posture:

I have reluctantly become aware that to the list of constituent factors collected some twenty years ago must be added violence, brutality, browbeating, harshness, teasing and tormenting. These loathsome practices, carried out unofficially and secretly by a small minority of callous unenlightened staff, are probably an important factor subjugating certain patients into an apathetic, cowed, mute and timorous state. I am amazed and humiliated that with all the evidence given one by patients, ex-patients, relatives and staff I did not identify it years ago.

Of the many scandals arising in hospitals for mental illness and mental handicap in the late 1960s and 1970s, none were in Scotland. This was partly attributable to the existence of the Mental Welfare Commission, a body introduced by the Mental Health (Scotland) Act 1960. The commissioners were mostly doctors, as well as one nurse and at least one lawyer, and they visited each Scottish mental institution twice per year. In *A Duty to Care*, a review of its first ten years, the Mental Welfare

Commission stated that over 700 allegations had been received. However, as commissioners did not get involved in any case arising from a clinical decision, the number of investigations was small, and reports were never published. Arguably a lid of administrative secrecy was kept on a jar containing the same ingredients as found south of the border.[133]

Had the mental hospitals got worse, or were the scandals simply exposing long-standing problems of institutional neglect? This was a moot point. 'Whistle-blowers' were typically young, educated members of staff, but to assume that problems would be resolved as nurses of obsolete mindset were replaced by more enlightened successors was naïve, and an indictment of those who had had devoted their careers to the service of the mentally ill. Practice may have been outmoded, but conscientious nurses were doing their best in difficult circumstances, and traditionally run wards at least provided basic care and comfort. Angela Ainsworth decided to become a psychiatric nurse following her childhood experience of visiting St Luke's near Middlesbrough, where her mother was admitted in 1971.

> Bristol Ward seemed enormous. The dormitory seemed jammed full of beds with flowery counterpanes on them and I remember that there was hardly any walking space between them. The ward staff were welcoming. Ten years later when I was a student nurse Ann Bowers was still the ward sister and remembered my name. I do not remember being frightened. All the other ladies were kind too. Most wore slippers and had no shoes. Mum said it was to stop people wandering off. There were several confused ladies there and my mum taught me to listen to them intently and be very gentle.[134]

A male nurse who started at Severalls in 1960 contrasted the older charge nurses favourably with their younger peers. The former had been sportsmen or bandsmen and knew how to play as a team; some were 'gentle giants' with great strength of character. Younger men who were being promoted were less skilled in managing people: whether colleagues, patients – or themselves. Among them were culprits of abuse:

> Punch. Hit. Knock and bash … There were a few, a pocketful of people who were out for mischief and would laugh and joke about it off the ward. These were largely younger charge nurses, my age, who shouldn't have been there. I think 85–90 per cent of the hospital used to sing along nicely, but there was this nasty little undercurrent, and I think a lot of the cruelty I saw was of the younger generation.[135]

Indeed, some of the malpractice exposed by the scandals may have been an unintended consequence of the liberalisation of mental hospitals. With shorter shifts and higher pay, nurses' working conditions improved substantially in the 1960s, yet standards of care did not necessarily go forward in tandem.[136] Indeed, improvement in the nurse-patient ratio may not always have been beneficial. Social loafing, a well-known phenomenon whereby individual effort reduces as responsibility spreads over a larger number of workers, may have been a factor: with fewer patients and introduction of domestic staff, two or three nurses could spend time chatting, and probably every hospital had shirkers who made minimal practical or therapeutic contribution. Brenda Wild,[137] who worked at Graylingwell over four decades, saw adverse outcomes of the softening of discipline; for example, a nurse sitting on a patient's bed reading a newspaper would have earned a severe reprimand from the matron in the past, but in a more permissive culture, thresholds of acceptable behaviour were lowered. Given an inch, some took a mile.

Feeling unfairly treated by the enquiries, nurses became more concerned with their job security. As Martin explained, the scandals led to a 'heightened union consciousness'.[138] Growing to over 10 million members, in the 1960s British trade unions were increasingly assertive in public and private sectors. Industrial action was avoided whenever possible by arbitration, but this was often bypassed by unofficial strikes. Unions were a parallel organisation in the workplace, and shop stewards, described as 'petty Napoleans' in a *Times* editorial in 1959, had great influence. Radical leaders such as Jack Jones of the Transport and General Workers Union, who had worked up from the shop floor, were seen as the authentic voice of employees. At the peak of the 'Cold War', many union activists worshipped the communist regime of the Soviet Union, but according to economist Stephen Milligan[139], the increase in strikes was due less to Marxist ideology than to understandable concerns about rampant inflation: the price of food and other commodities was rising inexorably.

The mental hospital was not the 'them and us' battlefield of the factory floor, partly because union officers were interspersed in the ranks, with charge nurses and sometimes nursing officers as branch secretary, and shop stewards throughout the workforce. Left-wing politics may have been a topic for the social club, but ideologues were unlikely to find favour on wards. The NHS was not a 'closed shop', but recruits were strongly encouraged by tutors and qualified nurses to join a union. In the past, union membership was higher among men because most shop stewards worked on the male side; female students were less likely to be approached. In the 1960s it became the norm for representatives of the RCN and COHSE to visit students in their introductory block at nursing school. Tim Mosses[140] remembers as the selling point for the union its protection should a patient make a complaint. Tom Chan[141] described COHSE as extremely strong at Park Prewett. One charge nurse spent most of his time on union activity; the ward staff accepted this as it created plenty of overtime. Anecdotal accounts suggest that the unions strove to preserve the status quo in the mental hospitals, often representing long-serving nurses against younger 'upstarts'. According to Tom Chan, when a charge nurse was reported for abusing patients by a student, the latter was suspended from his placement while the allegation was investigated. Staunchly defended by COHSE 'reps', the charge nurse was vindicated, while the student was ostracised.

Kinship was at least as powerful as union machination in the hospital culture. Family fiefdoms were embedded at every rung of the organisation, from domestic assistant to senior nursing officer. With its informal information channels, the institution was in the grip of gossip: a nurse's reputation could be destroyed by malicious rumour. Carmel Piris[142] remembered a girl in her class who received the prize for best student, despite not scoring the highest mark in the examination. This was attributed to her clandestine relationship with a senior male nurse. Tutor Bill Owen told all at the social club, and promptly resigned. Such nepotism was against the egalitarian and emancipatory principles of the trade union movement, but was perpetuated by a self-serving coterie of managers and staff tied by familial bonds.

Slow progress

Replacement of the asylum with a modern system of health and social care was not bounding forward as Powell had envisaged. A major obstacle was the administrative split between hospital and community in the National Health Service Act 1946. Indeed, the NHS was dubbed the 'National Hospital Service', and the large district general hospital with its many specialties and clinical experts reinforced professional power, aloof from the population served. While psychiatrists were spending less time in the old institutions, their increasing presence in the general hospital contributed to the medicalisation of mental disorder. In 1964 Severalls joined Essex County Hospital to form the St Helena Group Management Committee, a move that Russell Barton later regretted.[143] Such amalgamations seemed advantageous for reputation and resources, but the mental hospital was the poor relation and psychiatrists felt marginalised. Nonetheless, by the early 1970s more than half of the mental hospital committees had dissolved into group management centred on a district general hospital. In fact, psychiatry's share of NHS resources improved in the 1960s. While the number of mental hospital beds in England and Wales was falling (down to 103,000 by 1970), the number of consultant psychiatrists rose from 507 in 1960 to 810 ten years later,[144] as the DHSS pursued a ratio of one consultant per 60000 people[145]. Ministerial reports showed an overall increase in qualified nurses over the decade, although closer scrutiny reveals less impressive patterns (see Tables 6.3 and 6.4):

From 1960 to 1970 the proportion of qualified staff rose from under half to two-thirds. Yet much of this was simply due to relabeling of nursing assistants as enrolled nurses. Indeed, the number of RMNs was slightly lower in 1970 than ten years earlier. The marked disparity in trained staff between male and female sides was corrected by 1970, but 42 per cent of female qualified nurses were SENs, compared to 19 per cent of men. There is probably no single explanation for this, but as female patients would not have deserved less proficient nursing care, perhaps hospital management were persuaded by traditional 'breadwinner' assertions, if not a macho unionised culture. Overall, while the amount of qualified nurses increased, the RMN proportion actually declined. The figures above do not convey the persistence of understaffing in long-stay wards. This was highlighted by the Whittingham report, where a relatively high staff-patient ratio in acute wards contrasted with Ward 16, where a sister, deputy and four nurses struggled to cope with 126 chronic and geriatric patients.

Table 6.3 Full-time psychiatric nursing workforce[146]

Year	RMN			SEN			Nursing assistants			Students and pupils		
	Male	Female	Total	Male	Female	Total	Male	Female	Total	Male	Female	Total
1960	7,104	4,349	11,453	—	—	—	1,979	5,183	7,162	2,867	2,957	5,824
1965	7,148	5,039	12,187	827	1,789	2,616	1,585	4,416	6,001	2,885	3,382	6,267
1970	6,374	4,625	10,999	1,469	3,322	4,791	660	2,060	2,720	2,776	2,935	5,711

Table 6.4 Full-time qualified nursing workforce

Year	Qualified nurses (RMN and EN)			Total workforce (including nursing assistants and trainees)			Proportion qualified		
	Male	Female	Total	Male	Female	Total	Male	Female	Total
1960	7,104	4,349	11,453	11,950	12,489	24,439	59%	35%	47%
1965	7,975	6,828	14,803	12,445	14,626	27,071	64%	50%	55%
1970	7,843	7,947	15,790	11,279	12,942	24,221	70%	61%	65%

Acute psychiatric units in general hospitals were luring talented nurses from the mental institution. By 1970 there were ninety-four such units, although they were relatively small and accounted for merely 15.5 per cent of psychiatric admissions.[147] Based on his experience at a 170-bedded unit at the University Hospital of South Manchester, psychiatrist Neil Kessel argued that all mental health beds should be in a general hospital, with regional provision for specialist alcohol and forensic services. Kessel likened the system to the late eighteenth century, when Manchester Royal Infirmary, Dispensary and Lunatic Hospital all occupied the same block. He argued:

> When you are ill you go to a district general hospital. Mental hospitals, like the stately homes and the dodo, are museum pieces.[148]

However, as Kathleen Jones argued, the general hospital unit was not a residential but a clinical setting, with little provision for socialisation.[149] Dismissing sociological challenges to its legitimacy, psychiatry was becoming more biologically orientated, with the emergence of neo-Kraepelinian disease classification and a rapidly expanding pharmacopoeia. In retrospect, Jones regretted the demise of social psychiatry:

> While the optimism initially generate by the phenothiazines was later modified, the introduction of this apparently cheap, trouble-free method of treatment radically altered the nature of psychiatry, and virtually ended a promising relationship with the social sciences. The major drug companies promoted their products with lavish medical conferences, scholarships and research grants, and opportunities for travel abroad. Psychiatrists and general practitioners were bombarded with literature promising miraculous results from the prescription of this compound or that. There were no comparable inducements for the social approaches to mental illness.[150]

In 1971 the RMPA was elevated to the status of Royal College, achieving psychiatrists' goal of parity with other specialties of medicine. According to Anthony Fry, who became a psychiatric registrar at The Maudsley in 1968, his professional peers were hostile not only to radical critiques but also popular psychology such as transactional analysis and the humanistic therapy of Carl Rogers:

> Mainstream psychiatrists were wary of these dark forces, which they saw as at worst ridiculous and at best irrelevant to their central project.[151]

Four years after the report by David Clark and colleagues on the future of psychiatric nursing, in 1972 the government published the findings of a committee reviewing nurse education, chaired by historian Asa Briggs at the University of Sussex. This committee had been established by Richard Crossman in 1970, in response to concerns about the status of nursing in the NHS, and standards of training. The Briggs Report criticised the dispersal of nursing education (in 1970 there were 727 training schools in Britain) and the two-tier qualification. To reduce high turnover in the profession, the report argued that instead of recruiting students on academic record, motivation must be the key to selection. An eighteen-month foundation training in basic nursing skills was recommended for all courses, with the pupil nurses qualifying as SENs and the more academic students moving into their chosen branch for a further 18 months. Specialisation, according to the Briggs Committee, was not preparing students for holistic care and for community practice. The report was widely welcomed for emphasising the distinct role of nurses, who were presented as not merely doctors' aides but as practitioners in their own right. However, Clark was furious: his report had been ignored, and it seemed that training in social therapy had been taken off the agenda.[152]

While medical hegemony was being revived by advances in diagnosis and treatment, a multidisciplinary ethos was gradually developing in the mental hospitals. Belatedly, clinical psychologists were introduced, although they were spread thinly.[153] Bob Wycherly[154] had a humble baptism at Middlewood Hospital in Sheffield, where he was given a set of keys and a basic set of rating scales. For individual sessions with patients, Bob could only use the busy nursing office; later a hut was erected in the grounds. Psychologists had little autonomy; any therapeutic intervention required prior approval by the consultant psychiatrist. Except at prestigious teaching hospitals such as The Maudsley, they had limited influence.[155] However, various behavioural treatment regimes were supervised by psychologists from the 1960s onwards. At Graylingwell, for example, patients who had been 'dried out' in the alcohol unit participated in a treatment programme combining group therapy and the drug Antabuse, which caused severe headache and vomiting if a patient drank alcohol.[156] Aversion treatment was used for phobias, and for sexual deviance including cross-dressing and paedophilia. Patients who would now rightfully identify themselves as gay, accepted treatment for this as a mental illness:[157] electrical shocks were administered to homosexual men as they were shown pornographic male images.

The 1959 Mental Health Act and rapid turnover of patients necessitated greater input by social workers in the mental hospitals. Psychiatric social work training had begun as far back as 1929 at the London School of Economics, but most social work for mental patients was performed by unqualified mental welfare officers, normally based in local authority offices.[158] In the early 1960s the government began to invest more in social services, and a doubling of qualified social workers was projected. By the end of the decade most mental hospitals had a psychiatric social worker on site, enabling coordination of medical and social care.

John Greene, a pioneer of community psychiatric nursing, saw a clear distinction between the roles of the social worker and the nurse in the community; the latter encompassed psychological and physical care, and advising district nurses and others on symptoms of mental disorder. By the 1960s there were five community psychiatric nurses in Plymouth,[159] but in most parts of the country there were scant opportunities to work outside hospital in a nursing capacity. Many nurses were attracted to social work. Having spent time with psychiatric social workers at Denbigh, Andrew McCrae was considering career options as he neared completion of his RMN course in 1962. After fellow student Ron Lloyd saw an advertisement in the *Liverpool Daily Post* for social work trainees, both were recruited as mental welfare officers, on the strength of their nursing experience.[160] On their first day they were each given a large case book; no training was ever provided. Barry Hopper[161] was also drawn to psychiatric social work following nurse training at Graylingwell. Nurses like Barry were attracted by a relatively autonomous professional role away from the constraints and subservience of nursing. And there was better pay.

The Council for Training in Social Work, established in 1962, favoured a generic rather than specialised qualification. Social work became fashionable at the new universities such as Keele, attracting bearded intellectual types who buried their noses in Pelican paperbacks on critical sociological theory. Following the recommendations of the Seebohm Report, the Local Authority Social Services Act 1970 unified the various strands of social work into a single social services department in each borough. This meant that close working relationships with psychiatrists were broken, as Hugh Freeman regretted:

> With the huge increase in scale of the new social services organization, it proved impossible for the kind of intimate working relationships which the clinicians had previously enjoyed with those in charge of the local authority mental health service to continue. Though the weekly case conferences went on for some time, they seemed to be attended by a shifting population of social workers, often with little apparent knowledge of mental health problems or overt concern for them.[162]

Ten years after the 'water tower' speech, the old mental hospitals had changed irreversibly. Gone was the farm, the medical superintendent, matron and chief male nurse, while desegregation of male and female divisions was progressing. Wards were less cramped, although the population was declining considerably slower than expected by government policy. At West Park in Epsom, for example, the total of 1,862 occupied beds in 1960 fell to 1,688 by 1970[163] – not enough to make nurses fear for their future. Few would have taken notice of the Worcester Development Project: launched in 1968, this was the first complete closure plan for a mental hospital.[164] Powick, the former county asylum, would be replaced by a community-based service, with two new psychiatric units of 150 beds and sixty beds in Worcester and Kidderminster respectively. Admissions to Powick were to cease by 1973. This was an experiment specially funded by the DHSS to test the viability of mental health policy, but elsewhere, hospital managers were in no rush to empty their wards.

While the 1960s to early 1970s was a time of progress in psychiatric nursing, the period was tainted by scandals. This chapter makes difficult reading for anyone with a rose-tinted view of the mental hospitals, but it should be acknowledged that most nurses continued to care despite the adversity of their impoverished and stigmatised environment. American documentary filmmaker Frederick Wiseman, whose *Titicut Follies* displayed the brutal regime in a Massachusetts hospital for the criminally insane, gave an insightful retrospect on his controversial first movie:

> Nobody could make a film about Bridgewater and not show how horrible it was. On the other hand, I think the guards, in their own rough-and-ready way, were more tuned into the needs of the patients than the so-called helping middle-class professionals, the psychiatrists and the social workers.[165]

Failings of care were not simply due to an outmoded institutional culture. The enquiries revealed not only problems of old, but also the outcomes of liberalisation. Reform of psychiatric care was driven by ideals that were not always fulfilled, as positive therapeutic practice was harder to ensure than adherence to rules and routine. Dismantling of the old regime should be understood in the context of broader social change, as society embraced postmodern ideology and moral relativism. Critics of this long-term trend[166] in societal mores contrast the liberal assumption of innate human goodness with the Christian doctrine of flawed nature. Just as teachers were abandoning didactic authority in favour of child-centred learning, mental nurses became facilitators of patients' latent potential. For nurses in the mould cast by the likes of David Clark, this was a role performed with compassion and commitment, but for others the relaxation of rules and routines was an excuse to sit back.

Patients needed a push, but in subtle collusion with nurses they could remain in the stable environment of the ward. At Phoenix House, the rehabilitation unit at Long Grove, despite patients being taught decimal currency and social skills in preparation for discharge, Ian Norman[167] recalls them having little desire to return to their Cockney roots where it all went wrong many years ago. Nurses repeatedly found that these chronic schizophrenics from the East End, several with leucotomy scars, would contrive a relapse. Having disposed of the patients most amenable to discharge to families or the few hostels, the mental hospitals were left with a rump of severely institutionalised people who appeared totally dependent on nursing care. For the majority of nurses, the case for the mental hospital was never in doubt.

Notes

1 Powell E (1961): Opening speech. *Annual Conference of the National Association for Mental Health*.
2 Tooth GC, Brooke EM (1961): Trends in the mental hospital population and their effect on future planning. *Lancet*.
3 Ministry of Health (1962): *A Hospital Plan for England and Wales*.
4 In 1963 there were 144 mental deficiency hospitals in England and Wales, accommodating 59,980 patients.
5 Smith S (1973): Psychiatric units and relation to mental hospitals. In *Psychiatric Hospital Care: a Symposium* (ed. H Freeman).

6   Sainsbury P (1973): A comparative evaluation of a comprehensive community psychiatric service. In *Policy for Action: a Symposium on the Planning of a Comprehensive Psychiatric Service.*

7   Freeman H (1965): Day hospitals. In *Psychiatric Hospital Care: a Symposium* (ed. H Freeman).

8   Farndale WAJ (1961).

9   Weeks KF (1965): The Plymouth Nuffield Clinic: a community mental health centre. In *Psychiatric Hospital Care: a Symposium* (ed. H Freeman).

10   Denham J (1965): Community care – basic needs and geographical factors: what local authorities should be providing *now*. In *Psychiatric Hospital Care: a Symposium* (ed. H Freeman).

11   Day T (1993).

12   Personal communication (PN, 2015). Felicity is renowned for her book *The Unpopular Patient,* which reported her study of the attitudes and behaviours of nurses in medical and surgical wards towards patients who they disliked, undoubtedly inspired by her experience with general nurses at the St Thomas' psychiatric unit.

13   Wing JK, Monck E, Brown GW, Carstairs GM (1964): Morbidity in the community of schizophrenic patients discharged from London mental hospitals in 1959. *British Journal of Psychiatry.*

14   Oakwood, the former Kent County Asylum, was an example.

15   Personal communication (NM, 1998).

16   Gittins D (1998).

17   Barton R (1959): *Institutional Neurosis.*

18   Wing JK, Brown GW (1961): Social treatment of chronic schizophrenia: a comparative survey of three mental hospitals. *Journal of Mental Science.*

19   Wing JK, Brown GW (1970): *Institutionalism and Schizophrenia: a Comparative Study of Three Mental Hospitals 1960–1968.* Population figures at end of 1959.

20   Rees L (1965): Drug therapy in perspective (discussion). In *The Scientific Basis of Drug Therapy in Psychiatry* (eds J Marks, CMB Pare). 205.

21   Entwhistle C (1968): Overcrowding in mental hospitals (letter). *Lancet.*

22   Wilkinson D (1994): Douglas Bennett: in conversation. *Psychiatric Bulletin.*

23   Gittins D (1998).

24   Rapoport RN (1960): *Community as Doctor: New Perspectives on a Therapeutic Community.*

25   Clark DH (1965): Ward therapeutic community and effects on hospital. In *Psychiatric Hospital Care: a Symposium* (ed. H Freeman).

26   Clark DH (1965). 78.

27   Foucault M (1961): *Madness and Civilisation: a History of Insanity in the Age of Reason.* When first published in France in 1961, few in Britain had heard of the thirty-four year-old philosopher but by the time of its translation to English, Foucault had shaken the intellectual world.

28   Cooper D (1970): *Psychiatry and Anti-Psychiatry.* 96.

29   Cooper D (1970). 102.

30   Wansbrough SN (1971): The future of industrial therapy. *Lancet.*

31   Wing JK, Brown GW (1970). 90.

32   Cohen GL (1964): *What's Wrong with Hospitals.* 145.

33   Wall BA (1977).

34   Cohen GL (1964). 144.

35   Gardner J (1999).

36   Cohen GL (1964). 144.

37   Morris R (1998): *Shelton: Past and Present.*

38   Department of Health and Social Security (1969): *The Facilities and Services of Psychiatric Hospitals in England and Wales 1966.* Showing hospitals with high, medium and low rates of elderly admissions.

39   Whitehead A (1970): *In the Service of Old Age: the Welfare of Psychogeriatric Patients.*

40 Personal communication (NM, 2013).
41 Personal communication (NM, 1998).
42 Personal communication (NM, 1998). According to Carmel, this practice persisted in the 1980s.
43 Nolan P (1993).
44 John A (1961). *A Study of the Psychiatric Nurse.* 147.
45 Menzies IEP (1960): A case study in the functioning of social systems as a defence against anxiety: a report on a study of the nursing service of a general hospital. *Human Relations.*
46 Moss MC, Hunter P (1963): Community methods of treatment. *British Journal of Medical Psychology.*
47 Personal communication (PN, 2015).
48 Jones M (1968): *Social Psychiatry in Practice: the Idea of the Therapeutic Community.*
49 Martin DV (1968): *Adventure in Psychiatry.* 147.
50 Morrice JKW (1964): The ward as a therapeutic group. *British Journal of Medical Psychology.*
51 Department of Health and Social Security (1971): *The State Enrolled Nurse.*
52 Committee on Higher Education (1963): *Higher Education: Report of the Committee.*
53 Royal College of Nursing (1964): *A Reform of Nursing Education: First Report of a Special Committee on Nurse Education.*
54 Nolan P (1999). In 1962 Altschul wrote a textbook on psychology for nurses.
55 Peplau H (1988): *Interpersonal Relations in Nursing.*
56 Altschul A (1957): *Aids to Psychiatric Nursing.*
57 According to David Glenister, who spent many an hour in candid conversation with Altschul, Peplau's focus on one-to-one relationships was seen by Altschul as befitting the individualism of American culture; instead she wanted nursing to be understood and practised as a social endeavour.
58 Glenister DA (2008).
59 May AR (1965): Observations on training the psychiatric nurse. In *Psychiatric Hospital Care: a Symposium* (ed. H Freeman). 265.
60 Bray RE, Bird TE (1964): *The Practice of Psychiatric Nursing.*
61 Ackner B (ed. 1964): *Handbook for Psychiatric Nurses* (8th edition).
62 Glenister DA (2008).
63 Hopper B (2011).
64 Personal communication with Ian Norman (NM, 2014). The 'Red Book' was used in Ian's combined RMN and mental subnormality course at St Ebba's and Long Grove Hospital, which he completed in 1976.
65 Personal communication with Carmel Piris (NM, 1998). It was eventually removed in 1975, after years of disuse.
66 Communication *via* Ali Costelloe (NM, 2013). www.canehill.org.
67 Personal communication (NM, 2013).
68 Personal communication (NM, 2013).
69 May AR (1964).
70 Adams JS (2009). *Challenge and Change in a Cinderella Service: a History of Fulbourn Hospital, Cambridgeshire, 1953–1995.*
71 Adams JS (2009). 177.
72 Clark DH (1974). 53.
73 Clark D (1974): *Social Therapy in Psychiatry.* 124.
74 Hopper B (2011). 230
75 Personal communication (PN, 2014).
76 Personal communication (NM, 1998).
77 Personal communication (NM, 2012).
78 Ministry of Health (1966).
79 Ministry of Health (1966).

80   Department of Health and Social Security (1972): *Progress on Salmon*.
81   The medical superintendent role was finally abolished throughout the NHS in 1971.
82   Personal communication with Tom Harrison (PN, 2014).
83   Personal communication with Tom Harrison (PN, 2014).
84   Personal communication (PN, 2014).
85   Adams JS (2009). 215
86   Personal communication (NM, 2014).
87   Personal communication (PN, 2014).
88   Personal communication (NM, 2013).
89   Personal communication (NM, 2015).
90   Valentine R (1996). 106.
91   *Taking over the Asylum*. BBC Radio 3 (December 1999).
92   Personal communication – name withheld (NM, 2014).
93   Quoted in Adams JS (2009). 214.
94   Personal communication (NM, 2015).
95   Personal communication (NM, 2012).
96   Crofts F (1998).
97   Personal communication (NM, 1996).
98   Personal communication (NM, 1998).
99   Michael P (2003).
100 Gittins D (1998).
101 Beresford A (1965): Integrating nursing service and mixing the sexes in a psychiatric hospital. *Nursing Times*.
102 Hopper B (2012).
103 Unlike most other hospitals, not until the 1980s did male and female patients share wards at Tooting Bec.
104 Cohen GL (1964). 151.
105 Author of the classic history of nursing, published in 1960.
106 Robb B (ed. 1967): *Sans Everything: a Case to Answer*.
107 This tendency has been repeatedly illustrated by political masters determined to keep a lid on serious problems, as recently illustrated by suppression of complaints at a general hospital in Stafford, which eventually led to a national scandal and a damning investigation (the Francis Report, 2013).
108 National Health Service (1968): *Findings and Recommendations Following Enquiries into Allegations Concerning the Care of Elderly Patients in Certain Hospitals*.
109 National Health Service (1969): *Report of the Committee of Inquiry into Allegations of Ill-Treatment of Patients and Other Irregularities at the Ely Hospital, Cardiff*.
110 Crossman RHS (1977): *The Diaries of a Cabinet Minister* (volume III). 195.
111 Personal communication (NM, 2013).
112 Bowen WAL (1965): Need for inspection (or survey) of psychiatric hospital services. In *Psychiatric Hospital Care: a Symposium* (ed. H Freeman). 14–15
113 Discussion of Bowen's paper.
114 Jones DAN (1968): Mental hospitals: a suitable cause for concern. *Sunday Times Magazine*.
115 Martin JP (1984): *Hospitals in Trouble*. 115.
116 The Ministry of Health was reorganised into the Department of Health and Social Security (DHSS) in 1968.
117 National Health Service (1972): *Report of the Committee of Inquiry into Whittingham Hospital*. 10.
118 Martin JP (1984). For his role in exposing the abuse at Whittingham, Barry Askew was awarded Campaigning Journalist of the Year at the 1972 IPC National Press Awards.
119 National Health Service (1972). The nurse member was R Kempster, chief nursing officer at St Crispin Hospital in Northampton.
120 Personal communication (NM, 1998).

121 Personal communication (NM, 2013).
122 NHS (1972). 15.
123 Personal communication (NM, 1996).
124 Martin JP (1984).
125 NHS (1972).
126 NHS (1972). 41–42.
127 Martin JP (1984).
128 Personal commination (NM, 2014).
129 Personal communication (NM, 2013).
130 Communication *via* Ali Costelloe (NM, 2013).
131 Crammer J (1990). 174–175.
132 Barton R (1976): *Institutional Neurosis* (3rd edition). 6.
133 Martin JP (1984).
134 Personal communication (NM, 2015)
135 Gittins D (1998). 186.
136 The recent Stafford Hospital scandal followed a decade of massive investment by the Labour government.
137 Personal communication (NM, 2015).
138 Martin JP (1984). 193.
139 Milligan S (1976): *The New Barons: Union Power in the 1970s.*
140 Personal communication (NM, 2014).
141 Personal communication (NM, 2013).
142 Personal communication (NM, 1998).
143 Barton eventually left Severalls in 1970, when he was embroiled in conflict with the hospital management committee, other doctors in the group, and central government.
144 Brothwood J (1973): The development of national policy: some further aspects of mental health policy. In *Policy for Action: a Symposium on the Planning of a Comprehensive Psychiatric Service.*
145 Department of Health and Social Security (1971): *Hospital Services for the Mentally Ill.*
146 Based on data compiled by Glenister (2008) from Ministry of Health / DHSS annual reports (data on part-time staff excluded).
147 Brothwood J (1973).
148 Kessel N (1973): The district general hospital is where the action is. In *Policy for Action: a Symposium on the Planning of a Comprehensive Psychiatric Service.*
149 Jones K, Sidebotham R (1962): *Mental Hospitals at Work.*
150 Jones K (1993). 183.
151 Fry A (2008): *Never Mind the Mind: Maudsley Hospital 1968–72 – a Narrative.*
152 Adams JS (2009).
153 According to Spratley and Stern (1952), the first full-time psychologist appointed in a public mental hospital in Britain was Miss Eleanor Eattell at Hatton, back in 1943.
154 Personal communication (NM, 2001).
155 Buchanan RD (2010): *Playing with Fire: the Controversial Career of Hans J Eysenck.*
156 Hopper B (2011).
157 Otherwise they were committing a crime, until 1967 when the Labour government repealed legislation outlawing male homosexuality.
158 McCrae N, Murray J, Huxley P, Evans S (2004): Prospects for mental health social work: a qualitative study of attitudes of service managers and academic staff. *Journal of Mental Health.*
159 Nolan P (2005): The history of community mental health nursing. In *Handbook of Community Mental Health Nursing* (eds M Coffey, B Hannigan).
160 Personal communication (NM, 2011).
161 Hopper B (2012).
162 Freeman H (1984): Mental health services in an English county borough before 1974. *Medical History.*

163 Surrey Area Health Authority (1980): *The Provision of Services for the Mentally Ill*.
164 Hassall C, Rose S (1989): Powick Hospital, 1978–86: a case register study. In *Health Service Planning and Research: Contributions from Psychiatric Case Registers* (ed. JK Wing).
165 Robey T (2015): Art-house cinema. *Telegraph Magazine*, 10 January. Banned for twenty-five years, this remains the only film censored in the USA on grounds other than obscenity.
166 Marsh J (2012): *The Liberal Delusion: the Roots of our Current Moral Crisis*.
167 Personal communication (NM, 2014).

7   Irish days, Mauritian nights

Perhaps the most neglected aspect of the history of the mental hospitals is the cultural diversity of staff and its impact on institutional life. Local people became a minority, as a widening net was trawled to recruit to a relatively unattractive workplace. The Irish were prominent, but from the 1950s onwards the nursing staff was increasingly constituted by recruits from more distant shores. Some foreign nurses, despite arriving with little grasp of English language or understanding of the host society, ascended the hospital hierarchy, or moved into nurse education. Others ended their careers where they began: living on the hospital site and taking every opportunity for overtime, while rarely engaging with the community outside. Why did they come, and how did they experience the peculiar setting of the mental hospital?

Help from neighbours

Recruitment had always been difficult in the mental hospitals, but the problem became more serious after the Second World War. Having exhausted the north-east of England, Wales and Scotland, hospital managers in the south of England increasingly looked across the Irish Sea. Historically there was a long tradition of emigration from Ireland to Britain, which escalated after the potato famine in the mid-nineteenth century. By 1871 there were 672,000 Irish-born people in Britain.[1] They accumulated in cities such as Liverpool and Glasgow, typically in squalid, polluted districts, as described by German socialist Friedrich Engels in his study of the working class in Manchester.[2] Facing hostility from local people for taking jobs, Irish labourers and their large families did not fully integrate with the host society. Their Roman Catholicism was at odds with the prevailing Protestant order in Britain. With their chapels, separate schooling for children and Celtic culture, generations of Irish descendants retained a distinct identity.

While their husbands toiled in heavy industries, many Irish women gained employment in public services, and particularly in nursing. By the 1930s Irish accents were commonly heard in general, fever and maternity hospitals, and the county mental hospitals began to attract men too. During the Second World War their number increased, replacing regular staff pulled into the war effort. The post-war needs of British public services brought a large influx from Ireland, where jobs were few and far between. The Irish government, worried by increasing emigration, tried to control the outflow. In 1944 it established the Liaison Office in Dublin to handle recruitment by English hospitals, but this could be by-passed. By 1946 seventy percent of female nurses at Runwell were Irish.[3] However, with plenty of other work opportunities in Britain, mental hospital representatives sometimes promised more than they would deliver, such as free food and an unrealistically generous time off duty. As Gardner noted in his history of St Francis' Hospital at Haywards Heath,[4] some recruits resigned soon after arrival, apparently using the hospital merely as a platform to seek better-paid and less restrictive work. Nonetheless, foraging in the greenery continued, as matrons or sisters of Irish blood made use of family connections to tempt school leavers to join their compatriots in British mental hospitals.

Morah Geall[5] came to Hellingly Hospital in Sussex in 1950, aged eighteen. Her sister, who was working as a mental handicap nurse in England, gave her addresses of two hospitals. Having the necessary school certificates, Morah was accepted at both, but chose Hellingly instead of a general hospital at East Grinstead due to the slightly better pay. Her travel costs were paid on condition that she stay for six months. After spending a night with family friends in Dublin, Morah boarded the ferry to Holyhead and from there made the long train journey to London. At Victoria station she was met by her sister, and they took a train to Hailsham, a mile from the hospital. After walking in the dark they were met at the gate lodge by the assistant matron. Along the winding, tree-lined drive they passed a large building, which Morah thought must be the hospital, but was told that this was only the admissions unit. She was shown to the nurses' home, where a light meal was provided. On the next day Morah began a career of four decades at this institution perched on the South Downs.

Olive Slattery[6] was raised in Donegal, where career opportunities were very limited. In 1952, after responding to an advertisement in the *Northern Standard*, Olive was invited for interview for nursing in Britain, held at a hotel in the nearest town. Initially she thought that the interviewer was making fun of her as the questions seemed random if not absurd, such as: 'What is the opposite of perfume?' Olive was given puzzles to complete, and participated in a game of noughts and crosses. A letter arrived a few weeks later offering her a job at a fever hospital in Glasgow. On arriving she was welcomed by the largely Irish nursing staff, but she disliked the intensive aseptic procedures and strict discipline. She became familiar with some nurses at the nearby mental hospital and decided to join them. Olive found Gartnavel much more to her taste: although the work was hard, she liked the atmosphere there. The wages were also better, enabling her to send money back to her family.

Despite a steady flow from across the Irish Sea, staff shortage persisted. Mental hospitals desperately sought new sources of labour on the Continent. A few young people were attracted from France and the war-ravaged lands of Eastern Europe. The Ministry of Labour paid travel expenses for recruits from countries such as Austria. So-called aliens were employed as assistant nurses until they mastered English sufficiently to start nurse training, and they were not allowed to converse in their own language except in the nurses' home. Some hospitals in the south-east, such as Hellingly, attracted large numbers of French girls, although many did not complete their training. Their abilities were often grossly underestimated. At Warneford, for example, Judith Watson[7] recalled several refugees from Lithuania and East Germany, who were never given responsibility merited by their professional or scientific background. Such nurses could communicate with the foreign patients who had appeared after the war, some of whom bore tattooed numbers on their arms, identifying them as survivors of Nazi concentration camps. Of all European nations, most fruitful were Spain and Italy, the former under the military dictatorship of General Franco, and the latter in economic and political turmoil.

Carlos Forni's[8] Spanish mother and Italian father met at Bexley Hospital. His mother came to England in 1955 from Madrid, intending to learn English before returning to Spain to work in banking. In the following year his father, aged twenty and living in impoverished Ferrara in northern Italy, wrote to authorities in England for work, and was offered a job at Bexley. Neither parent spoke English on their arrival. They married in 1959, after Carlos was born, and eventually they bought a house for their growing family in Dartford. His father work in the daytime, while his mother did night duty. Their social network entirely comprised hospital staff, mainly fellow Spaniards and Italians. Carlos' first visit to the hospital was for a patients' dance, when he was eight years of age. He was not frightened but fascinated by the strange people, with odd clothing and behaviour: women with facial hair, missing dentures and clumsy movements. In 1977, when aged eighteen, Carlos followed in his parents' footsteps at Bexley, initially working as a volunteer with elderly patients. His mother and father worked there until retirement, a few years before the hospital closed. Their standard of living had improved substantially since their early years at Bexley, when days were long and pay was poor.

Recruitment campaigns were not supplying enough workers to run the wards, to wash the incontinent, or to watch the suicidal; indeed, the viability of some hospitals was at stake. As human wells dried up, hospital managers broadened their horizon to the colonies of the Caribbean, western and southern Africa, the Indian subcontinent and the East Indies. The composition of mental hospital staff was about to change dramatically.

Ports on the hill

In the early twentieth century a few African and Asian people lived in areas such as the east end of London, and the established black communities in Liverpool and Bristol. In response to severe post-war labour shortages, Britain tapped its imperial legacy. A seminal event was the arrival of SS *Windrush* from the Caribbean in June 1948, when 500 West Indians disembarked at Tilbury Dock.[9] Bus conductors, public lavatory attendants and other menial jobs were undertaken by men from the colonies of Jamaica, Barbados and Trinidad. Two thousand West Indians arrived in 1953, rising to 30,000 in 1956, mostly settling in parts of London and the Midlands. As Commonwealth subjects, they were afforded citizenship rights by the British Nationality Act 1948, but they experienced much prejudice. Indigenous working class people feared that the immigrants would take their jobs and houses, while some complained of immoral behaviour bringing down the tone of their neighbourhood, and of indolent incomers drawing public assistance. Trade unions often supported a colour bar in factories.[10]

Black nurses began to appear in mental hospitals in the mid-1950s. Some received a frosty reception. Nurses at Storthes Hall opposed the arrival of twenty-nine probationers from Nigeria and Jamaica; in 1954 the Cefn Coed branch of COHSE argued that the employment of six young women from Barbados should not have been necessary, as local people would be attracted to such work if pay and conditions were improved.[11] As well as enduring the cold climate, nurses from the colonies were susceptible to European diseases to which they had no immunity. Gardner[12] records the death of a Nigerian nurse, aged twenty, from acute bronchial pneumonia; her distraught and angry parents were physically restrained at the inquest.

The large number of West Indians settling in the Birmingham area was reflected in the hospital workforce. Mary and Sophie Slevin,[13] sisters from County Monaghan in Northern Ireland who came to All Saints in the late 1950s, found such nurses polite and gregarious, although not always able to develop a rapport with patients, and their unease in performing intimate care tasks was not helped by some patients preferring white nurses to care for them. According to Mary and Sophie, the West Indian nurses insisted on using their own cups in tea breaks, avoiding any cutlery or crockery used by patients due to their belief that mental illness was contagious. Respectful to senior nursing staff and deferential to doctors, they took their training seriously, and some were promoted to charge nurses and ward sisters within a few years of qualification.

As gender segregation of staff was relaxed in the 1960s, courtships occurred between West Indians and local nurses. Outside the tolerant atmosphere of the mental hospital, white women who fraternised with black men were often ostracised. Although interracial marriage became common long before its acceptance in wider society, engagement to someone of other ethnicity was a delicate announcement for a nurse writing home, as depicted in the popular fiction of Catherine Cookson:

> Dear Ma ... there's something I should tell you, but I can't write it down.[14]

After gaining eight school certificates in Kingston in Jamaica, in the late 1960s Herman Wheeler[15] was working as a research assistant in a malarial laboratory. Seeing advertisements for nurse training in England, he contacted Rubery Hill Hospital, and was assured that he would receive an excellent training that would help him to a position of seniority back in Jamaica. Nothing was mentioned about this being a psychiatric hospital. Herman travelled to London in his best suit, but he lacked the overcoat and hat donned by other passengers on landing at Heathrow. As soon as the cabin door was opened, Herman shivered, never having felt such cold. He found his way to the hospital on the outskirts of Birmingham, and presented himself for work on the next day. The chief male nurse was a Scot with a heavy accent, incomprehensible to Herman, who had expected everyone to speak like presenters on BBC World Service. Sent to a geriatric ward with seventy patients, Herman toiled in making beds and polishing floors, work that would have been performed by servants in Jamaica. When his training began, Herman asked the principal tutor if he could move to a ward where he could learn more about nursing. He was invited to become a member of the nurse education committee, and his forthright views led to the hospital employing twenty domestic workers, so that nurses could spend more time with patients. Herman knew that he had irritated the senior ranks, but he was undeterred from criticising deficiencies in the hospital. He was upset by discriminatory treatment of black patients, who were given enormous doses of medication; he suggested to some of these men that they return home.

A pioneering project involving Nigerian nurses began at Hollymoor in Birmingham in the mid-1950s. It centred on the work of Dr Thomas Adeoye Lambo[16] who had qualified in medicine in England, before returning to his native land to take charge of the newly built Aro psychiatric hospital in Abeokuta. Prior to independence from Britain in 1960, the Nigerian government attempted to introduce a modern psychiatric system, but institutionalisation of mental health care was viewed with suspicion by Nigerians, who preferred to seek help from native herbalists. Lambo saw that the best way forward was to integrate traditional religious practices with Western ideas about mental health. He embraced village support, combined with modern treatments and therapies. Local farmers were encouraged to employ patients as labourers, and native healers to work alongside medical practitioners. With his strength of personality, Lambo played a key role in reducing stigma towards the mentally ill and their families, persuading Nigerian society of the need for proper care and treatment.

It was during a placement at Hollymoor that Lambo had appreciated the valuable contribution of mental nurses. He had observed that while patients feared talking to doctors, nurses spoke in familiar terms and did not claim to know more about them than they did about themselves. Lambo wanted to bring the best of British mental nursing into the system he was devising in Nigeria. He founded a nurse training college in Nigeria and invited a senior nurse and a tutor from England to run it.[17] He also arranged for Nigerians to do mental nurse training at Hollymoor, where he instructed the English nurses in aspects of Nigerian culture and suggested how they could acquaint the visitors with the host community. Twice each year, five or six Nigerian nurses arrived at the hospital. On completion of their training, the hospital management committee arranged farewell parties, and contact was maintained with the Nigerians after they returned home. Over time, Nigerian nurses trained in England assumed teaching roles in Lambo's college.

The wave of migration from the Indian subcontinent began in 1955, when 7,800 arrived in Britain. They accumulated in northern mill towns and fading hubs of the textile industry such as Leicester. Like the Caribbeans, normally young men came first, bringing their families later. While black migrants brought the enticing rhythms of reggae and ska, Asians flavoured British life with the culinary delights of the curry house. There was no rapid transformation in people's attitudes towards those of different culture, but a gradual process of adapting to a new social reality.

> The way in which the British viewed the outside world could never be quite the same after they had accepted into their midst thousands of newcomers from overseas, and similarly, the easy assumption that Britishness itself was a matter of racial inheritance was no longer acceptable in a multi-racial society.[18]

As highlighted by social historians such as Dominic Sandbrook and David Kynaston, no topic was as controversial and emotive during the late 1950s and 1960s as immigration. In 1962 Macmillan's government acted on public anxieties by imposing restrictions on unskilled migrants. However, there was dispensation for the NHS, which had 25,000 nursing vacancies in 1961; efforts to raise standards of care in hospitals for mental illness and mental handicap were hampered by severe understaffing. Nursing was not necessarily the first career choice of immigrants from the colonies, but the NHS offered an opportunity for a professional qualification, with full board and recreational facilities. For black or Asian nurses, there would be no need to navigate the market for rental accommodation that did not exclude 'coloureds'.

Beyond the relative sanctuary of the mental hospital, underlying racial tension was never far from the surface. Public unease at the growing number of immigrants led to an outspoken intervention in 1968 by Enoch Powell. In his infamous 'Rivers of Blood' speech to West Midlands Conservatives, Powell warned of the danger of mass immigration, predicting riots and eventual enslavement of white people. Instantly dismissed from the Conservative shadow cabinet, Powell argued that he was representing the views of his constituents in Wolverhampton, where local people felt swamped by foreigners; such opinion was indeed evident in the local newspaper.[19] Around this time another surge of immigration arose following decolonisation in East Africa, where a merchant Asian class was sent packing by despotic leaders of newly independent Uganda and Tanzania. The 1971

Census recorded over 650,000 people originating from the West Indies, India or Pakistan.[20] By then, it was often said that the NHS would fall apart without its foreign doctors and nurses.

On leaving school in Hong Kong, Tom Chan[21] enquired at the British Consulate for work in Britain. In the 1960s there was a troubling political situation in the colony, with communist China flexing its muscles, and an uncertain economic future. Park Prewett Hospital in Hampshire was offering places for nurse training, and having gained a work permit Tom travelled to Britain. On the train from Waterloo he was struck by the grimy buildings, which surprised him as this was the capital of the Empire. In his experience in Hong Kong, British people were of high social class and wealth, but he soon realised that the colonial administrators were not representative of the general population. At Park Prewett he sat a screening test, set by the psychologist Mr Staunton. Those who passed became RMN students; failures did pupil nurse training. About half of Tom's cohort was from overseas. He observed that the foreign trainees were not only more educated than those of the host country, who struggled with calculations, but also the tutors. In a session on measuring alkalinity and acidity, Tom corrected a tutor who wrote 'PH' on the blackboard, instead of 'pH'.

Perhaps the most notable foreign import to mental nursing was from a small island in the Indian Ocean. Under control of France until 1810, Mauritius had a rigidly hierarchical social structure, with a vast populace of black slaves from Madagascar and the African mainland, various artisans occupying the middle ranks, and an elite class of landowners, merchants and a professional class of French descent.[22] After abolition of slavery in 1833, the British brought indentured labour from India to work on the sugar plantations. Education offered a glimmer of hope for poor children, and pupils clamoured for entry to the Cambridge Examination Certificate or the Oxford Examination Board.[23] Yet many, despite their academic achievement, failed to secure a permanent job in their homeland. When Mauritius gained independence in 1968, the first prime minister was a London-trained doctor, who made improvement of health services a priority. An agreement was made with the British government to facilitate training of Mauritian nurses, and interviews were arranged annually in the capital, Port Louis. However, many of those who travelled did not return: not surprisingly, understaffed NHS hospitals wanted to keep those they had trained.

Jean McFarlane, professor of nursing at University of Manchester,[24] observed that nurses from Mauritius were generally calm, courteous and hard workers who liked to do the job properly. Jean was intrigued by their response to patients. Many could not accept that some patients were mentally ill; by Mauritian standards, there was no need for them to be in hospital. In their homeland they had seen

In the late 1960s and 1970s, around 40,000 young people came to British hospitals from this colonial outpost. One of those who stayed was Teeranlall Ramgopal (Ram),[25] who came from the small town of Rivière des Anguilles. On leaving school, Ram would have struggled to get a job in the two nearby hospitals, the Civil and the Queen Victoria; both had a mostly British clinical staff, with merely a few Mauritian nurses. In 1970, attending interview for training in England, Ram was astonished by the amount of fellow applicants in the waiting room. The interview was conducted in English by a white British nurse; Ram later learned that she was matron in a hospital in Port Louis acting on behalf of the British government. Ram thought that he had done well, although he was admonished for using the slang 'yeah' instead of 'yes'. Almost a year later, he received a letter confirming a place at Stafford Hospital. Although he had not heard of the town, Ram was ecstatic and became the envy of his friends. While his parents were pleased for him, they worried that he might not come back.

On 14 August 1971, Ram set off from Plaisance Airport, where 300 friends and relatives bid him farewell. This was the first time he had flown; he found Frankfurt Airport (where he changed to another flight) daunting, and he was overwhelmed by the human throng at Heathrow. On the train to Stafford, he was surprised by the green countryside. On arrival he was given tea in the hospital canteen, but then stayed in his room in the nurses' home for two days, eating biscuits and drinking tap water. Tiredness, hunger and homesickness overwhelmed him and he was very grateful when some Malaysian nurses knocked on his door and invited him for a curry – his first real meal in England.

Ram began general nurse training in September. On entering the wards, he met the only Mauritian doctor in the hospital, who was polite but not friendly towards him. This man appeared to have learned from other doctors that nurses were not to be seen as his social equals. Ram met some male nurses doing a general hospital placement as part of their psychiatric nurse training. He found that these nurses had a good sense of humour and an ease in relating to people. Ram decided that as soon as he had gained the SRN certificate, he would apply for psychiatric training at nearby St George's Hospital. Initially he found St George's frightening, with its high walls, locked doors and aggressive patients. Soon, however, Ram came to enjoy the conviviality between staff and patients, which he preferred to the stilted atmosphere of the general hospital.

people with much worse mental disturbance who were looked after by relatives and friends. Not all Mauritians adjusted well to nursing in Britain; some returned home before completing their training, while others qualified but changed to different types of work. According to Ian Norman,[26] there was a sense of exploitation among nurses from Mauritius at Long Grove:

Some Mauritian nurses I knew felt that they had been taken advantage of by the hospital, which appeared to offer them a professional nursing career – and then on arrival in Blighty finding themselves on the SEN programme rather than the RMN one.

SEN training emphasised basic nursing care and ward routines, and some Mauritians found this demeaning: they were expected to perform tasks below their social status at home, as a nurse at Horton remarked:

We didn't expect to have to shave patients, or empty commodes.[27]

Many Mauritian enrolled nurses eventually qualified as RMNs, but it took them much longer than white colleagues to reach this level. Meanwhile, they resented being paid less than colleagues while taking on similar responsibilities. To some extent, working overtime compensated for this disadvantage. Mauritian nurses were appreciated for their willingness to work on holidays and weekends, and to cover staff shortages on other wards. As implied by the title of this chapter, many chose night duty, working alongside similarly nocturnal compatriots.[28]

From monastery to mental hospital

By the 1960s, over one-third of the workforce of some hospitals in England was from Ireland. Most Irish recruits had no prior experience of mental nursing, but a few had worked in institutions run by Catholic charities. When co-author PN entered nurse training at Tooting Bec in September 1962, he and one other of the six Irish in his cohort had come from religious orders (there was also an Englishman who had left the Jesuit priesthood, and four Indian nuns). In a study in the 1990s, PN and fellow scholars[29] interviewed fourteen people who had left monasteries or convents and later entered mental health work. An important skill acquired by such workers in their previous calling was self-contemplation (as emphasised in mental health nurse training today, one must understand oneself before one can understand others). With a spiritual orientation, the nurse of monastic background could look beyond mere appearance to consider the patient's plight in a deeper existential context.

In an increasingly secular society, those leaving religious orders were reluctant to divulge their past to others for fear of stereotyping or ridicule. Interviewees had been drawn to such servitude by the promise of structure and meaning to their lives; most had enjoyed the silence, the music and chanting, wearing a habit, and the rewards of pastoral work. However, for a variety of reasons, they had become disillusioned with monastic life. As well as the strict rules, they did not always find other members of the community to be kindly or good role models; some had felt themselves fraudulent when treated with reverence by local people. Difficulties were often experienced on leaving the religious order: a confused identity, feeling that family had been let down; some suffered from depression or turned to alcohol. Yet while their search for truth was frustrated, they developed a strong social conscience, eventually leading them into the caring professions. Four of the interviewees went into psychiatric nursing, where they found the work spiritually and materially fulfilling. They gained personal insights through attending to the suffering of others, as this nurse reflected:

> It was part of my own recovery, my own interest in the way that humans can transform themselves. I still felt I had to honour my vow to God that I would serve people.[30]

Recruits of monastic background were well prepared for the institutional detachment of psychiatric nursing, and those from Catholic orders in Ireland could feel at home in Britain alongside so many kinsfolk.

Tony Quinn[31] came from Limerick to Tooting Bec Hospital in 1963, encouraged by an aunt working there as a ward sister. Tony had little notion of what the job entailed, and he was awestruck by the size of the buildings, and the myriad of nationalities, accents and diets. Initially Tony shied from starting conversations for fear of his strong Irish accent not being understood, and he was reluctant to answer the telephone. He was grateful for the guidance of COHSE representative, Bernard Morgan, who helped him to adjust to life in England and to appreciate the importance of psychiatric nursing. The majority of nurses from Ireland, in Tony's opinion, were good carers, irrespective of their knowledge and skills. He attributed this to their religious education and upbringing in small communities in which people looked after each other. However, the physician superintendent, also an Irishman, was arrogant and aloof; nurses satirised him as a feudal lord, riding roughshod over the peasants. Meeting colleagues from other parts of the world, asking them how they came to England, their hopes, and what they thought of working at the hospital: for Tony this was an education in itself. He found a vibrant social life at the hospital, and like many nurses he met his spouse (Angela, a Greek émigré) at a staff dance.

The Irish emigrants may have missed the tight community bonds of home, but some felt liberated from Catholic moralism. At All Saints, Mary and Sophie Slevin[32] came across a few young Irish patients who had been dispatched to England after giving birth out of wedlock, their babies having been taken for adoption. The stress of forced emigration, and loss of a child, caused profound mental distress. With their own experience of religious stricture, the Slevin sisters tried to comfort these women, and were sensitive to the misery that they were enduring.

Imelda Bures,[33] an Irish nurse who married a Czech colleague at Netherne, told of the antics of young nurses raised in the insular and strict Catholic culture in Ireland, whose sudden freedom sometimes produced scenes akin to *Lord of the Flies.* She recalled how four nursing students found an old ECT machine in the dump, and tested it on a goat from the hospital farm; the poor animal died. Irish humour was always appreciated, but in the late 1960s there was a dark cloud on the horizon. 'The Troubles' in Northern Ireland became a very emotive issue, compounded by acts of terrorism spreading to the British mainland.[34] The conflict had enormous impact, and many nurses would have known civilians or servicemen who died in shootings or bombings. Irish nurses sometimes faced an unfair expectation that they should apologise for the deeds of their countrymen and coreligionists. For occupational survival, Ireland was a taboo topic, enabling Protestants and Catholics to maintain good working relationships in mental hospitals. According to Peter Walsh,[35] any religious bigotry of the west of Scotland was left at the gate of Woodilee; indeed, he suggested that the problems of Ulster could have been resolved in a day by the pragmatism and camaraderie of psychiatric nurses.

Fiona Nolan[36] left home, a beef farm in Enniscorthy, County Wexford, in 1984. Her intention was to do nurse training in Britain so that she would qualify for a grant to attend university (she could not afford to study at an Irish university). Initially she took a summer job as a domestic at Cell Barnes mental handicap hospital in St Albans, where her aunt and uncle worked. A few months later, aged eighteen, she started nurse training at Banstead Hospital, where two of her school friends had started nurse training in the previous cohort. Half of her cohort of twelve students was Irish. During the introductory block of six weeks in the nursing school Fiona spent a day at an acute female ward. This was a terrifying experience, not helped by Fiona's consciousness of her rural Irish brogue and her inability to understand the unbridled Cockney of patients.

Challenges for foreign nurses

Mental hospitals, particularly in southern England and the Midlands, began to rely heavily on foreign nurses, who they employed in increasing numbers. Yet the obvious challenges presented by cultural and linguistic differences received scant attention in nursing literature. Psychosocial perspectives on psychiatric nursing, such as by David Clark[37] and by David Towell,[38] skirted around this issue. Eamon Shanley, a tutor in Edinburgh, candidly described the difficulties faced by such nurses – and the impact on patients.[39]

> In many wards the indigenous staff members are in a distinct minority. Overseas staff have little in common with the patients and their values, norms, attitudes and patterns of social interaction may differ. This seems to disregard the effect, whether therapeutic or indeed harmful, of the patient's social environment or his well being.

Shanley considered five factors in the performance of foreign nurses. First, their expectations of nursing were likely to differ from reality. African and Asian recruits had little prior awareness of British hospitals and the differences between general, mental illness and mental handicap. Indeed, recruitment tactics were brazenly economic with the truth, as many ex-nurses from abroad attest to omission of any reference to 'mental' in information provided. Many newcomers were shocked on reaching their destination. For those who had been misled into believing that they would be working in a modern general hospital, the mental institution was an unwelcome surprise: so many disabled people living in bleak, antiquated buildings was not how they had envisaged Britain. Unrealistic ideas could lead to disillusionment and resentment at being used as cheap labour in a stigmatised setting.

The Briggs Committee's report on nursing[40] noted that for some migrants nurse training was merely a gateway to Britain and the hope of a better life, but their continued residence in Britain depended on their status as a student; unless able to pay their way in another field of study, they would need to return home. Indeed, attrition of foreign and native nursing students contrasted sharply: according to one report in the 1970s, the rates were 10 and 35 per cent respectively.[41] Mental nursing recruits were like some early twentieth-century Europeans who crossed the Atlantic to America, passing the Statue of Liberty, only to be held indefinitely on Ellis Island. The mental hospital was the port of entry, but there they stayed.

Shanley's second factor was limited contact with the host culture. Typically foreign recruits started work on the day after arrival, and having little need to venture to nearby towns and amenities, they spent almost all of their time on site, including days off and holidays. Their only window to British society was the television set in the nurses' home. Shanley argued that the authorities should do more to help immigrant recruits to integrate, perhaps by requiring a period of living outside the hospital, enabling them to acclimatise to British life and hence develop better awareness of their patients' circumstances. However, Shanley acknowledged in his third factor the reaction of the host community to immigrants. Racist attitudes were not necessarily blatant, but there was a lurking prejudice that conferred a lower status to people of African or Asian background. To some extent, therefore, the mental hospital was a ghetto.

The fourth factor was language. Many immigrants had a poor grasp of English, obviously restricting their therapeutic potential. Russell Hackett, a nurse at Hellingly, recalled communication problems arising with the large influx of foreign workers in the 1960s.[42] Once he found a patient cleaning the television set with soap and water; after swiftly disconnecting the power supply, Russell asked the patient why he was doing this. The patient pointed to a Mauritian member of staff, explaining it was the member of staff who had told him to do so. With his strong Oriental accent, Tom Chan may have struggled to make himself understood to patients at Park Prewett, but he was not the only one. On M1, his first ward, the staff was of very mixed origin, including Mauritians and Italians. Nowadays such diversity would be expected, but in the 1960s some families complained about foreign nurses' ability to talk to patients. Hospital management committees rejected such criticisms as ignorant or racist attitudes[43], but there was legitimate concern about the effects of linguistic and cultural differences on caring relationships.

Finally Shanley considered job security. On qualifying there was no guarantee of appointment, and as unemployment increased in the 1970s the government changed the law to ensure local people had an opportunity to apply for vacancies. Each job was to be advertised locally for at least three weeks, and the nurse from overseas had the additional requirement of obtaining a work permit. Overall, Shanley concluded that such nurses were not being adequately prepared for their role. Communication difficulties and cultural misunderstandings were barriers to the ideals of the therapeutic community model, with its emphasis on intensive human relationships. Foreign nurses, and consequently their patients, were being neglected by health authorities and the nursing profession.

In 1980, Velvendar Godfrey (Vel) was one of a cohort of mostly Malaysian nursing students starting at Runwell Hospital, which had a relatively small number of foreign staff. Like many other recruits from the former colonies, Vel had felt deceived by the recruitment process. The agency that had visited her school in a rural area near Taiping implied that she would be coming to a general hospital in London, but instead Vel found herself in a psychiatric hospital in a backwater of Essex. She perceived that Malaysian nurses were treated as 'second-class citizens': on qualifying they were posted on the geriatric wards, while white nurses went to the acute wards. Vel attributed this to the Malaysians being 'an unknown quantity'.[44]

Similar issues arose with doctors. In his book *Psychiatry in Dissent*, Anthony Clare lamented the failure to attract medical graduates trained in Britain or Ireland to a career in psychiatry; by 1972, half of NHS psychiatrists were from abroad.[45] A Sri Lankan psychiatrist explained the adversity they faced:

> Having chosen a field he is least interested to work in, befuddled by the terminology of dynamically orientated psychiatry, perplexed by the anxiety-provoking interview of an acute psychiatric admission ward, lacking fluency in the English language, let alone familiarity with the English culture and idiom, the postgraduate tries hard to put on a bold front, masking his chronic anxiety created by apprehension as to when he will succeed in obtaining a job of his choice.[46]

The RCN, giving evidence to a Committee of Inquiry into the Regulation of the Medical Profession, expressed concern about communication problems faced by nurses in working with foreign doctors, making particular reference to psychiatric hospitals.[47] Colloquialisms were often misinterpreted as evidence of psychotic disturbance, such as a patient referring to butterflies in her stomach.

While struggling to adapt to a different culture, many doctors from the Indian sub-continent received little in-service training, and had a low success rate in examinations for membership of the Royal College of Psychiatrists. Understandably their motivation may have been blunted.

Multicultural harmony

While Shanley's paper was a considered account of the challenges faced by nurses from abroad, a consistent message from interviewees for this book is the interracial harmony in the mental hospitals. British nurses accepted that the hospital needed staff, and that foreigners were doing work shunned by local people. In 1973, in Mike O'Connor's[48] training cohort at Park Prewett, three of the fifteen were local people, and one other white British; all others were from Africa or Asia, including Ghana, Philippines, Malaysia and Mauritius. For Mike this was a culture shock after his schooling in Alton, Hampshire. However, while there were some Mauritian charge nurses, the 'officer class' was all white. At the tender age of sixteen, Mandy Everett[49] came from Manchester in 1978 to work in the voluntary service at Cane Hill, where she was given a room in the ground floor of the domestic block. Sharing her corridor were Spanish cleaners, who conversed in their own tongue, but they took Mandy under their wing. Upstairs were cleaners and nursing assistants from the Philippines; on the second floor were men of the estates department, some from northern England like Mandy; the nursing staff was dominated by Scots and Spaniards. When Peter Walsh[50] started at Woodilee Hospital near Glasgow in the mid-1970s, there were several nurses from Mauritius and the Philippines, and a few West Indians; the COHSE secretary was Jamaican. Peter attributes the respect shown for colleagues of different cultures to the need for nurses to support and protect each other in potentially hazardous circumstances.

Some migrant groups grew into established communities in the mental hospitals. At Netherne the dominant nationalities were Irish and Spanish, and intermarriage was common. Mary Gutierrez,[51] an auxiliary nurse from Ireland who married a Spaniard, was once asked for a favour by colleague Paco Espinosa. In the evenings Paco hunted by torchlight for snails, which were considered as a delicacy in his culture. He sometimes worked at a Spanish restaurant in Purley, and on this occasion he was asked to help the chef at short notice. Having collected hundreds of common gastropods from the chalk terrain of Netherne in a carrier bag, he asked Mary to deposit them in a barrel in a ward cupboard until later, when he would take them for steeping in black soda. Unfortunately Mary forgot to put the lid on the container, and consequently the walls and shelves were plastered with slime from the escaping prey.

According to several informants, Netherne was known for its 'Spanish Mafia'. Many from the Iberian peninsula were gipsies, and with their irreverence for authority, they were sometimes seen as a threat by the management. One Irish nursing officer was known to prohibit more than two Spanish nurses working on the same ward. Imelda Bures[52] observed that some Spanish nurses exaggerated their language difficulties to avoid documentation. They also made their presence felt on the football field. Dermot Hennessy[53] played alongside several Spanish players in the Netherne team that won the prestigious London Mental Hospitals Sports Association Cup in the 1970s. As well as midfield maestros, the defence featured members of the hospital 'heavy squad', which was called to deal with violent incidents.

Cultural diversity was celebrated at the staff Christmas party and other annual events, when nurses prepared their national cuisine and wore traditional costumes in a wonderfully colourful spectrum of humanity. People of all backgrounds used the social club, although social circles naturally formed around shared origin. At Park Prewett, Tom Chan[54] and foreign colleagues preferred to play table-tennis, while the club was mostly frequented by white staff. Janet Herd,[55] a general nursing student who had a three-month placement at Warlingham Park in 1971, observed that the mostly Irish and Mauritian staff worked well together and socialised afterwards in the commodious club. According to Janet, the Mauritians were not averse to alcohol but never drank to excess (unlike an overindulgent Irish charge nurse who always propped up the bar).

When Tim Mosses[56] started RMN training at Bexley in 1973, three-quarters of his cohort was foreign, including Indian, Ceylonese, Oriental, Africa and Mauritian students. On the last day of the introductory period at the nursing school, they all went to the social club, except for some female Oriental students who preferred to revise in the nurses' home. This was not because they did not like their peers, but simply because they would not normally go to a bar.[57] A pop band The Crimson Berries, which played regularly at the Bexley social club, comprised a multicultural mix of an Indian, African, English and two Oriental members of staff, performing contemporary songs by the likes of Slade. New musical flavours were infused in the hospital atmosphere. At Cane Hill in the late 1960s, nursing student Peter Robinson[58] often heard the sound of flutes in the evening. On investigation he found some Rastafarian workers testing the acoustics. One of them repeatedly sang 'Rudi don't fear, no boy, Rudi don't fear'; years later Peter discovered that this was from a song *Tougher than Tough* by Jamaican reggae singer Derrick Morgan. Ian Norman[59] remembers Latin flamboyance on the dancefloor at Long Grove discos, often initiated by the popular song *Y Viva Espana*; meanwhile the Mauritians gambled on three card brag in the nurses' home.

The only racial animosity reported by informants for this book occurred during industrial action. Fiona Nolan[60] recalled a bad atmosphere when foreign nurses were accused of exploiting staff unrest for their own pecuniary gain. As a staff nurse at Horton in the winter of 1987 to 1988, she participated alongside most of the nursing staff in a strike resulting from a local dispute. Minimal ward staffing was provided, and COHSE declared an overtime ban. Double and treble pay was offered by management to any willing strike-breakers, and several nurses from Trinidad made a lot of money from the collective withdrawal of their colleagues. The 'blacklegs' (in union slang) probably did not care about the insults when they received their pay packet.

The propagation of foreign nurses was uneven across Britain. According to Allan Hicks,[61] St Lawrence's in Cornwall had two groups of staff: Cornish and southern Irish. Many of the latter had been recruited during the Second World War when male nurses joined the county regiment. They worked up the ranks and by Allan's time the Irish occupied all senior nursing ranks: principal nursing officer, three senior nursing officers and four of the six nursing officers (the other two were Cornish). Apart from the Irish, there were few outsiders: one male nurse from Birmingham, two Chinese nurses (one of whom Allan married – see the box that follows) and an Indian nurse tutor.

Mary Hicks (née Mui) qualified as a psychiatric nurse in Hong Kong. Her training was entirely at Castle Peak, a large institution with 100-bed wards in the New Territories. The UK curriculum and examination applied, with all teaching in English. On the wards Cantonese was spoken, but nursing notes were in English. Two years after qualifying, in 1980 Mary applied for jobs in Canada, Australia and England advertised in the *Nursing Times*; her intention was to work in each country before returning home. The first job offer was at St Lawrence's in Cornwall, and once Mary had confirmed her registration status the hospital obtained her visa and sent travel directions. After the 16-hour flight she got a train from Paddington to Bodmin. On this late Sunday afternoon in December, the station was very dark and with all her belongings in tow, Mary was glad to be met by a senior nursing officer in his car. In her tiny room in the nurses' home, Mary burst into tears: there was nobody around and she felt adrift. Unable to sleep due to jet lag, she stared at the walls and ruminated. In the morning she went to the main building for induction and on the Tuesday started on the 'sick ward'.

Mary was one of few foreigners at St Lawrence's: there was a Malaysian and two Mauritian nurses, and a Mauritian canteen worker. Everyone was friendly. She met some school leavers who were waiting to start nurse training, and was invited to three family Christmas meals. However, Mary found her time off duty tedious. The nurses' home was often deserted, as many nurses only used their rooms for sleeping between late and early shifts, otherwise living out. In the small sitting room Mary could not relate to the soap operas on television. She wrote letters and her daily highlight was going to the mail room. There was a payphone in the nurses' home but ringing Hong Kong was prohibitively expensive. As the bus service to Bodmin was poor, Mary dined in the hospital canteen. She gained weight on the stodgy jam roly-poly and rice pudding. After fourteen months Mary left for a job in London, but shortly before leaving she met Allan, a final-year student. They married, and Mary cancelled her world tour.

Cultural patterns may have been discernible among nurses of particular origin such as Hong Kong or the Caribbean, yet each person is unique and their response to their surroundings differed accordingly. It would be folly to view human experience only through the prism of culture. Individual agency tends to be overlooked in generalisations made about people of cultures of traditional community cohesiveness, yet some people came to Britain to escape from stringent social mores.

In rural Malaysian society, a young woman could not go out alone or freely choose a partner. At Runwell, by contrast, there was a lively social club with weekend discos, where Velvendar Godfrey[62] frequently got drunk on Martini or 'snowballs', and had a series of intimate relationships. An attractive young woman, Vel was constantly pursued by male staff and particularly English men. However, fellow Malaysian students disapproved of her behaviour. Vel found them boring, and had no desire to recreate tropical village life in her English bolthole. Meanwhile her older sister, a pupil nurse at a London general hospital, regularly came to Runwell parties. Through social contacts this sister had become friendly with American soul band The Drifters, who were touring Britain. While her sister was seeing one of the band members, Vel had a brief romance with the band's producer, but she was deterred by the regular snorting of cocaine after gigs: this was going too far.

For about a year Vel had an English boyfriend, a porter at Runwell. On hearing that she was seeing someone else, he tried to strangle her. The police were called but Vel chose not to press a charge, feeling that she had wronged him. In another incident Vel was at the social club when an outsider asked for her address in the nurses' home. Without thinking Vel gave a random number. The man went to this room, and in anger at being tricked, he punched the innocent white English girl who opened the door. The police asked Vel for his name but she genuinely did not know it. This left a simmering atmosphere: other young women were jealous of Vel for the attention she got from men, and now she had caused this incident and failed to help the victim. Two days later, on returning to the nurses' home after work, she was surrounded by a group of English nurses who jostled and hit her. Ostracised by Malaysian colleagues, resented by English women, but an alluring presence for the men, Vel left her mark on Runwell.

At St Luke's near Middlesbrough, Angela Ainsworth[63] was part of an exclusively local intake in the early 1980s, as was Neil Brimblecombe[64] at Hill End in Hertfordshire, although several of the qualified nurses were of earlier Mauritian influx. Co-author NM did not see any foreign students during his training at Ravenscraig in the west of Scotland (1987 to 1990), but there were two Mauritian charge nurses. Such geographical variations continue, but there are probably few NHS services today that are entirely staffed by English, Welsh or Scots. Furthermore, as society becomes more diverse, the demography of patients has also changed dramatically. Whereas mental hospital patients in the 1970s were mostly local white people, the psychiatric admission units of today are an ethnic kaleidoscope, although there are concerns about the disproportionate number of black men detained under the Mental Health Act. Communication with patients could be a difficulty for white staff, particularly doctors from affluent middle-class background. Jo Brand[65] recalled an incident in the 1980s, when she worked in the emergency clinic at The Maudsley. A Rastafarian man was brought in by police, expressing severe delusions. He was aggressive, calling Jo a *bombo clat* (Jamaican dialect for a blood cloth or sanitary towel, but a commonly used curse). Psychiatric registrar Louis Appleby (who later became the government's national director of mental health), misunderstood this as the patient fearing he had a blood clot. Many black young men, in Jo's experience, were erroneously diagnosed as schizophrenic.

The history of the NHS is aligned to a history of economic migration. For a foot in the door, incomers were lured to nursing, and it was the understaffed mental hospitals where they accumulated in greatest number. Indeed, the multicultural mix in these hospitals preceded the peri-millennial phenomenon of demographic globalisation by at least two decades. Why did it work so well? The mental institution was a tolerant environment, where to be different was the norm. Although at first glance nurses from far-flung places such as Nigeria, Sri Lanka, Trinidad and Malaysia had little in common with their patients, they shared a sense of 'otherliness' to wider British society. Despite the majority of nursing staff in some hospitals being of different ethnicity to the mostly white patients, this cultural mismatch was scarcely considered in pre-registration or in-service training: a nurse was a nurse irrespective of background. Also, expectations of nurses from overseas were low. In the past, such nurses were not always credited for their ability, although this may have been more due to ignorance than to racism. Immigrants in Britain are often praised by the political establishment for working hard, and by implication harder than the indigenous workforce, but any differences in caring qualities or productivity would be speculative. Foreign nurses, it seems, fitted in to an established routine, and worked unpopular shifts (at enhanced rates of pay). In so doing, they performed a vital role eschewed by the native population.

Until at least the 1970s the mental hospital was a separate community, where nurses were trained, worked, slept and socialised. A high proportion of foreign nurses lived on site, where they developed a strong identification with the hospital. Few special requests were made for cultural or religious customs. By contrast, today there are equality and diversity officers to promote respect for minority groups, with somewhat hectoring posters on noticeboards. In modern society racial discrimination is prohibited and socially unacceptable – particularly in the NHS with its heavy reliance on workers of black and Asian ethnicity. Yet some nurses look back on friendships transcending race and culture in a warmer and more genuine spirit than exists now. Organisations, in good intentions, take the credit away from employees' inclination to work in harmony with people different to themselves. Arguably, diversity has been distorted as a political mantra. Indeed, the growth of identity politics in Western society was criticised by liberal Archbishop of Canterbury Rowan Williams for detracting from the common good.[66] Mental nursing, perhaps more than any other type of work, shows that we are more similar than different.

Notes

1   Best G (1979).
2   Engels F (1845/2009): *The Condition of the Working Class in England.*
3   Gardner J (1999).
4   Chatterton CS (2007): *'The Weakest Link in the Chain of Nursing?' Recruitment and Retention5in Mental Health Nursing, 1948-1968.*
5   Personal communication (NM, 2013).
6   Personal communication (PN, 2014).
7   Personal communication (NM, 2014).
8   Personal communication (NM, 2013).
9   Sandbrook D (2006): *Never Had it So Good: a History of Britain from Suez to The Beatles.*
10 Kynaston D (2009): *Family Britain 1951–57.*
11 Carpenter M (1985): *They Still Go Marching On: a Celebration of COHSE's First 75 Years.*
12 Gardner J (1999).
13 Personal communication (PN, 2014).
14 Cookson C (1971). *Colour Blind.* In this story, Bridget writes home tentatively of her marriage to an African sailor.
15 Nolan P, Hopper B (2000): Revisiting mental health nursing in the 1960s. *Journal of Mental Health.* Soon after qualifying, Herman became a nurse tutor.
16 After qualifying in medicine in Birmingham in 1952, Thomas Adeoye Lambo went to The Maudsley, where he was reputedly the first black African psychiatrist to be trained in Britain. He became renowned for his work on ethnology and epidemiology of mental illness.
17 Azu-Okeke O (1992): Experiments with Nigerian village communities in the dual roles of Western psychiatric treatment centres and homes for indigenous Nigerian inhabitants. *Therapeutic Communities.*
18 Sandbrook D (2006). 208.
19 Sandbrook D (2006).
20 Sandbrook D (2006).
21 Personal communication (NM, 2013).
22 Houbert J (1981): Mauritius: independence and dependence. *Journal of Modern African Studies.*
23 Jayawardena C (1968): Migration and social change: a survey of Indian communities overseas. *Geographical Review.*
24 Personal communication (PN, 1996). Jean McFarlane was the first professor of nursing to be appointed in England. She became a life peer in 1979 (Lady Farlane of Llandaff).
25 Personal communication (PN, 2014). Typically having long multi-syllable forenames and surnames, some Mauritians took British names such as 'Jeff' or 'Steve'.
26 Personal communication (NM, 2014).
27 Valentine R (1996). 96.
28 At St Clement's in east London, co-author NM worked with a Mauritian nurse who worked every shift under sun and moon: he would do an early or late shift on the ward, plus the opposite shift on the staff bank, and he would spend nights at another psychiatric unit in Hackney. Allegedly he was paying off an enormous gambling debt.
29 Crawford P, Nolan P, Brown B (1998): Ministering to madness: the narratives of people who have left religious orders to work in the caring professions, *Journal of Advanced Nursing.*
30 Crawford P, Nolan PW, Brown B (1998).
31 Personal communication (PN, 2015).
32 Personal communication (PN, 2014).
33 Personal communication (NM, 1996).
34 Most notoriously the Birmingham pub bombings in 1974. Six Irishmen were jailed for life, but their convictions were eventually overturned in 1991. In 1992 psychiatric

nurse David Heffer was a random victim of an IRA pub bombing at The Sussex pub in central London; he died of his injuries, aged 30.

35 Personal communication (NM, 2014).
36 Personal communication (NM, 2013).
37 Clark DH (1974).
38 Towell D (1975): *Understanding Psychiatric Nursing: a Sociological Study of Modern Psychiatric Nursing Practice.*
39 Shanley E (1980): Overseas nurses – effective therapeutic agents? *Journal of Advanced Nursing.*
40 Department of Health and Social Security (1972): *The Briggs Report: Report of the Committee on Nursing.*
41 *Nursing Times* (13 November 1975): Seeking a better deal for overseas students.
42 Trimingham A (2008).
43 Co-author NM attended a closure ceremony at Harperbury, a mental handicap hospital adjacent to Shenley Hospital, where local newspaper clippings from the late 1960s showed managers accusing visitors of racism for complaining about the number of foreign nurses.
44 Personal communication (NM, 2014).
45 Clare A (1976): *Psychiatry in Dissent: Controversial Issues in Thought and Practice.*
46 Perinpanayagam MS (1973): Overseas postgraduate psychiatric doctors. *News and Notes* (supplement to the *British Journal of Psychiatry*).
47 Clare A (1976).
48 Personal communication (NM, 2013).
49 Personal communication (NM, 2013).
50 Personal communication (NM, 2014).
51 Personal communication (NM, 1996).
52 Personal communication (NM, 1996).
53 Personal communication (NM, 1996).
54 Personal communication (NM, 2013).
55 Personal communication (NM, 2013).
56 Personal communication (NM, 2014).
57 Personal communication (NM, 2014).
58 Communication via Ali Costelloe (NM, 2013).
59 Personal communication (NM, 2014).
60 Personal communication (NM, 2013).
61 Personal communication (NM, 2013).
62 Personal communication (NM, 2014).
63 Personal communication (NM, 2014).
64 Personal communication (NM, 2015).
65 Personal communication (NM, 2015).
66 *Daily Telegraph* (27 March 2012): Rowan Williams: fixation with gay rights, race and feminism threatens society.

8   Holding the fort

Investment in public services faltered in the 1970s, as successive Tory and Labour administrations struggled to keep the lights on. In the oil crisis of 1973, Ted Heath's government imposed a three-day working week in industry, and the decade was marked by crippling dock, railway and miners' strikes, with a series States of Emergency declared. Facing rampant inflation, workers understandably demanded pay rises, and chants of 'What do we want? Twenty per cent' typified trade union demonstrations. Bailed out by the International Monetary Fund, Britain took refuge in the European Economic Community.

This was the context for the first major overhaul of the NHS since its inception. Costs were spiralling upwards in a system of cumbersome and ineffectual leadership. The reorganisation in 1974 abolished hospital management committees and regional boards, integrating hospitals and general practitioners in a new network of regional and area health authorities. To improve collaboration, area health authority boundaries were coterminous with those of county councils (in London, two or three boroughs), and subdivided into districts for operational purposes. Despite compromise with professional interests, the new structure appeared more amenable to rational planning and implementation of policy.[1]

As voluntary committees were replaced by an army of appointed bureaucrats at regional, area and district levels, it seemed that mental hospitals would remain the poor relation. Most chairmen, medical directors and administrators of the new bodies were unfamiliar with the needs of psychiatric patients. As the epicentre of the health service in each district, the general hospital consumed most of the resources, but a benefit was the further growth of acute psychiatric units. For example, Avon Health Authority planned a total of 500 psychiatric beds in the general hospitals of Southmead, Frenchay, Weston-Super-Mare and Bristol Royal Infirmary; the institutions of Glenside and Barrow would be left to a declining population of long-stay patients.[2]

Enoch Powell having predicted that the amount of mental hospital beds would halve by 1975, the official figures for that year are thus of particular interest.[3] Although the reduction had been slower than anticipated, the population had dropped by more than a third. In an ageing society, the proportion of admissions of people aged over sixty-five was rising (22 per cent in 1975), and the elderly accounted for almost half of the mental hospital census: of the total of 87,012

Table 8.1 Mental hospitals in England with over 1,500 beds (31 December 1975)[4]

Hospital	Capacity	Residents	Qualified nurses	Total nursing staff
Winwick	1,806	1,711	341	841
Rainhill	1,768	1,632	439	903
St Bernard's	1,675	1,541	293	616
Prestwich	1,582	1,438	340	766
High Royds	1,542	1,484	301	668
Shenley	1,508	1,385	398	670
Whittingham	1,505	1,394	343	753
Claybury	1,505	1,346	357	688

patients in the 104 mental hospitals with over 200 beds, 42,478 were aged over sixty-five. After soaring in the 1960s, the rate of admissions had stabilised. There was no longer any institution with over 2,000 beds, and occupancy had fallen to an average of 88 per cent. Yet in some ways the old hospitals were busier than ever. Staffing levels had improved, with the nursing workforce in England more than doubling from 24.5 per 100 patients in 1964 to 54.8 in 1975 (although this included unqualified workers; the rate for nurses of RMN or SEN status was 28.5).[5] In the same period medical staffing trebled, while there was also a burgeoning of psychologists and other therapists.

In 1975 the government issued its policy document *Better Services for the Mentally Ill* (DHSS, 1975), which urged locally based hospital and community mental health services. It proposed a reduction in mental hospital beds to 0.5 per 1000, which amounted to a thirty-bed ward for a district of 60,000 people. To drive care in the community forward, local authorities were to provide for all patients whose needs were more social than medical (as was assumed for the majority of long-stay patients). Instead of relying on generic social services departments, specific social workers would link with consultant psychiatrists' teams. A major obstacle was the impossibility of transferring savings from the reduction in hospital beds to local authorities. Acknowledging the lack of infrastructure to develop residential care, the government introduced the Joint Finance scheme in 1976, incentivising collaboration between health authorities and social services. However, with competing demands from other client groups such as the elderly and mentally handicapped, local authorities were reluctant to take responsibility for highly dependent patients currently receiving all their care from the NHS. Meanwhile, as a condition for the government's massive loan, the International Monetary Fund imposed conditions on the ailing British economy. In local authorities, money was becoming too tight to mention.

Faulty towers

The best medical and nursing care could not always prevent untoward incidents, and an occasional suicide was accepted as tragic but inevitable. Warlingham Park was a hospital with a good reputation, but an unusual spate of fourteen suicides occurred there in 1974 and 1975, compared to an annual average of one in the preceding ten years. An enquiry by Croydon Area Health Authority included a Queen's Counsel lawyer, a consultant psychiatrist and an area nursing officer.[6] The committee began by consulting specialists on suicide, including Peter Sainsbury at the MRC psychiatric research unit at Graylingwell Hospital, and data were sought on suicides elsewhere. Information received from thirteen mental hospitals showed that the annual DHSS statistics grossly underestimated the incidence of suicide: the official record of eighty-six such deaths in 1974 was probably half of the true total.

The enquiry focused on the admission wards, where the HAS had recently raised concerns. After reconfiguration, these wards were shared by five consultant psychiatrists, and this required nurses to attend multiple ward meetings. Although the resident population at Warlingham Park was steadily falling (in 1975 alone, from 586 to 529), the rate of admissions had risen, apparently due to the progressive policy of returning patients to the community as soon as possible. The community psychiatric nursing service was hopelessly understaffed for monitoring discharged patients, and psychiatrists tended to err on the side of caution by readmitting patients deemed at risk. Overworked nurses in the admission wards focused on severely disturbed or violent patients, while the quietly depressed received less attention. Absconding was not difficult in a hospital renowned for its 'open doors'. Gate porters had been withdrawn in 1970, and the extensive grounds, surrounded by a low fence with suburbs and woodland beyond, gave ample opportunity for a determined patient to disappear.

Low morale among nurses was compounded by recruitment problems. Following the critical HAS report the management agreed to restrict medical responsibility in the admission wards to two consultant psychiatrists, but this change was not made until July 1975. Unlike in other enquiries, there were no claims of abuse, and the committee produced a report sympathetic to the hospital, praising the staff as devoted, caring and forward-looking. Recommending a substantial boost to the nursing establishment, the report presented a clear message: for nurses to perform their role effectively, they needed sufficient strength and support. Moreover, the Warlingham Park highlighted the tension between liberty and safety.

> Society cannot both demand the pursuit of liberal treatment, and always expect to find a scapegoat if tragedy occurs.[7]

It was not only patients that were at risk in an open institution. For people with drug or alcohol addiction, the psychiatric hospital became a pit-stop in their cycle of dependency. In a state of intoxication or acute withdrawal symptoms, addicts could be volatile. Co-author PN was profoundly affected by the killing of a colleague by a drug addict. Daniel Carey, from County Kerry, was an enrolled nurse who was popular with patients. On 2 August 1974, Danny was assisting in a transfer from an open to a closed ward, when the patient took out a knife and inflicted several stab wounds on Danny. He died almost immediately, in the arms of a colleague.[8] Incidents like this were very rare, but the risk was raised by a high turnover of patients, with whom nurses were not always familiar.

Mental nursing had hazards, but the most vulnerable were the patients, as illustrated by a widely publicised enquiry at St Augustine's Hospital near Canterbury. In April 1974 two members of the nursing staff, frustrated by the lack of response to concerns they had raised about patient care, wrote a document titled 'A Critique Regarding Policy'. As well as distributing this in the hospital, they sent copies to the Secretary of State, the regional, area and district health authorities, and the HAS. The committee of enquiry was chaired by a lawyer who had led a recent enquiry at South Ockendon (a mental handicap hospital in Essex); its psychiatrist member was Alex Baker, and the nursing representative was John Greene.[9] The enquiry was conducted in a legalistic manner, with 168 witnesses formally interviewed and thorough scrutiny of all wards involved in the allegations.

The main author of the critique was William Brian Ankers, a postgraduate student at the University of Kent, who started work as a nursing assistant at St Augustine's in July 1972 while writing his thesis on organic chemistry. In September 1973 he gained his PhD, but continued to work at St Augustine's until the end of 1974. By then he had gained two and-a-half years of experience on the male long-stay wards. The co-author was Olleste Weston, who came to St Augustine's in 1970 for RMN training. Some years earlier, Weston had withdrawn from training at a mental handicap hospital due to his dissatisfaction with the standard of care. In his own words an idealist, Weston did not readily fit into the nursing culture, but he qualified in November 1973 and subsequently became a staff nurse at Heather Ward. At this long-stay ward he worked with Ankers, but resigned on circulation of the critique.

Ankers and Weston criticised a lack of policy for long-stay patients, limited therapeutic activity on the wards, and poor standard of care; they did not present specific allegations of mistreatment and malpractice. The document was dismissed by the senior hospital administrator as outdated and exaggerated, and doubts were cast on the experience and abilities of the two complainants. Irked by this reaction, in February 1975 the authors produced 'Part II: The Evidence', a more strident attack on the running of the hospital. Unlike the moderate wording of before, the sequel was embittered in tone. It was a litany of allegations of neglect and abuse, with page and after page of incidents of patients being deprived of their rights, insulted, over-medicated and sometimes assaulted by nurses, while their money and cigarettes were misappropriated. Nobody was named, but identities would have been obvious to anyone working in the hospital. For example, an enrolled nurse was described as follows:

> The regular SEN on one ward had the appearance of a member of the Gestapo. Coming on duty she swaggered into the wards and with legs

outstretched and hands on hips surveyed the state of the ward and the inmates with an arrogant and pitiless stare. She was ill-tempered with patients and made it clear that she thought them members of an inferior species. In once heard a young nurse ask her what was the matter with a certain patient. 'Oh him,' she replied in a loud, disdainful way, 'He's a schiz! Once a schiz – always a schiz!' The person whom this remark concerned heard it clearly.[10]

Another enrolled nurse had a habit of addressing a patient as 'dirty old man', causing him much distress. It was apparent to the committee that some nurses, as described by Ankers and Weston, lacked the appropriate skills and values for a position of power over vulnerable patients. The enquiry heard from patients, including a man aged eighty-three who had served in the war:

> If I had known I was coming here I'd have got one of those Prussian guards to stick a bloody bayonet through me.[11]

The committee released its report in March 1976, and it made front-page headlines. The enquiry supported the first critique and found most of Part II an accurate portrayal of the long-stay wards. St Augustine's was a medium-sized mental hospital, with 929 patients in November 1975, the resident population having dropped by 400 in the past five years.[12] However, long-stay wards continued to house around fifty patients, with staff deficient in number and qualification; enrolled nurses were often in charge. According to Jayne Love, who was at St Augustine's during the enquiry, ethically dubious activities were accepted norms at the time. While studying at Canterbury Art College, Jayne was a nursing assistant at the hospital, which was still known locally as 'Chartham' (its pre-NHS name). On an acute ward Jayne spent many a shift in the nurses' office, which was like a greenhouse in the middle of the ward, drinking sherry with the qualified staff. One patient, observing their merriment, looked in to ask 'Are you having a nice time in there?'[13]

Much blame was attached to the nursing management. Just as the best nurses tended to work in acute or specialist areas, the most progressive nursing officers were not attracted to the long-stay or geriatric units. Trained in the era of custodial care, change was not in the vocabulary of some senior nurses. According to Allan Hicks[14] at St Lawrence's in Bodmin, the post covering night duty was reserved for nursing officers approaching retirement, enabling them to leave with a higher pension. As a student, Allan was sent on errands to the offices of the principal and senior nursing officers, usually finding them sitting in comfortable armchairs smoking or drinking tea; he doubted whether they did anything of value. Mike O'Connor[15] remembers a surfeit of nursing officers at Park Prewett: these shadowy figures in dark suits visited wards infrequently and then only to speak to the charge nurse. As the St Augustine's report asserted: 'those with a managerial role must manage'.[16]

The input of doctors in the care of long-stay patients was heavily criticised in the St Augustine's report. On Hawthorn Ward, where Ankers worked in the last six months before his resignation, a consultant psychiatrist expressed a typically nihilistic attitude to the committee:

> There are far too many patients in a ward of this nature, being patients of the type they are, senile dements, terminal cases that have come to the end of their life and really have very little to do but sit, and so demented that the nurses cannot communicate with them.[17]

Doctors made fleeting appearances on the wards and nurses had no access to the medical notes. This may have preserved the esoteric status of psychiatry, distancing it from the intuitive, experiential knowledge of nurses, but it also conveyed a rigid class divide. A main recommendation of the enquiry was that nurses and doctors must work together, as part of a multidisciplinary team.

> One profession can no longer be dictated to by another.[18]

In the aftermath of the report, Ray Rowden, a charge nurse at St Augustine's, wrote in the *Nursing Times* on the pomposity of doctors and its deleterious effect on medical-nursing relations:

> Many doctors believe that holding the odd meeting in the ward constitutes team work. These meetings allow all staff to meet the consultant and so often a sham for democracy.[19]

In the same edition, WB Ankers commented on the verdict of the enquiry. While satisfied that the report had accepted most of the critique, he did not agree that maltreatment was excused by lack of resources; in his view, this was primarily a problem of attitudes. Nursing, Ankers argued, needed to act more like a profession.

> For too long nurses have deferred to doctors, allowed themselves to be stifled by nursing hierarchies, tolerated what they know to be intolerable conditions, and have not been prepared to blow the whistle when they see things that are wrong.[20]

At Woodilee near Glasgow, Peter Walsh[21] observed that hospital managers were reluctant to change the traditional hierarchy. Younger charge nurses disliked restraining, secluding or 'knocking out' patients with tranquillisers, and they wanted more say in the treatment regime, but nursing officers regarded these as medical issues. When the ward doctor arrived the nurses were expected to stand in respect. In 1980 Peter moved to Banstead, where nurses were more involved in clinical decisions, and regularly attended ward rounds. However, deference to medical authority persisted. On one occasion when the doctor entered the ward office to write his notes, Sister Sue Austin stayed sitting, as there another chair was free. She was asked to move, but refused. The doctor stormed off, returning with chief nurse Michael O'Shaughnessy, who told her to show due respect. Sister Austin kept her cool and simply asked why she should give up her seat when she was busy. As a witness, Peter saw that the chief nurse was unable to justify his instruction. This courageous act was discussed for months afterwards.

The *Nursing Times* highlighted recent improvements in organisation and care at St Augustine's. Nurses working in these institutions knew that the public image was distorted, and that the great majority of staff looked after patients with calm compassion. However, the broader message from the enquiry was that such insular institutions could never be an ideal environment for patients, as Martin described:

> It must simply be recorded that one of the lessons of St Augustine's is that large, closely knit institutions, mainly staffed by conscientious professionals, find it very difficult to accept and react positively to criticisms, however well intentioned and well funded.[22]

Such lessons were hard to take, because they would lead to the terminal decline of the mental hospital, which was as much home to the staff as to patients. The enquiries undoubtedly undermined public confidence in the inherently caring endeavour of hospitals within the NHS. In retrospect, the combination of poor leadership and the actions of an unscrupulous few reinforced the case for rundown and replacement of an outmoded institutional system. Scandals continued throughout the 1970s, and mental hospital managers were all on notice that they could be next. No hospital had long-stay or psychogeriatric wards that ran perfectly. Care was provided in a way that may have looked impersonal or inhumane to an outsider, but the workload was so high on some wards that corners had to be cut. In some cases, as described by Henry Marsh, wards and patients were temporarily smartened for visitors' appreciation.

> I was surprised one morning, when spooning gruel into an old man's edentulous mouth, to see the nursing officer come into the dining room. He told me that I had the afternoon off, though he gave me no reason. He had brought with him a large laundry bag full of worn but clean old suits, some of them pinstriped, and much underwear. The patients were all doubly incontinent so we kept them all in pyjamas as it was easier to change them, but my fellow nurses and I were told that all the patients were now to be dressed in suits and underwear. So our poor, demented patients were all dressed up in sagging, second-hand suits, and put back in their geriatric chairs and I went home. When I checked in for the late shift the next day I found the patients all back in pyjamas and the ward back to normal.[23]

The charge nurse later said that the visiting commission were impressed by the suits, and that the nursing officer had not wanted Marsh around as he might have said the wrong thing.

A certain remit

The cloud of scandals had a silver lining, as the nurse–patient ratio improved dramatically. Would this enable nurses to perform a more therapeutic role? In 1972 a book written by Annie Altschul, head of the nursing department at University of Edinburgh, would become a classic of psychiatric nursing literature. For her observational study, Altschul gained access to the wards of the Royal Edinburgh Hospital with pen and paper to hand. After any nurse–patient contact lasting at least three minutes, she asked the nurse to reflect on what happened. Many of these interactions may have been supportive or otherwise useful to the patients, but the nurses failed to describe any therapeutic intent.

> It has proved impossible to obtain any picture of the treatment ideologies which prevailed among nurses, or of any theoretical basis, upon which nurses acted in their dyadic interactions with patients.[24]

Altschul concluded that nurses needed to learn techniques of interpersonal communication, and to apply therapeutic principles in a more purposeful relationship with patients. This was the first study in Britain of psychiatric nursing by a psychiatric nurse, and the first to investigate the role beyond mere activity measurement. Meanwhile, another study was being conducted at the pseudonymous 'Eastville' (actually Fulbourn). In 1967 postgraduate sociology student David Towell approached David Clark for permission to investigate the impact of the therapeutic community model on nursing. Completed in 1973, his doctoral thesis was published two years later by the RCN as *Understanding Psychiatric Nursing*, with a foreword by Clark.[25] In this seminal text, Towell described the trials and tribulations of applying social therapy in a mental hospital. Nurses, according to Towell, tended to seek a good nurse–patient fit, whereby patients accepted that they were ill and irresponsible. By contrast, they rejected patients labelled with personality disorder, who often challenged nurses' authority. Most nurses relied on doctors for instruction rather than fulfilling their therapeutic potential in the care and treatment of patients. Others, influenced by the anti-psychiatry movement, criticised the medical model but often from an unsophisticated perspective: doctors were not preventing nurses from engaging with patients. Indeed, British psychiatrists were relatively free of the ideological bias that prevailed in other countries:[26] most were pragmatic pluralists who accepted a need for social, psychological and biological treatment.

Psychiatry was on the defensive in the 1970s, challenged by staunch critics from inside and outside the discipline. In 1973 American psychologist David Rosenhan produced an explosive paper *On Being Sane in Insane Places*,[27] which seriously undermined the scientific credibility of psychiatric diagnosis. Rosenhan described the experiences of a group of pseudo-patients who got themselves admitted to various psychiatric hospitals after stating that they repeatedly heard the word 'thud' in their heads. Almost all were diagnosed as schizophrenic. Despite behaving normally throughout their stay, their activities were pathologised in the nurses' notes, with entries such as 'engages in writing behaviour'. Most of the dummy patients were discharged as paranoid schizophrenics in remission. One hospital contacted Rosenhan, refusing to believe the same errors could be committed by their clinicians. In response Rosenhan promised a further group of fakes over a fixed period, and records revealed that of 193 admissions, forty-one bogus cases were suspected. In fact, Rosenhan had not sent anybody.

Another damaging blow for professional prestige was the cinematic success in 1975 of *One Flew over the Cuckoo's Nest*. Among the horrors of this dramatised life in an American state asylum, the dreaded ECT was prescribed for punishment, but the most notorious character was not a psychiatrist but a nurse. Played by Louise Fletcher, Nurse Ratched was the archetypal 'battle-axe'; a cold, heartless character who dominated the ward. She made the merest comforts a privilege for patients, which could be withdrawn as punishment. Nurse Ratched was not representative of psychiatric nurses, although probably all mental hospitals had one or two of her kind. This film was shown in nurse training, to a receptive audience. The nursing culture was evolving, as a younger generation disparaged the 'old guard', who retired with their memories of better times. The character of psychiatric nursing recruits reflected broader trends in society, with a theme of irreverence to tradition and establishment values. Informality was the rule: mufti, mixed-sex wards, and nurses and patients on first-name terms. This was not simply a slackening of discipline but a philosophy of care. Instead of helping people to be better patients, nurses were to make the lives of patients as 'normal' as possible.

In the 1970s a guiding philosophy on long-stay wards was 'normalisation'. This was described by Wolf Wolfensberger at the Canadian National Institute on Mental Retardation as a means of enabling people with disabilities to follow the same patterns of everyday living as other people; disability was reconceptualised as a social condition.[28] Aware of the tendency for professional distancing and reinforcement of the sick role, Wolfensberger encouraged deployment of care workers without formal training. Normalisation was influential but it was not always applied sensibly; often it was misinterpreted as imposing social norms on people, or as a rationale for leaving patients to look after themselves. Nonetheless, normalising principles helped to transform the social atmosphere of the mental hospital. Uniform was seen as a barrier between staff and patients, and was steadily abandoned in psychiatric nursing. Most male nurses were glad to be free of the institutional suit. In its place, a personal clothing allowance was introduced. At West Park, for example, instead of the 'identikit' grey jacket and trousers supplied by the hospital tailor, vouchers were issued for the John Collier menswear shop in Epsom.[29] Male and female recruits continued to receive white coats and dresses for physical care, but eventually geriatric wards were the only place where these were worn.

For the imperative of rehabilitation, in the 1970s psychologists became more involved in the long-stay wards. While nurses accepted a psychologist's supervision just as they complied with medical authority, their enthusiasm for behavioural treatment varied, as found by Bill Reavley, psychologist at Graylingwell:

Most of the clinical work was with outpatients. Our work with inpatients was not so successful. Not all nurses were keen on behavioural approaches and it was not possible to have consistency in application of positive reinforcement programmes.[30]

Mark Rudman,[31] who started nursing at Whitecroft Hospital in the Isle of Wight in 1976, found that a superficial focus on behaviour detracted from developing meaningful relationships with patients. The currency of the token economy was brass washers, which were redeemable at the Whitecroft shop, and mostly used for tobacco; Mark recalls instances of rehabilitated patients attempting to use them for purchases outside the hospital. This treatment was no panacea for the severe social disabilities of long-stay patients, and initial improvements rarely endured. Nurses' commitment was crucial, but with its demands for observation and recording, a behavioural treatment regime added to the burden of running long-stay wards, and inevitably there was sabotage.

In nurse training schools, meanwhile, interpersonal skills were promoted over blunt behaviourism. According to Mike O'Connor, tutors at Park Prewett in the 1970s encouraged students to take active interest in the unique perspectives and life stories of each patient, and not to frame all behaviour by psychiatric diagnosis. However, as Mike observed, there was a deep moat between theory and practice: ward staff had little interest in the ideals emanating from the 'ivory towers'. None of the charge nurses or nursing officers at Park Prewett came to the nursing school, and a solitary clinical teacher had negligible impact.[32] Anti-academic attitudes prevailed among older nurses: in their view training ended on qualification; from then onwards experience was all that mattered. Few nurses read nursing journals except to peruse job advertisements.

Illustrating the mismatch between the professionalism taught in the nursing school and students' experience on the long-stay wards was the drug round. At Woodilee, Peter Walsh[33] recalls that nurses followed the prescription card but did not sign for dispensing medication, and often a little extra was given to patients on the nurse's discretion. In a rehabilitation ward a charge nurse gave Largactil (blue label) to Protestant patients and Melleril (green label) to Catholics; a 'big one' or 'wee one' was given, depending on the patient's mental state. Some wards were so quiet at night that Peter suspected that the patients had been doped with Mogadon or Welldorm. John Kelly[34] remembers a stint in his training in Ward 9 in the old block at Hartwood, where he administered the medication assisted by a 'trusty', who was allowed to pour and give out the syrups, sometimes adjusting the dose for patients who were restless or noisy.

In training at Gartloch near Glasgow in the late 1970s, Kay Baggins was impressed by the liberal teachings of senior tutor Jack Lyttle, but on a long-stay ward she was dismayed by indignities imposed on patients.[35] The dormitories were upstairs and locked in the daytime, and Kay recalls that as the men came downstairs in the morning, the charge nurse whacked each of them on the back of the head with a rolled-up newspaper, saying 'Morning, Jim' (or whoever). The old ritual of patients queuing naked for a bath in water already used by several others persisted. As Iain Tulley[36] described, nurses at Hartwood maintained an authoritarian stance. On a summer coach outing to the seaside at Troon, the men from Ward 8B were each dressed in tweed jacket, shirt and tie, despite the warm, sunny weather. Although they were all taking Largactil, no sun cream was applied and they got badly burnt (a side effect of tranquillisers). The group walked along the promenade and then stopped at a pub for a pie and pint. Before returning one nurse stood by the coach and another at a public toilet, each counting the men. The latter nurse was from another ward and did not know the patients. After all forty-six patients had boarded the coach, this nurse was seen holding a man by the collar and dragging him out of the toilet. He had mistaken a member of the public for a patient! Letting him go, the nurse brushed himself off, and they all laughed about it on the way home.

The GNC decreed that any part of a hospital failing to provide a suitable learning environment would be denied students. 'Teaching wards' were required to have up-to-date nursing policies and procedures, with adequate staffing to supervise students. As recalled by Tom Walsh,[37] placements in several 'back wards' at West Park were discontinued. Sunlight is the best disinfectant, and the absence of students compounded the poor standards of care in failing wards. Students feared getting a job on such a ward on qualifying, while the most proficient were earmarked for the new admission unit at Epsom General Hospital.

By nature and nurture, psychiatric nursing was becoming less regimental and more psychosocially orientated, but patient's experiences are equivocal on such change. For example, John McCusker, a final-year university student, was admitted to a mental hospital in 1972 with depression and persecutory delusions. He was given hefty doses of Stelazine and thirty sessions of ECT, but had little therapeutic interaction with staff.

> I found the nurses flippant and impatient, and often authoritarian. They were used to dealing with awkward customers and you had to do what you were told. It was easy to get branded as a troublemaker. The drugs made me sleepy and I wanted to lie down at lunchtime, but they saw that as laziness. They would threaten me with a locked ward if I did not get up and walk around.[38]

A study by psychologists of nursing staff attitudes[39] showed that authoritarian traits correlated with gender, age and level of qualification. Women, older nurses and unqualified staff had a tendency to prioritise orderliness on the wards. As the largest group of staff at ward level, nursing assistants had great impact on patients' experience of care, but many lacked finesse in their communication style, and were quite bossy with patients. In their daily tasks, nursing assistants showed little willingness to change time-honoured rituals such as serving tea in a large urn with milk and sugar already added.[40] Compared to RMNs, the study showed that enrolled nurses were less inclined to seek a rapport with patients, regarding care as a primarily physical process. Despite progress in the attitudes of RMNs, the ranks constituting the majority of care staff were lagging behind.

Meanwhile the therapeutic premium from RMN training was not always cashed, as such nurses were typically in charge of a ward, burdened with administrative tasks. Psychiatric nursing, despite greater emphasis on interpersonal skills, was struggling to develop as a distinct therapeutic enterprise. In his book *Psychiatric Nursing Observed*, Desmond Cormack observed that the medical model continued to dominate over psychosocial approaches,[41] and this was to the regret not only of nurse educators but also some psychiatrists. At Fulbourn, the demise of social therapy began in 1976 after Martin Roth was appointed as the first professor of psychiatry at Cambridge University. Most of the new consultants were in tune with Roth's pathological model of mental illness, and they stopped attending the daily meetings with patients and nurses.[42] David Clark retired in 1983, having witnessed the rise and fall of the therapeutic community.

In 1982 the GNC introduced a new syllabus, spurred by the Jay Report on mental handicap nursing.[43] Having examined the training and role of nurses in this field, Baroness Jay was not convinced that mentally handicapped people required nurses at all. Instead, they needed educational and social support for living in the community, and this was increasingly provided by social services and other agencies. The shift from NHS to local authority provision was much more advanced than in mental health care. Whereas mental handicap had been demedicalised as a disability, mental illness was by definition a medical domain. Nonetheless, the GNC reacted swiftly to the Jay Report, fearing demise of a whole branch of nursing. The RMN syllabus was greatly influenced by Annie Altschul, who had become a professor of nursing at Edinburgh in 1976. A shining beacon in establishing nursing as a therapeutic discipline, rather tahn a mere ancillary to medical treatment, Altschul urged psychiatric nurses to build their own theory and clinical practice. Her textbook *Psychiatric Nursing* ran to a sixth edition in 1984, and later training manuals such as by Jack Lyttle and Phil Barker carried her baton forward. The revised syllabus was significant in three ways. It gave prominence to interpersonal skills and to psychological and social models of care; it asserted a distinction of mental health from physical health nursing, and it was the first to be designed without input from the Royal College of Psychiatrists.

As a ward sister at Coney Hill, Patricia Burdett[44] was offered a post as an unqualified teacher in the school of nursing at Gloucester Royal Hospital, due to staff shortages. Patricia went on to gain the Further Education Teacher's Certificate through an evening course at Gloucester City College of Technology, which qualified her as a clinical teacher to guide students in practice. To become a registered nurse tutor, it was necessary to take a full-time, one-year course leading to the Postgraduate Certificate in Education, but this was unavailable locally. The nursing school had two intakes of ten to twelve students, in March and September, for the three-year RMN course. The entry threshold was five O-level school certificates, but an applicant with lower attainment could be accepted on passing the General Nursing Council (GNC) entrance test. Two other courses were run: the two-year SEN training, and a fifteen-month course for nurses with the SRN certificate who wanted to move into psychiatric nursing. The range of clinical experience for students was left to the discretion of the school, and usually included elderly care, acute admissions, rehabilitation, substance abuse and one general nursing placement. Courses were advertised in the *Nursing Mirror* and *Nursing Times*, as well as in local newspapers and job centres. According to Eric Chitty,[45] senior tutor at Moorhaven, scheduled courses were not always run due to inadequate recruitment. The teaching staff was low in number and mediocre in quality: tutors tended to keep their jobs until retirement, thus creating few opportunities for new personnel who could prepare students for a role quite different to that known to older colleagues.

While the national syllabus was followed, nurse training was strongly influenced by the particular interests of tutors. Some schools emphasised social and psychological therapies, while others were more orientated to psychiatric illnesses and practical nursing procedures. Jim Vaughan,[46] senior tutor at Barrow Hospital in Bristol, arranged sessions by policy analysts, health economists, management theorists and organisational psychologists, so that students understood the broader context of nursing.

In 1982 co-author PN was appointed as senior tutor for psychiatric nursing at Bath School of Nursing, based at Roundway Hospital in Devizes. As the courses were beginning to be less medical in design and more tuned to the needs of nurses, PN had the awkward task of informing the medical director, Michael Bird, that his teaching services (amounting to four or five hours per week) would no longer be required. Bird asserted his firm belief that nurses could not be trained without the guidance of doctors, but PN explained that changes in the nursing curriculum were being made across the country and not simply at Roundway. After regaining his composure, Bird shrugged and walked away, remarking: 'There goes my holiday money'. He had received £500 per month for teaching nurses, a considerable amount at the time, and hard to justify when the school could not afford core books and journals.

All on the house

Although the scandals portrayed an unhappy scene, a good time could be had in the mental hospitals. Many nurses enjoyed being in a place free from the stultifying norms of society, where patients and staff alike could express themselves. One woke in the morning to birds singing in the tall trees of the hospital grounds, and opened the curtains to a green vista – quite serene on a sunny day. A short walk and one arrived in the ward office, met colleagues in handover, and then spent a few hours in unhurried cajoling of patients, tuning in to their idiosyncrasies and avoiding unnecessary conflict. There were daily chores such as the medication round and the nursing notes, but there was usually time to play snooker or watch television. Finishing the shift in early afternoon, and after returning to one's room for a rest, one might take the hospital minibus to the nearest town for some provisions, or a punt at the bookmaker. The evening was spent in the social club, irreverently dissecting hospital politics and the latest gossip over a few pints of beer. Perhaps to add to the nest egg or compensate for a bad day at the races, one could always work a late or night shift.

In a gallery of odd and amusing behaviour, the job was never like a dull day in the office. *Spectator* columnist Jeremy Clarke recalled his time as a nursing assistant and trainee in the 1980s at Goodmayes, where he found that the normal rules of society did not apply to patients or staff:

> If you live in a large mental hospital, these parameters widen drastically, or even disappear altogether. And after a time one comes to relish and prefer the greater variety of behaviour, and the daily surprises occurring within the crenelated walls, and life outside becomes insipid.[47]

Some of the most popular nurses were those who were laid-back and who laughed in the face of adversity. They were the bridge between psychiatry and the patients, and in social class often closer to the latter. When co-author NM started nurse training, a nurse told this tale, reserved for novices.

> On an official visit to Ravenscraig, the mayor was met at the gate by the medical superintendent. It was a fine day and the mayor was interested in a patient who was tending the pristine flowerbeds. The doctor introduced him: 'We are very pleased with Harry; he keeps the gardens very tidy for us.' 'So I see,' said the mayor, shaking Harry's hand. After chatting briefly, the mayor turned to catch up with the medical superintendent, but Harry stopped him to ask: 'Please sir, they are keeping me here for no reason. There's nothing wrong with me. Could you help to get me out?' The mayor politely offered to have a word. Fifty yards further up the drive, as the mayor was making his tentative enquiry, he was suddenly struck on the head by a large stone. As he was helped to his feet, he saw Harry gesticulating: 'You won't forget, will you?'

Family networks kept a steady flow of workers at the mental hospitals. Tim Mosses' parents worked at Bexley Hospital, and six of their children followed in their footsteps. One of Tim's sisters remained a nursing assistant throughout her career, but he and the others qualified as nurses (another sister was a general nurse). None were academically minded, and may have found themselves in 'dead-end' jobs, but Bexley offered stable and rewarding work. At the age of sixteen, Tim was told by his father that Eric, the chief male nurse, wanted him as a cadet nurse. He spent the next two years in the industrial therapy unit, before starting RMN training in 1973. Well into the 1980s, Tim recalls, nobody in Bexley believed that the hospital would close.[48] Like most of his peers, every evening Tim went to the social club, run by retired charge nurses George and Noreen Walsh. As well as a bar there was a television lounge and a snooker room, and squash courts were added at the rear. Regular events were held for the various sports teams, a photography club, old-time dance club, and there were fortnightly discos. One would need several pints to get drunk on the Whitbread's 'Trophy' or other insipid keg brew, but it was cheap. When the Bexley club temporarily closed after a fire, Tim and others ventured to a nearby pub, and were shocked by the prices.

Not every hospital had such facilities. Peter Walsh told of the frantic efforts of staff at Woodilee to enjoy a drink after work. Nearby Kirkintilloch was a dry town,[49] and pubs bordering the district closed at 9 p.m; 'carry-out' was offered but this was more expensive than drinking inside. Eventually in 1970 the first pub opened in Kirkintilloch, and Peter described the daily 'Wacky Races', when nurses went off duty to form a procession of 'old bangers', hurtling along the country lane for two miles to reach The Antonine in time. The ritual was for each nurse to order eight pints to share with three colleagues, one of whom would buy another round before last orders at 9.50 p.m. This was before the campaign against drink-driving; Peter remembers the return journeys as less dangerous than the sober rush to get there. Parties were frequently held in rooms of the nurses' home, where guests were expected to lay a supply of alcoholic drinks on the table for general consumption. This was not an ideal setting for revelry, the building containing a ward on the ground floor, but in 1977 a social club was opened in the barn of the hospital farm. This had a games room upstairs, with a pool table and darts. For a lunch break on the forensic ward, Peter and colleagues sometimes went to the club, having a sandwich and three pints of lager before returning to work. This relieved tension, but left a long and lethargic stretch until the night shift arrived. Some of the older nurses at Woodilee had serious alcohol problems. A shock reverberated around the hospital when two charge nurses were sacked for being drunk on duty, although they were reinstated on appeal. One of the reprieved charge nurses had told Peter that he could not get up in the morning without a half-bottle of whisky.

Starting at West Park in 1978, Tom Walsh[50] and fellow Irish students went to the social club every evening, often staying well into the early hours. 'It was great fun in those days,' he reminisced. Towards the end of the month, when he was out of money, he would go to the canteen on his way back to the nurses' home, where a free breakfast was provided by a sympathetic catering staff on night duty. Despite fond memories, by the early 1980s the hospital social club was past its heyday. More nurses were living out, leaving behind an increasing proportion of staff from abroad, many of whom did not drink. For young British students the hospital club seemed drab and institutional, with its dwindling clientele of old-timers. At Fulbourn in the mid-1970s, Louise Hide[51] was an avid reader of Foucault and anti-psychiatry, and enjoyed the company of fellow students with left-wing views. They avoided the social club, instead socialising in the nurses' home, smoking 'spliffs' and listening to avant-garde music. The Whitecroft bar had little appeal for Mark Rudman:

> I do not recall the social club being a particularly lively affair. There were organised coach trips and so on, but the club bar itself was generally quiet, frequented by a small number of staff who perhaps played snooker or pool. I remember it as being a rather 'sad' place, which closed early when the bar steward had had enough or there was no custom.[52]

During John Kelly's training at Hartwood,[53] in 1978 the male nurses' home was converted to social work offices. The men were allocated a floor of the female nurses' home, where many a wild party was held. As the training school was on the ground floor, John sometimes got up five minutes before classes started at nine o'clock. A 'trusty' with a master key cleaned the men's rooms in the nurses' homes. He had a list of nurses on night duty so not to disturb them, but he often tidied around a nurse lying in with a hangover.

Moving to Fair Mile in 1975, Jayne Love[54] became aware of a group of final-year students who became *sannyasins* (disciples of Indian mystic Bhagwan Shree Rajneesh). The movement promoted 'free love', dynamic meditation and encounter groups. Adherents dyed their clothes orange, and Jayne remembers the students wearing beads on the wards. Some went to the ashram at Poona on the west coast of India, the centre of the movement. On returning, one young nurse of affluent background bought a house for himself and fellow travellers, who changed their names and wore malas on duty, to the disdain of older staff.

The mental hospital thrived on absurdity. For a dare at Whitecroft, according to Mark Rudman,[55] a charge nurse rode a motorbike around the hospital corridors. Pranks were a regular feature of hospital life, and as Mark describes, this was mostly harmless fun:

> Most memorably for me was the good-natured opportunity to send a new staff member or student to borrow the 'Oxometer'. After a 'wild-goose-chase' starting with the senior nursing officer, the victim was sent to every ward until it emerged that the mythical device was designed to 'measure bullshit by the yard'.

As the uncertain future of the mental hospitals began to cause anxiety, many nurses extolled the virtues of institutional care for patients, while also appreciating the perks of the job. There was good money to be made: one could double the income of a nurses' salary with overtime, while rent on hospital accommodation was minimal compared to private lodgings. It was possible (if not necessarily permissible) to get by without buying food. Nurses on duty often had their meals from the ward trolley, although patients were served first. Some members of staff found the ready supply of goods too tempting. Mary Gutierrez, Tony Tramalgini and Imelda Bures[56] told of the exposure of widespread staff misappropriation at Netherne in the early 1980s. Managers brushed this under the carpet, until an Italian member of domestic staff was caught stealing an expensive delivery of meat. Under questioning, this person 'spilled the beans', and the police were called. Checks on staff homes were announced, leading to mass burning of food and commodities around the estate. Detectives, however, found a freezer full of hospital meat in a nurse's house: he was sacked, but got his job back due to flaws in the evidence. Meanwhile, on holiday with her Spanish husband in rural Andalucia, laundry manager Maureen Gomez[57] was astounded to find bundles of towels for sale in a local market, marked 'Property of Netherne Hospital'.

Compound fractures

As the workforce expanded, COHSE gained new members, and it wielded considerable power in the running of mental hospitals. Managers knew that nurses were difficult to replace, and understaffing remained a problem in some institutions, compounded by recruitment problems and staff sickness. Brookwood Hospital in Surrey had a long history of shortages, and in 1975 this caused conflict between COHSE and the management. The union instilled a 'workers' council' to run the hospital in parallel to the official organisation. In this febrile atmosphere allegations were made about an experienced and popular charge nurse, followed by counter-allegations against the two student nurse complainants. Surrey Area Health Authority decided to appoint two committees of enquiry: one to investigate patient care, and the other to focus on industrial relations. The aforementioned charge nurse was sacked before the enquiry, but no staff member agreed to give evidence on the circumstances leading to his dismissal. An atmosphere of fear had deterred staff members from speaking out. According to one witness, student nurses were told that by tutors they should never accuse anybody of a wrongdoing unless there was another witness. While noting genuine concerns with understaffing, the report criticised COHSE for obstructing a concerted effort to improve conditions for patients. Yet while describing bad practices, the report acknowledged a generally high standard of care in the hospital. Commentators suggested:

> Perhaps a hospital such as Brookwood is like a man who is basically in sound health but has a raging toothache.[58]

Tom Chan, who worked at Brookwood in the years of discontent, remembers overtime as readily available. While it was obvious that tired nurses could not provide the best care, staffing shortages prevented managers from restricting nurses' working hours. Some nurses seemed to be constantly on duty, day and night. Whereas an early shift was busy, the late shift was more relaxed and on night duty the nurse could sleep through, rising an hour or so before handover. In opposing curtailment of overtime in the late 1970s, COHSE was rightly representing its members, but this seemed to prioritise the income potential of nurses over patient care. Amidst the scandals, public sympathy could not be guaranteed.[59]

Although the RCN was characterised as a general nurses' union, it had some presence in mental hospitals. Jayne Love[60] remembers the sister of her ward having several meetings with Ray Rowden, the RCN steward, in the St Augustine's enquiry. Mike O'Connor was in a minority choosing the RCN at Park Prewett; he saw this as more in tune with nursing as a profession.[61] At Scalebor Park, where Philip Barton-Wright started SEN training in 1979, the RCN representative was a charge nurse on the alcohol unit, and the COHSE equivalent a charge nurse on an admission ward. Like most of his peers, Philip joined COHSE, having heard that the RCN were 'management lackeys'.[62] A fundamental difference between the RCN and the conventional trade unions was its opposition to strikes or any withdrawal of patient care. Underlying tension between these organisations rose to the surface as the Tory government, elected in 1979, attempted to overhaul the public sector. Industrial action spread in the 1980s, as the mostly COHSE-affiliated workforce took to the streets to demonstrate on causes local and national. John Kelly[63] remembers Hartwood nurses standing at the brazier in support of the miners' strike in the early 1980s. A picket line dissuaded colleagues from going to work, while minimal staffing was maintained for basic care; John recalls managers supporting the protest. The main rival for COHSE was not the RCN but the National Union of Public Employees (NUPE), which was making ground in the nursing workforce. COHSE had the advantage of being focused on health care workers, but NUPE had a broader base and had run many effective campaigns for better pay and conditions in the public sector.

It would be unfair to portray the RCN as too posh for psychiatric nurses. The RCN campaigned for better pay across the nursing profession in the 1980s, led by Trevor Clay. Nurses often grumbled about conditions but were not politically active, and in Clay's view they were apathetic to their lack of influence on how the NHS was run. Appointed as general secretary in 1982, Clay immediately began to agitate for a pay review body, which resulted a substantial increase across the board. He encouraged nurses to be more assertive, to confront managers at all levels, and to engage in policy decisions that affected them and their patients.[64] However, Clay acknowledged that nursing was a heterogeneous profession with a variety of interest groups, divided by branch, and also by status: the number of enrolled and auxiliary nurses had outgrown the full registrants. Clay's activism, however, broadened the appeal of the RCN: by the time of his retirement in 1989, membership had surged to 285,000.[65]

Unlike unions in industry, COHSE was often in a position of protecting managers against the lower ranks of staff, as illustrated in an enquiry at Winterton Hospital in County Durham in 1979. A party for a member of night staff who was leaving was held in a patients' quiet room in the early hours of the morning, when the staff took their break. This was a boisterous affair, with plentiful alcohol. A ward sister, who had been drinking heavily, used medication and a seclusion room to keep patients at bay, allowing the party to continue. Some off-duty nurses remained on the ward at 6*a.m.* While most of the party-goers kept quiet afterwards, one staff nurse reported the unprofessional actions of the sister to a nursing officer. An area health authority committee of enquiry failed to gain staff cooperation, and concluded that some of the thirty-five witnesses were lying. Here again was a picture of poor leadership and deficiencies in care, maintained in a culture of misplaced loyalties and intimidation. While the unions purportedly represented the workers, hierarchical favour was apparent, with charge nurses having established influence and connections that easily trumped the word of a junior complainant.

A bone of contention for unions was the closure of wards by stealth, and the threat this presented to future employment. In his history of Long Grove, Tony Day[66] described a militant response to the area health authority's decision to close Oxted Ward, which the TGWU and COHSE cast as a cynical financial decision.

The management pressed ahead, resulting in a walkout by 180 domestic, laundry, portering and estate workers.

> Local newspapers carried a weekly update of the saga, often with a head and shoulders picture of a man with a mop of tousled hair, a furrowed brow, and a bushy beard. Maurice Smith, Long Grove Branch Secretary of the Transport & General Workers Union, devoted all his time to representation of his fellow ancillary workers, and was at the centre of many disputes. It is said, by one of those on the opposite side of the fence at the time that Maurice 'had the whole Epsom Cluster completely in his grip'.

In November 1981 there was a violent incident after a social club committee meeting at Long Grove. As the meeting was inquorate, it could not approve plans for a major refurbishment of the club bar, and a fight broke out as members were leaving. Hospital administrator Jim Chalmers immediately suspended Maurice Smith and three other men. Despite demonstrations and walkouts, Smith was not allowed to return until three months later, and he never regained his power. Meanwhile, the health authority closed another five wards at Long Grove. A new social club committee was formed in June 1982, and Jim Chalmers issued an ultimatum: either he received the accounts, or the police would be called. The accounts were not forthcoming and the club was closed. Unions won some battles, but were losing the war.

Another dispute at Long Grove was over the proposed opening of a psychiatric intensive care unit, which the staff feared would be used for dangerous patients from Broadmoor. This was an issue that had first been raised at Prestwich in Manchester, where opening of a regional secure unit in was vehemently opposed by COHSE. This development followed the Butler Report in 1975, which criticised the lack of progress in introducing regional secure units for mentally disordered offenders, as first recommended by official report in 1961. The situation had worsened in recent years, due to the liberalisation of mental hospitals, open door policy and psychiatrist's reluctance to accept patients with propensity for destructive behaviour. Consequently, hospital orders from the courts resulted in men and women being sent to the special hospitals of Broadmoor, Rampton, Moss Side or the recently built Park Lane, with their risk often exaggerated to fulfil admission criteria.[67] Hundreds more were kept in prison, with limited attention to their mental health needs. There was a yawning gap between the high security of the special hospitals and the mental hospitals, which had no security. The government responded to the Butler Report by issuing central funding for interim regional secure units, as a stop-gap until permanent facilities could be built.

In each region of England, secure units were hurriedly instituted in converted wards of the old hospital buildings. The first was at Prestwich (Manchester Region) in September 1976, followed by Knowle (Wessex) in January 1977. Rainford Ward at Rainhill was typical: a ground-floor ward with several side-rooms and a high perimeter wall was selected, and structurally modified to create a 14-bed unit for both sexes, with a double-door security lobby. A nurse–patient ratio of 1.5:1 was instilled. A modest supplement was paid to nurses in the new unit, but this soon caused difficulties. When a patient was deemed suitably stable to move from the secure unit to an ordinary ward, the unions agitated. Nurses elsewhere in the hospital could not cover for staff shortages in the secure unit, because they lacked the special training and remuneration. Despite their physical integration, the units became isolated from the main hospital, and as the pay lead was insufficient to attract staff, in some cases temporary closure was necessary[68]. Problems also arose with the type of patients sent by the courts. Clear criteria were presented for admission: the patient must be mentally ill (not psychopathic), and dangerous to self or others as a result of that illness. In reality, while the most common diagnosis was schizophrenia, patients with personality disorder were also received. Psychiatrists complained of their clinical autonomy being overridden by the area medical officer's insistence on a patient's admission.

The unions flexed their muscles on the issue of offender patients. At Rainhill they 'blacked' transfers to an open ward, and parole was postponed for several months until staff opposition softened.[69] The strongest reaction was at the first unit at Prestwich, which opened after protracted negotiations about the nurse–patient ratio and salary supplement. However, when Elton Ward became the new secure unit, the local branch of NUPE withdrew catering, portering and other ancillary services. Apparently a rumour had circulated that notorious 'moors murderer' Myra Hindley was to be transferred there. Senior shop steward Geoffrey Wilson argued:

> This is the wrong site for the unit. We're in the midst of housing and children and the centre of Manchester is only 20 minutes away.[70]

Ironically, unions were resisting a major investment that potentially prolonged the life of the mental hospitals Meanwhile, obsolete practices and abuses had been exposed at the former state institutions for the criminally insane, now known as the special hospitals. In 1980 Rampton was subject of a shocking television documentary and a government enquiry. Investigation on a ward at Broadmoor found potent tranquillising medication being used at two or three times the maximum recommended dosage, ECT given 'straight', and a patient secluded in a cell smeared with faeces from a previous occupant.[71] Shamed by cases of wrongful treatment taken to the European Court of Human Rights, the government was pressed into reducing the population at Broadmoor and Rampton by ensuring that regional health authorities created sufficiently large, purpose-built secure facilities. The first permanent regional unit, with 30 beds, was opened in 1980 by Northern Regional Health Authority in the grounds of St Luke's Hospital in Middlesbrough. This was followed by a sixty-bed unit at Towers Hospital (Trent Region) in 1983, and although local community opposition was a problem, similar provision was eventually made throughout England.

Meanwhile at Long Grove, the unions eventually agreed to the proposal of an intensive care ward (not a regional secure unit) on condition that nursing officers retain responsibility for any of their patients transferred there. When management reneged on this, staff throughout the hospital went on strike for five hours. Divisional nursing officer Eddy Black received threatening telephone calls, and his home was ransacked with suspicions of staff involvement; fellow managers' cars were vandalised in the hospital grounds. Serious overspending in the hospital necessitated staffing cuts, and night nursing was reduced. Tension was heightened after a consultant psychiatrist supported the unions in the *Surrey Comet*, blaming the health authority for mismanagement and underfunding. Long Grove was wallowing in the mire.

Nurses were beginning to assert themselves on treatment policy, but this could be risky. While nursing leaders strove for higher professional and academic credentials, the free-thinking of the new breed of nurses irritated some service managers. One of the first conscientious objectors to psychiatric treatment was Les Parsons, an exemplary third-year student nurse at Broadland School of Nursing in Norfolk. In 1982 Parsons refused to participate in administration of ECT due to its suspected long-term damage to the brain.[72] ECT was certainly controversial, and Parsons had read widely on the topic. However, he was dismissed. The decision was upheld by an industrial tribunal, whose role was to ensure that proper procedures were followed, and not to adjudicate on the efficacy of any treatment.

Later in that year a student nurse at Shenley was sacked for similar reasons. Dee Kraaij alleged that ECT was administered incorrectly and inhumanely, with failings in premedication and aftercare. In her appeal she acknowledged the benefits of the treatment in patients with endogenous depression, but claimed that it was disproportionately applied to female patients of low social class. Speaking in her defence, Larry Gostin from MIND stated that ECT was an empirical treatment with no established evidence; he had heard several psychiatrists complain of its excessive use. Labour ex-minister David Ennals sought an amendment to mental health legislation to allow nurses to opt out of assisting with ECT, but this was defeated in parliament. In another case, Paul Walsh, senior nursing officer at Wexham Park Hospital in Slough, was sacked for refusing to administer an injection prescribed for a lucid female patient against her will. Walsh was suspended and the seventy-bed psychiatric unit was closed for two months due to mass resignation of nursing staff. The hospital managers described Walsh as 'a loose cannon', and he lost his appeal at the European Court.

Stepping out

The Seebohm Report on social work had resulted in removal of specialised social workers from the mental hospitals, but this created opportunities for nurses. In the few areas where they existed, community nurses dealt with patients already in the psychiatric system, their work delegated by consultant psychiatrists. They visited discharged patients at home, checking their medication compliance. Depot injections were administered to schizophrenic patients to prevent relapse. Modecate, a viscous substance given weekly or fortnightly, was literally a pain in the arse, but it allowed patients with chronic schizophrenia to live outside the hospital.

The community was a very different working environment for nurses. The first course in community psychiatric nursing was introduced by Chiswick College in 1973, and three years later a one-year course was started in Manchester. The latter was designed by Paddy Carr, who played a major role in the development of community psychiatric nursing in Britain. Paddy[73] had worked as a porter at Parkside in the late 1950s before going to University of Manchester to study psychology. He left this course halfway through, disillusioned by the dominance of statistical methods, and started nurse training at Parkside. After qualifying in 1963 he worked as a staff nurse for a year before leaving for general nurse training in Oxfordshire. On gaining the SRN certificate he worked at Cowley Road Hospital in Oxford, where he was rapidly promoted to night superintendent, but he was not attracted to nursing management. In 1968 he went to Keele University to study law and sociology, graduating in 1972. He applied for a DHSS research fellowship, and was funded from 1972 to 1975 for a PhD at University of Manchester, investigating the role of nurses in acute psychiatric wards in district general hospitals.

While observing nurses in the psychiatric unit at Withington Hospital, Paddy often spent time with the community nurses. In 1975 he was headhunted by Manchester Polytechnic, who had been approached by the Joint Board of Clinical Nursing Studies to design and run a course in community psychiatric nursing. Paddy was aware of the determination of community nurses and managers in Manchester to keep institutional attitudes out of the new teams. The nurses who fitted the bill were typically older with long experience but adaptable and able to use their initiative. However, it was obvious to Paddy that resocialisation was necessary in preparing hospital-based nurses for the community. Launched in 1976, the course titled Psychiatric Nursing in the Community presented a multifaceted role, and practitioners from other disciplines such as district nursing contributed to teaching. As the course included two placements, Paddy forged links with psychiatric services across the country. Most of the placement areas had already established community nursing, but in some places nurses on the course were expected to start the ball rolling. Paddy was approached by Churchill Livingstone to write a manual on community psychiatric nursing. Having more of an academic than a clinical background, Paddy brought in Tony Butterworth (who had left his nursing officer position at Withington to join Paddy at Manchester Polytechnic), and Brian Hodges, a visiting lecturer at the college on mental handicap. Published in 1980, for many years this was the CPN's 'Bible'.[74]

As community psychiatric nursing expanded, a group of practitioners and course leaders created a national association. One of the founders was Paddy, who had started the North West Community Psychiatric Nursing Association. In 1976 this merged with a similar southern body to form the Community Psychiatric Nursing Association (CPNA), with an initial membership of 120.[75] Paddy, then head of Nursing Studies at Manchester Polytechnic, was appointed as legal advisor (he was later elected as president). A main aim of the CPNA was to instill standards for CPN training, and it lobbied for a mandatory specialist qualification for community practice. Early CPN courses were criticised for being too generalist, with physical health content to the expense of developing skills in psychotherapeutic interventions. Nurses needed preparation for treating people with social phobia, depression and other common mental disorders, amidst a health promotion role. However, as Paddy argued, the strength of nursing was in its pragmatic, holistic approach.

A pioneering service was in Salford, where community nursing had begun modestly in 1973, with three hospital-based nurses visiting discharged patients who had missed their outpatient appointments. In 1979 all of the CPNs moved into general practice surgeries, where they took referrals directly from family doctors. By 1984 the eighteen CPNs received just 16 per cent of their referrals from psychiatrists.[76] The Salford service was not the norm for community psychiatric nursing, but everywhere the profile of patients was changing, with a shift from psychosis to neurosis. The caseload of the community nurse was beginning to reflect the general morbidity of the community. In primary care CPNs enjoyed a more equal relationship with doctors than they had experienced with psychiatrists. However, a discussion document by the Royal College of Psychiatrists in 1980[77] expressed concern about CPNs' detachment, urging their reintegration in mental health teams.

According to the CPNA, the number of community nurses at or above charge level grade rose from 1,667 in 1980 to 2,758 five years later.[78] Although in retrospect CPNs were at the vanguard of modern mental health practice, in the early 1980s it remained a minority pursuit. Jim Newlands was one of the first nurses at Hartwood to do CPN training; most fellow charge nurses declined the offer as they thought community nursing was a 'fad'.[79] For younger nurses, such as Mike O'Connor at Park Prewett,[80] prospects of a career beyond the old institution were appealing. This part of Hampshire was served by a community nursing team, but Mike was aware that it would take a long time to become a CPN: qualification in general nursing and promotion to charge nurse level were prerequisites for working in the community.

Mike's experience at Park Prewett reveals significant changes at the hospital in a short period of time. Unlike Tom Chan, who was barracked in the mental hospital accommodation in 1968, five years later Mike was welcomed with a room in the nurses' home at the new Basingstoke General Hospital, which was built on a large section of the Park Prewett grounds[81]. The nursing school had also moved to the general hospital, and these clean, modern buildings seemed haughtily superior to the dreary, red-brick sprawl. After moving to a newly built psychiatric unit in Doncaster, in 1974 Tom[82] had returned south for a charge nurse post at Brookwood, where in 1982 he become one of the first CPNs. Despite their lengthy experience, in the community Tom and colleagues felt like fish out of water. It took six years before he was given a place on CPN training. At least they looked the part: with their smart attire and attaché case, CPNs were far removed from the drudgery of the wards. Perhaps in envy of the new elite, hospital nurses remarked scurrilously that on a working day a CPN was most likely to be found in the aisles of Marks & Spencer.

Sanctuary redefined

The 1980 annual conference of Mind (the renamed National Association of Mental Health), titled 'The Future of the Mental Hospitals', showed little consensus on mental health policy. Speakers were polarised: some willed the end of the old asylums as soon as possible, but others were horrified by the fate of patients abandoned in the community. Patrick Jenkin,[83] the first Secretary of State for Social Services in Margaret Thatcher's government, acknowledged that most mental hospitals would remain in use over the next decade, but envisaged closure of at least thirty within a few years. A trenchant critic of the rundown was Kathleen Jones, head of the Social Administration and Social Work Department at the University of York. She reminded the audience that by the 'golden year' of 1975 the mental hospitals had not halved in population, that the wards had not been substituted in general hospitals, and that advances in medication had not enabled discharge of long-stay patients en masse. Jones did not mention the actual reduction in mental hospital beds (down to 76,364 residents in England at the end of 1979[84]), or that general hospital units had become a core component of mental health services, or that while long-stay patients accounted for two-thirds of the residents of large mental hospitals, their number was also declining. For Jones, 'nearly twenty years of neglect and public opprobrium has left (the mental hospitals) smaller, but no less hard-pressed'.[85]

Yet many Mind delegates did not share Jones's idealism of the mental hospital as a place of sanctuary and social therapy. Ex-patients were increasingly vocal about the darker side of the system. The conference report featured several anecdotes and poems about the indignity of life in the mental hospital, as in this prose by PJ Hughes:

> Over in the corner, a man and woman sit. 'Buy me a cup of tea, love', she begs. He pours tea from his cup into a saucer and grudgingly pushes it towards her. Around them buzzes the old woman of the ashtrays. Her licked fingers are wiped in each ashtray and sucked expertly.[86]

Jones, however, blamed government policy for relegating the mental hospitals to a state of disinvestment and demoralisation.

> There is the hard core of patients still in mental hospitals – the chronic, the violent, the dementing elderly – whose condition has not improved in the past twenty years. In some ways it has worsened: hospital-bashing has made its mark. Our mental hospitals have run down in more than one sense. Doctors now often come from another culture and are not easy to talk to; nursing morale has suffered badly; and the extensive social programmes of twenty years ago – the education, the art therapy, the sports – have often been replaced by the mechanical provision of endless television.[87]

Immediately following Jones' critique, Donald Dick painted a more promising picture: psychiatric hospitals had moved on from the scandals and were providing a vital role in the transformation of mental health services.[88]

> This is a time of great excitement and great success in psychiatry. There has been a broad running stream of development over the last 25 years which promises to lead further still. There are some pools that have been left behind, and some of them are stagnant, but conditions in most contemporary psychiatric hospitals are vastly better than they were 20 years ago. Hospitals today are brighter, better decorated and better furnished places with more realistic amenities and a more relaxed environment, but above all the purpose of the people within them has changed. A hospital used to be judged by its cleanliness, its orderliness, its tranquillity, its capacity to make custody bearable. Nowadays a hospital is judged on its activity, its advocacy on behalf of its patients and on whether it is easy for patients to leave if they wish. The staff are judged by whether or not they allow vulnerable people to slip into a lifelong career as mental patients.

Dick himself was the judge, having visited eighty mental hospitals as director of the HAS.[89] As a psychiatrist at Herrison Hospital in Dorset, Dick had seen care in the community work, with dozens of schizophrenic patients discharged to supported accommodation. In 1976, at a King's Fund conference celebrating the centenary of St Crispin Hospital in Northampton, Dick had asked:[90]

> Do we really need buildings? The shortage of money should stretch imaginations.

Sanctuary, Dick explained, was not a place but a sense of being. It was more important to focus on individual patients' needs, not where care is provided. Nonetheless, it seemed that many patients would need continual nursing support. David Clark described a continuum between dependency and independent living in Cambridge, ranging from fully staffed hospital wards to a variety of group homes run by voluntary organisations. The rehabilitation programme at Fulbourn included 'hostel wards' without staffing at night, and a cottage and flats in the grounds where ten patients lived without nursing supervision. The industrial workshop at Fulbourn had a workforce of 150 patients, of whom 30 lived out. However, as in most areas, there was limited involvement by social services in Cambridge.[91] Meanwhile, psychiatrists highlighted the phenomenon of the 'new long-stay' patients as a rationale for retaining the mental hospitals, albeit of reduced size.

The politics of mental health presented a schism between the defence of conventional services by public sector workers and their trade unions, and the radical ideology against psychiatry and its oppressive institutions. Mind evolved into a libertarian campaigning group, and in 1975 it appointed as legal director American human rights lawyer Larry Gostin, whose book *A Human Condition* was a blueprint of rights for psychiatric patients. Mind was heavily involved in the drafting of the new legislation, and most of Gostin's recommendations were enacted in the Mental Health Act 1983 (and the similar 1984 Act in Scotland).

The 1983 Act continued the process set in train by the previous statutes of 1930 and 1959. The three main forms of formal admission were retained, but with shorter duration and enhanced rights of appeal. The initial period for the treatment order (Section 3) was reduced from one year to six months. The assessment order (Section 2) was for twenty-eight days, and emergency order (Section 4) for seventy-two hours. Application for admission would be made by an 'approved social worker', a role requiring social work qualification and additional training for conducting assessments under the Mental Health Act. In an emergency situation on a psychiatric ward with no medical presence, Section 5(4) allowed a nurse to detain an informal patient for up to six hours, allowing time for a psychiatrist to arrive and conduct an assessment. A readily accessible tribunal system was established for patients, and any facility used for detaining patients would be inspected by the Mental Health Act Commission.

Although a progressive statute, the Mental Health Act focused on patients in hospital, with little reference to the community. As Kathleen Jones argued, it was easier to constrain the negative than to enforce the positive. Neither the NHS nor local authorities were required to develop mental health services in the community by the Act, which appeared in the context of economic recession. Thatcher's government cut grants for local authorities and introduced rate-capping, particularly affecting Labour-controlled boroughs with high levels of social need. The council coffers ran dry in once-proud towns and cities that were now desolate scenes of closed mills and factories, with mass unemployment followed by depopulation. As psychiatric patients would be at the back of the queue for local authority funding, perhaps they would be better staying in a place where they would not worry about their next meal.

Government policy, however, was not for turning. As stated in the document *Care in the Community* in 1981, the NHS would not in future be the primary provider for the type of person in long-stay psychiatric wards. Health authorities were urged to plan disposal of outmoded institutions, releasing funds for community care. In June 1983 South West Thames Regional Health Authority proposed a way forward for its mental health services. Each district would devise a range of services including community teams, residential care and day hospitals, using funds released from the closure of an entire hospital in the Epsom Cluster. The death knell was sounded for Long Grove. The regional health authority document was criticised by Surrey County Council for its presumptions of local authority responsibility and lack of costing analysis. The trade unions were more dismissive. Jack Dromey of the TGWU argued that the envisaged community services were not viable within existing resources. His union produced a glossy leaflet for public consumption titled *The Future of the Epsom Hospitals: a Better Future or Chaos?* The proposal was denounced by COHSE as a 'real estate agents' charter',[92] but nonetheless, in November 1983 it was approved as regional policy.

At this time, few of the former county asylums had a definite schedule for closure. If long-stay patients were deemed too disabled and institutionalised for returning to the community, and thus allowed to stay for the rest of their lives, it could take twenty years or more to close the hospitals. Alongside staff insecurities there was widespread suspicion in society about community care policy as an unholy alliance of capitalist Thatcherites and ideological zealots ignorant of the real problems of the mentally ill. Yet the mental institutions, whether or not people believed it, were in terminal decline. From day to day nurses carried on their work as before, but senior nursing officers, who were managing the process of vacating and merging wards, were alert to the future. As patients were shunted from one ward to another, with their nurses in tow, it became harder to deny the reality. Whereas earlier ward closures had provided space for occupational therapy or other facilities, whole ward blocks now stood empty. A brooding silence enveloped great swaths of the estate. Inside, there was no longer a cacophony from wards fore and aft, but echoes in the corridors.

Notes

1 Carrier J, Kendall I (1998): *Health and the National Health Service.*
2 Early DF (2003).
3 Department of Health and Social Security (1977): *The Facilities and Services of Mental Illness and Mental Handicap Hospitals in England 1975.* After the NHS reorganisation in 1974, figures were collated separately for England and Wales.
4 DHSS (1977). All staffing figures are whole-time equivalent.
5 DHSS (1977).
6 Croydon Area Health Authority (1976): *Report of the Committee of Inquiry: Warlingham Park Hospital.* The nursing member was Roy Macrae, SRN, RMN.
7 Croydon AHA (1976). 13.
8 Personal communication with Tony Quinn (PN, 2014). The colleague was Tony's wife, Angela.
9 By then, Greene was decorated with an OBE (Order of British Empire).
10 SE Thames RHA (1976). 156.
11 SE Thames RHA (1976). 166.
12 South East Thames Regional Health Authority (1976): *Report of Committee of Enquiry St Augustine's Hospital, Chartham, Canterbury.* The peak was 1,678 patients in 1956.
13 Personal communication (NM, 2015).
14 Personal communication (NM, 2014).
15 Personal communication (NM, 2013).
16 SE Thames (1976). 128.
17 SE Thames RHA (1976). 37. Comment by 'Dr X'.
18 SE Thames (1976). 126.
19 Rowden R (1976): St Augustine's aftermath. *Nursing Times.* As a RCN steward, Rowden represented some nurses in the enquiry, although most of those facing allegations were COHSE members.
20 Ankers WB (1976): A good report, but … *Nursing Times.*
21 Personal communication (NM, 2014).
22 Martin JP (1984). 35.
23 Marsh H (2014). 116. Marsh was a nursing assistant in 1976 at a large mental hospital near London.
24 Altschul A (1972): *Patient–Nurse Interaction: a Study of Interaction Patterns in Acute Psychiatric Wards.* 191.
25 Towell D (1975).

26 Clare A (1976).
27 Rosenhan DL (1982) On being sane in insane places. In *Social Research Ethics* (ed. M Bulmer).
28 Wolfensberger W (1972): *The Principle of Normalization in Human Services*.
29 Personal communication (NM, 1997).
30 Personal communication (NM, 2015).
31 Personal communication (NM, 2014).
32 Personal communication (NM, 2013).
33 Personal communication (NM, 2014).
34 Personal communication (NM, 2014).
35 Personal communication (NM, 2015). Jack Lyttle became principal tutor at the nursing school in Greenock, where he taught co-author NM.
36 Personal communication (NM, 2015).
37 Personal communication (NM, 1997).
38 McCusker J (1981): Mental hospitals – a view from the inside. In *The Future of the Mental Hospitals: a Report of MIND's 1980 Conference*.
39 Scott DJ, Philip AE (1985): Attitudes of psychiatric nurses to treatment and patients. *British Journal of Medical Psychology*.
40 In co-author NM's experience at Ravenscraig, a diabetic patient was given the same sugary brew served to everyone else.
41 Cormack D (1983): *Psychiatric Nursing Observed*.
42 Adams JS (2009).
43 Department of Health and Social Security (1979): *Report of the Committee of Enquiry into Mental Handicap Nursing*.
44 Personal communication (PN, 2014).
45 Personal communication (PN, 1982).
46 Personal communication (PN, 1984).
47 Clarke J (2014): Low life. *Spectator*.
48 Personal communication (NM, 2014). Dry in alcohol, but by annual rainfall, the wettest town in Britain.
49 Personal communication (NM, 2014).
50 Personal communication (NM, 1997).
51 Personal communication (NM, 2015).
52 Personal communication (NM, 2014).
53 Personal communication (NM, 2014).
54 Personal communication (NM, 2015). See *A Life in Orange*, an account by Tim Guest of being raised as a child in this cult (2004).
55 Personal communication (NM, 2014).
56 Personal communication (NM, 1995).
57 Personal communication (NM, 1995).
58 Kirkpatrick A, Feldman P (1983): Is anyone out there listening? Official enquiries into psychiatric hospitals. *Hospital and Health Services Review*.
59 The scandals were becoming 'old news' by the turn of the decade, but they made a deep imprint on the public imagination, gaining mention in the popular BBC television comedy series *Yes Minister*.
60 Personal communication (NM, 2015).
61 Personal communication (NM, 2013).
62 Personal communication (NM, 2014).
63 Personal communication (NM, 2014).
64 Salvage J (1985): *The Politics of Nursing*.
65 Casey N (1994): Trevor Clay (obituary). *Independent*.
66 Day T (1993). 47.
67 Blugrass R (1978): Regional secure units and interim security for psychiatric patients. *British Medical Journal*.

68 As at the Wessex unit. Faulk M, Taylor JC (1986): Psychiatric interim regional secure unit: seven years' experience. *Medicine, Science and the Law*.

69 Higgins J (1981): Four years' experience of an interim secure unit. *British Medical Journal*.

70 Morris P (1978): The scandal of the Prestwich secure unit. *Nursing Times*. Fears of a 'mini-Broadmoor' at Royal Earlswood (hospital for mental handicap) in Surrey provoked opposition from fourteen members of parliament. At the Bethlem Royal, amidst genteel suburbs of south-east London, the health authority minimised the risk of a negative media campaign and public anxiety about murderers and rapists being let loose on the neighbourhood by inviting a major celebrity to the opening ceremony of a secure unit. Jimmy Savile was on good form, conducting the brass band while smoking a fat cigar. According to a senior nursing officer in the staff bulletin, Savile 'lived up to his reputation by paying much attention to the children who were there'. At the time, Savile hosted the popular television series *Jim'll Fix It*. Decades later, after his death, Savile's contact with mental hospitals was scrutinised as hundreds of incidents of sexual abuse came to light. Staff bulletin report quoted in Bean C (2014): *Investigation into the Contact that Jimmy Savile had with the Bethlem Royal and Maudsley Hospitals: a Report for the Board of Directors of the South London and The Maudsley NHS Foundation Trust*.

71 Gostin LO (1986): *Institutions Observed: Towards a New Concept of Secure Provision in Mental Health*.

72 Vines G (1983): Sacked nurse takes ECT case to Europe. *New Scientist*.

73 Personal communication (NM, 2015).

74 Trustees of the CPNA. www.trusteescpna.co.uk. Tony Butterworth chaired a national review of mental health nursing, published in 1994, and be became a leading figure in nursing policy.

75 Godin P (1996): The development of community psychiatric nursing: a professional project? *Journal of Advanced Nursing*.

76 Wooff K, Rose S, Street J (1989): Community psychiatric nursing services in Salford, Southampton and Worcester. In *Health Service Planning and Research: Contributions from Psychiatric Case Registers* (ed. JK Wing).

77 Royal College of Psychiatrists (1980): Community psychiatric nursing: a discussion document by a working party of the Social and Community Services Section. *Bulletin of the Royal College of Psychiatrists*.

78 White E (1993): Community psychiatric nursing 1980 to 1990: a review of organisation, education and practice. In *Community Psychiatric Nursing: a Research Perspective* (volume 2; ed C Brooker, E White).

79 Personal communication (NM, 1996).

80 Personal communication (NM, 2013).

81 Several other district general hospitals were built on mental hospital land; e.g. at Oakwood in Kent.

82 Personal communication (NM, 2013).

83 Jenkin P (1981): Mental health and mental illness services in the 80s. In *The Future of the Mental Hospitals: a Report of MIND's 1980 Conference*.

84 Jones K (1993).

85 Jones K (1981): Re-inventing the wheel. In *The Future of the Mental Hospitals: a Report of MIND's 1980 Conference*.

86 Hughes PJ (1981): Saturday morning in the Whittingham Hospital café. In *The Future of the Mental Hospitals: a Report of MIND's 1980 Conference*. 68.

87 Jones K (1981).

88 Dick D (1981): The place of the mental hospital in services which should begin at home. In *The Future of the Mental Hospitals: a Report of MIND's 1980 Conference*.

89 Progressive improvements in the wards were evident when co-author visited the recently close Horton in 1998. Partitioning was demonstrated in several stages by

estates men who had built the fixed wooden dividers. The earliest type offered little privacy, with four beds enclosed by a low side-screen. Later types were 6 feet high with the top foot of obscure glass (the ward ceiling was several feet higher). Lastly there were fully enclosed units, with 7.5 feet walls and a door.

90   Smith JP (1976): The changing role of the large psychiatric hospital. *Nursing Mirror.*
91   Clark D (1981): The long term psychiatric patient and the future. In *The Future of the Mental Hospitals: a Report of MIND's 1980 Conference.*
92   Quoted by Day T (1993). 51.

9   End of the asylum

Intended to demonstrate the first closure of a mental hospital in Britain, the Worcester Development Project was making slow progress. When the acute psychiatric units at Kidderminster and Worcester eventually opened in 1978, admissions to Powick ceased, leaving a residual population of 343. Of these, 56 per cent had been admitted over ten years ago, 71 per cent had schizophrenia, and 79 per cent were aged over sixty-five. The Department of Health was troubled by the expense of the Worcester experiment, as the health authority was investing in new services in the community while the old hospital continued to consume resources with its army of care and ancillary staff and mounting costs of heating, maintenance and repairs. Furthermore, the project showed that care in the community would continue to be costly: people with chronic mental disorder made heavy demand on health and social services.[1] Policy-makers had overestimated the need for acute beds, while underestimating the needs of chronic and psychogeriatric patients. A unit for elderly mentally ill opened in Worcester in 1983, but there was no room for Powick patients. Over a period of eight years since the doors closed for admissions, 181 patients passed away in the Victorian wards, while just twenty-nine were discharged. The surviving denizens proved remarkably stubborn: Powick still had 114 patients in 1986.[2] By then, it had lost the race.

The first of the old asylums to close was on the fringe of London. Closing a hospital was an enormously complex process, but the least problematic situation was where more than one large institution was run by the same authority, allowing patients and personnel to be shifted from one to the other. The south-east of England was divided into four regional health authorities, each with its share of the former county mental hospitals, whose patients 'belonged' to a multitude of district health authorities, a new tier of the NHS introduced in 1982. With a high proportion of patients originating from parts of west London north of the Thames, Horton and Banstead were placed under the responsibility of Riverside District Health Authority. As Banstead was relatively isolated, the authority decided to concentrate resources at the Epsom hospital.

Peter Walsh,[3] on qualifying at Banstead in 1983, was appointed as a staff nurse on a rotation system. He worked on several wards, each time for three months, but he was also on a holiday cover rota, which entailed running wards while charge nurses were away. Banstead had a tightly knit staff, with strong characters on both union and management sides. In 1985 a dispute between the COHSE branch and the hospital management escalated from an overtime ban to a demonstration outside the main gate. Peter participated on a picket line, which barred any vehicles bringing non-urgent supplies, while minimal staffing was maintained on the wards. Police stood by but intervened when a male member of staff repeatedly crossed the road with his placard. According to Peter, the presence of journalists discouraged any aggression.

The nursing school at Banstead had closed in Peter's last year of training. When Fiona Nolan[4] started nurse training in 1984, she moved into the nurses' home at Banstead, but attended the Lorna Delve School of Nursing at Horton. Fiona recalls that many of the nurses were in denial about the future, and were as institutionalised as the patients. The buildings were rapidly decaying as all but essential maintenance was withdrawn. Having previously worked at Cell Barnes, a mental handicap hospital, Fiona was shocked by the grotty, cockroach-infested wards and corridors.

In 1985 Peter was promoted to charge nurse on the 'hospital ward' for patients with physical illness. Nine months later he took charge of a female psychogeriatric ward. Managers were concerned by evidence of high mortality when older people were transferred from institutions, so Peter's mission was to prepare the patients for a smooth transfer to Horton. The eventual exodus lasted three days, as wards moved en bloc to Epsom. Fiona remembers a 'funereal atmosphere' as windows were boarded and doors locked.[5] After serving from 1877 to 1986, Banstead was demolished and replaced by a prison.[6]

The many vacated wards at Horton were refilled, taking the hospital back up to full capacity. The staff also doubled, as resident nurses at Banstead moved into the four-storey home at Horton. The Banstead nurses were given a hostile reception, which surprised Peter as they were securing the future for Horton, while their own hospital had been sacrificed. On arriving at O Ward, Peter recalls the bloody-mindedness of their hosts. The wards were unheated, and nurses learned to put an ice cube on the thermostat to get the radiators to come on. The system at Horton was unfamiliar, and Peter could not understand the meal ordering procedure.

> It was Hell. We were told we would have a 'befriender' from the staff. They sent a patient to show us what to do.[7]

Separate identities persisted for many years. The management began to integrate staff, which alleviated some of the tension, but there was lingering resentment about Banstead staff taking over. Banstead PNO Michael O'Shaughnessy became the chief nurse, deputised by his Horton counterpart Michael Freeman. Freeman blustered but was no match for O'Shaughnessy, who was feared by staff. Similarly, Kevin O'Brien became the COHSE leader at Horton. Peter found Horton lackadaisical: nursing officers were rarely seen on wards, and standards were lower. Banstead nurses, including Peter, were rapidly promoted.

The closure of Banstead drew much sceptical comment in medical journals. It was not readily apparent how such a huge institution had been replaced by services in the community, but this was partly because such facilities were dispersed over a wide area. New inpatient units had been established at St Mary Abbot's Hospital in Kensington, on the third and ninth floors of Charing Cross Hospital, a purpose-built mental health unit with six wards at St Charles' Hospital off Ladbroke Grove, psychogeriatric services at Chiswick Lodge, and the former Gordon Hospital for Diseases of the Rectum and Colon was converted for psychiatric use in Westminster borough.[8] Responding to negative press, the district general manager of Riverside noted that the writers of a critical report by Mind had not visited the new services:

> Our strategy, which has been six years in the planning and which aims to provide a better life for every one of Banstead's residents, has succeeded in that aim … By all means let us talk about the problems we face in implementing our mental health programmes, but let us also give credit to the hard work and enthusiasm of the many hundreds of staff who have achieved the replacement of Banstead.[9]

A smooth crossing

A success story for the transformation from hospital to community care was in Devon, as described by David King.[10] When he was appointed as chief administrator for Exeter district following the NHS reorganisation in 1974, King's immediate concern was the unsatisfactory conditions at Exminster and Digby mental hospitals, which he feared could be scandalised. Indeed, several complaints were received, in one case leading to a criminal investigation. King focused on upgrading of wards, but later realised that this was throwing good money after bad. Senior managers had minimal influence on the running of the mental hospitals:

> How often over the years we had gathered in the Board Room at Exminster for lengthy discussions – for example, to negotiate alterations to the shift systems so that nurses no longer worked 12 hours at a stretch, or to get the last meal of the day for patients served later than 4.30 in the afternoon. The joint meeting of management with the trade unions was usually preceded by each side meeting separately to prepare its ground and anticipate what the other might have in store.[11]

After several inconsequential working parties, in 1983 the newly formed Exeter District Health Authority announced a radical plan to close all of its institutions for mental illness and mental handicap within four years. While the mental hospitals were gradually contracting, there was a pervasive belief that they would survive in some form, but the health authority displayed a timetable showing how every ward would be replaced by new services in the community. The programme was carefully planned, with a single leader for each project instead of the cumbersome multidisciplinary system of management. Opposition was inevitable. In 1986 a meeting of the Royal College of Psychiatrists, held in Torbay, ended with an overwhelming vote against government policy. While many of their peers feared loss of authority and fragmentation of services, psychiatrists in the Exeter district were more optimistic, and their influence was valued by the senior management team in their efforts to persuade staff of a brighter future.

Through delicate consultation, the trade unions were brought on board. The secretary of the largest COHSE branch in Exeter was a member of a national committee led by Terry Mallinson. Beginning his working life in a Yorkshire coalmine, Mallinson had qualified in both psychiatric and general nursing, before his full-time appointment as a COHSE regional secretary in 1962. He was secretary to the COHSE working party that produced the enlightened report *The Future of Psychiatric Services*,[12] but sadly he died before its publication, at the age of forty-nine. Mallinson's deeply felt concern for psychiatric patients helped to dissuade union representatives from a narrow course of self-interest. In the Exeter hospitals, the confrontational tone of meetings was dropped as the unions contributed to a consensus for care in the community, and against turning back the clock. Resistance to change was overcome, as the unions saw the importance of their role in supporting staff through the challenges ahead. Instead of distant authorities making all of the decisions, nurses could be masters of their own destiny. A major issue was job security, and to ensure goodwill it was agreed that there would be full redeployment. Some of the most trenchant critics of hospital closure were keen converts to community care.

One of the nurses who made change happen in Devon was Iain Tulley.[13] Like Peter Walsh at Woodilee, Iain had felt stunted by the culture at Hartwood, and having read of revolutionary developments in mental health services in England, he too moved south. In 1985 he applied for a job in Devon as a resettlement nurse, at charge nurse level, and was interviewed at Exminster Hospital. Although there were community teams in the Torbay area, these did not deal with rehabilitation, and Ian needed to be creative to find suitable accommodation and care for long-stay patients. After a year Iain was appointed as a senior nursing manager, responsible for developing community services in south Devon. Iain corroborates David King's depiction of a well-managed hospital closure programme, with clear objectives, proper funding, and clinicians kept on board.

Exminster Hospital was shut in 1987, and when the first portion of land was sold to housing developers in the following year, the proceeds were channelled into services in Torbay. Reprovision in Exeter was boosted by the sale of Digby Hospital on the outskirts of the city; a shopping mall now stands where thousands of people spent lives in red-brick Victorian wards. On the grounds of Wonford House, a former private asylum later incorporated in the Exe Vale group, the Royal Devon and Exeter Hospital was built. Facing seemingly insurmountable challenges in replacing their outmoded institutions, health authorities around the country saw Exeter as a model.

The new economy

With tardy progress in collaboration between health and social services, Margaret Thatcher's government asked Sir Roy Griffiths, managing director of Sainsbury's supermarket chain, to write a blueprint for the organisation and funding of care in the community. Griffiths had good form; in 1983 he had produced an influential report on senior management in the NHS. He suggested that if Florence Nightingale was carrying her lamp through the corridors of the NHS, she would be looking for the person in charge. A passionate believer in the NHS, which he regarded as the finest piece of social engineering of the twentieth century, Griffiths was critical of how it was run. Division of labour was arbitrary, powerful professions decided what they would do and not do, and productivity was rarely considered by either managers or clinical personnel. Griffiths focused on how the workforce could be reorganised to fulfil the potential of the NHS. Rejecting management by consensus, Griffiths proposed a single leader, acting as chief executive officer. His report led to the introduction of general management principles and practices: a district general manager was appointed in each district health authority in 1984, and the principal nursing officer and deputies were reduced to an advisory role. Managers with a background in commerce received a cool reception in the NHS, and they needed all of the skills of running a large organisation to survive.

Such development must be understood in a wider context of radical neo-liberal politics and global corporate expansion, as the old order of both public and private sectors was challenged by technological advances, individualistic consumerism and the pursuit of efficiency. Inspired by the Enlightenment philosophy of Adam Smith, Thatcher was a devout believer in natural market forces. Neither tradition, nor state command-and-control, could hold back the tide of an increasingly globalised society. Indeed, the most prominent issue for organisation theorists in the 1980s was management of change.[14] Professional groups and trade unions remained influential, but power increasingly lay in the hands pulling the purse strings.

Griffiths[15] developed the theme from his management critique in his enquiry into community care, which was not really working in the 1980s. Old problems persisted: the NHS and social services had different remit and responsibilities, funding mechanisms, planning cycles, geographical boundaries, ideologies and cultures. There were strong disincentives to joint-working. Health authorities tended to hang on to their budgets, using Joint Finance for marginal, ad hoc projects. Local authorities were unwilling to adopt the long-term financial commitment for discharged psychiatric patients, and the situation was not helped by spending cuts imposed by the Conservative government. Beyond a few exemplars of collaboration, achievements were limited.[16]

In 1985 a report by the Audit Commission revealed wide variation between local authorities in England and Wales in the resourcing of community care, and confusion of responsibilities. Piecemeal planning and delivery of services in the community was hindering resettlement of the most disabled patients who remained in the mental hospitals, and those who had already left were not always receiving adequate support. Many discharged patients from London were dispersed to faded coastal resorts, which became a dumping ground for social misfits. The surfeit of bed-and-breakfast houses in towns such as Hastings offered cheap temporary accommodation for local authority 'clients', including the mentally ill. Banished from such premises in the daytime, psychiatric refugees spent staring at the sea from a promenade bench, in bad weather congregating in the public library. Some proprietors packed several residents into each bedroom, with little privacy or comfort. Elaine Murphy[17] described such conditions as a reprise of the private madhouses of the eighteenth century.

Somewhat surprisingly, the Griffiths Report in 1988 proposed that local authorities take the lead responsibility for community care. A care manager (ideally a social worker) would assess each person and plan a package of care, not necessarily delivered directly by social services, but by private and voluntary sectors wherever appropriate. Housing and welfare benefits would be channelled through the local authority, with NHS input restricted to health care. However, psychiatrists were sceptical about the capacity and commitment of local authorities to cater for people with mental health problems. While in favour of decentralisation, Thatcher's government was troubled by Griffiths' recommendation of giving power to local authorities, many of which were regarded as bastions of socialism. Nonetheless, the proposals were enacted two years later.

Pursuing a 'seamless service', the NHS and Community Care Act 1990 differentiated the responsibilities of health and local authorities, and although the care management system was not applied until April 1993, other provisions began earlier. In 1991 specific mental health funding was made available for social services to prioritise investment in facilities for people who would previously have received all care and hospitality from NHS psychiatry. The Mental Illness Specific Grant was only to be used for new services jointly planned by the NHS and local authority; a portion of the central government grant to the local authority would then be ring-fenced for care of people with mental disorder.

The NHS and Community Care Act redrew the entire landscape of health and social care. In 1991 an internal market was created in the NHS, separating the functions of purchaser and provider. Hospitals and community health services were allowed to become self-governing NHS trusts, accountable to the Department of Health but free from district health authority control. By 1993, most NHS providers had gained trust status. Market forces replaced centralised command and control. Competition was expected to improve efficiency in the NHS, which Thatcher described as 'a bottomless financial pit'.[18]

With its cost-cutting and privatisation agenda, the Tory government was suspected of closing the mental hospitals for economic and political reasons, with little concern for the patients. Yet British policy was not an isolated case. The USA had led the way in deinstitutionalisation, but the most radical policy was in Italy, where a law passed in 1978 prohibited admissions to mental hospitals, which were to be replaced by fifteen-bed units in general hospitals and a range of community clinics. The Italian experiment was lauded by some, but regarded by others as a disaster; several hospitals survived the statute due to yawning gaps in care in the community. The first country to open a system of public asylums, Britain was at the vanguard of a global movement to close them.

A statutory framework was evolving for the nebulous entity of community care. Introduced in 1991, the Care Programme Approach (CPA) clarified psychiatric illness as a health service responsibility. A keyworker (typically a CPN) was appointed for each patient, but this caused confusing overlap with the role of the local authority care manager. The Department of Health clarified the care manager as broker, and the keyworker as a direct provider. The CPA required the various agencies to work together, and for practitioners to attend multidisciplinary review meetings. Some of the most severely disordered patients were the most reluctant service-users, and there was a danger of them slipping through the net, potentially bringing the whole policy of care in the community into disrepute.

On new year's eve, 1992, a psychiatric patient climbed the lions' den at Regents Park zoo. Ben Silcock was severely mauled, as was the policy blamed for his neglect. Facing a deeply sceptical and fearful public, the ideal of care in the community was desperately in need of proof that it worked – or that it existed. The well-managed programme of mental hospital closure in Exeter showed that patients could be successfully discharged to a new range of services in the community, with full employment opportunities for nurses. Yet government policy, since its announcement decades earlier, had never been supported by robust clinical evidence. The Worcester experiment had demonstrated the challenges but no clear benefits for patients, while Exeter had been described from a managerial and possibly biased perspective. Were patients really thriving outside the sheltered environment of the mental institution, or were they languishing in squalor? A strategic document for closing Shenley Hospital illustrates the authorities' concern about stepping into the dark:

> The earliest indications of long-stay hospital closures have been mixed as has resettlement been patchy across Britain. Some people have achieved a quality of life denied them for years in an institution; others, though, have found themselves in an uncaring community with inadequate support services and have drifted into poverty, isolation and homelessness … The historical cycle of neglect, reform, and then again further neglect of services for mentally ill people has been well documented. Thereby in the context of full scale reprovision of existing hospital services into community-based care and reforms instituted by this move must not be allowed to lead again into neglect.[19]

The most rigorous study of the impact of community care was in north London. In 1983 North East Thames Regional Health Authority had announced its plan to close two of its mental hospitals over a ten-year period. The Team for Assessment of Psychiatric Services (TAPS), founded by research psychiatrist Julian Leff at the MRC, was contracted for a prospective evaluation of the reprovision programme on patients, staff, families and the public. A major component of the study was an assessment of outcomes in long-stay patients one and five years after discharge, with a battery of standardised assessment instruments measuring patients' mental state, social behaviour, basic living skills, physical health, environment and attitudes.[20] When TAPS began, Friern and Claybury each had around 900 patients.

On completing nurse training in 1990 and intending to move to London, co-author NM applied for a post at Claybury, which the *Nursing Times* advertisement portrayed as a stone's throw from the heart of the metropolis. He was astonished by the map sent for the interview, which seemed to depict a whole town, with church, social club, workshops, tennis courts and bowling green, circuitous lanes and a grid of streets in the centre. Deterred by the remoteness of this institutional setting, NM did not attend the interview, but two years later he was shown around by Ruth Benbow, a colleague of previous Claybury employ. By then this large Victorian asylum was at an advanced stage of rundown. Ascending the main drive, they passed several blocks with boarded windows. Claybury had retreated to its core, but the wide central corridors, with names such as Church Street, were full of life; motorised carts passed en route to or from the laundry or kitchens. Ruth took NM upstairs to the rehabilitation ward where she had worked for many years. In this high-ceilinged cavern, with its overpowering institutional odour, chronic schizophrenic patients cadged cigarettes, while nurses in aprons calmly carried on their routine.

In 1990 the regional health authority decided to postpone closure of Claybury indefinitely, due to tardy progress in developing services in the catchment area. Resources were concentrated on the closure of Friern, which consequently accounted for most of the patients in the TAPS evaluation. Assessments were completed with 671 ex-patients of Friern or Claybury one year after discharge, and the results were promising. Overall, there was stability in mental and physical health, and decline in negative symptoms, which the researchers attributed to the more stimulating environment outside the institution. Indeed, social activity improved, as did everyday living skills; the discharged patients were mostly satisfied in their new homes. After five years fifty-four of the patients had died, which was almost double the general population mortality rate. This was troubling, but it is well known that people with schizophrenia have lowered life expectancy, probably due to a combination of unhealthy lifestyle and the long-term effects of antipsychotic medication. Five of the deaths were suicides. Five years after discharge, 235 of the study cohort participated in further assessment. Social and clinical improvements were mostly sustained, and there was no evidence that psychiatric patients were contributing to an increase in vagrancy or violent crime. Public fears were not realised.

Training for a new era

In a study of 1984 to 1987 cohorts at five nursing schools in south-western England, co-author PN explored students' reasons for entering psychiatric nursing. One woman had previously worked in a pub, where she had been intrigued by the habitually solitary customers.

> Those I really felt sorry for were the ones who came in just after opening time, asked for a half of shandy, sat by themselves and were still there at closing time. I have known one old gentleman spend the whole evening staring at the floor, totally oblivious to what was going on around him. On several occasions, he left the pub without even touching his drink.[21]

A common theme was a desire to help estranged human beings. Reflecting on their experiences, most of PN's interviewees felt that they had developed personally, but they criticised the training. They found much of what they were taught in nursing school barely evident in practice. Tutors were remote from the wards and morale among nurses was low. Half of the sample did not intend to stay in psychiatric nursing. This was a group of articulate, assertive students who did not think that their chosen profession could fulfil its caring potential, or present satisfactory career prospects.

As recommended by the Briggs Committee, radical change to nurse training was afoot. In 1983 the GNC for England and Wales and counterpart for Scotland were replaced by the United Kingdom Central Council for Nursing, Midwifery and Health Visiting (UKCC), and boards of nursing for the four countries of the United Kingdom. The UKCC aimed to raise academic standards, thereby preparing for nurses for more autonomous practice, and enhancing the status of the profession in a multidisciplinary system. While striving to free itself from medical hegemony, nursing was restrained by its lack of esoteric knowledge and skills. An eclectic mix of theory was borrowed from other disciplines, mainly medicine and psychology.

Since the 1960s, nursing theorists had been busily devising theoretical frameworks to guide practice. In Britain, the Roper, Logan and Tierney[22] model of nursing was prominent in training in the 1980s. In this formulation, Nancy Roper, Winifred Logan and Alison Tierney at the University of Edinburgh directed nursing to twelve activities of daily living: maintaining a safe environment, communicating, breathing, eating and drinking, eliminating, personal cleansing and dressing, controlling body temperature, mobilising, working and playing, expressing sexuality, sleeping, and dying. Each activity related to the 'nursing process': a logical trajectory of assessing, planning, implementing and evaluating care.[23] Unlike the sophistry of American theorists, Roper, Logan and Tierney presented a straightforward, practical approach unencumbered by philosophical discourse. In his acclaimed nursing manual *Mental Disorder: its Care and Treatment*, Jack Lyttle[24] used the model as a vehicle for individualised care. While doctors diagnosed and prescribed treatment, nurses devised and followed a care plan based on a nursing model.

In practice, however, nursing theory failed. Writing in the *Nursing Times*, co-author NM[25] described how the nursing school and general hospital had attempted to integrate theory and practice by applying the Roper, Logan and Tierney model throughout clinical settings, yet care plans had deteriorated into a template for students to complete. The apparent strength of the model as an explicit tool of the nursing process made it prone to routinisation; the twelve activities of daily living were etched on clipboards on patients' beds, with a narrow range of stock phrases. Eventually nursing models were abandoned, but the baby was thrown out with the bathwater[26].

The nursing process helps nurses to think clearly about what they are trying to achieve, in partnership with the patient. It underpinned a quality improvement project at Tooting Bec, where Bill Lemmer[27] was appointed as a nursing officer in 1983. Succeeding from a retired sister, Lemmer had a specific remit for in-service training of the 130 nursing assistants, but he saw the futility of the existing scheme. Nursing assistants provided most of the care, but despite a two-week course and refresher week, there was little evidence of their learning being applied in practice. Task-orientation persisted. The daily routine ran at least two hours ahead of social norms: elderly patients (who accounted for seventy per cent of the Tooting Bec population) were woken at 5.30 a.m. by the night staff, and were back in their nightdresses by 6 p.m. Thus the morning workload of the daytime nurses was relieved, and in return, the night staff arrived to a ward with patients already asleep in bed. Enrolled nurses and nursing assistants were frequently sent to other wards to cover shortages. Lemmer observed an incident that typified nurse–patient relations:

> A lady is pushed in a chair across a room at such speed that she misinterprets the nurse's action for aggression. The nurse offers no verbal explanation for this action. The lady strikes out at the nurse with her elbow and, turning slightly in the wheelchair, manages to punch the air behind in the direction of the nurse. The nurse – focused on her task of getting the patient from A to B so as to return to dress and convey the next person from bed to breakfast table – has demonstrated institutional behaviour, where concern with the task has become, imperceptibly and without conscious thought, more important than concern for the person.[28]

A series of HAS inspections in the mid-1980s found not a single psychogeriatric ward at Tooting Bec with a satisfactory standard of care. As a CPN in south London, Fiona Couper was appointed by the Nightingale School of Nursing at St Thomas' Hospital to train nurses for community work,[29] and she recalls her impression on arriving at her new base at Tooting Bec. Compared to The Maudsley, it was like stepping into the abyss. Scary patients lurked in the corridors: some shouting or screaming, others mute. The enormous wards had long, gloomy dormitories with few staff around. The caged iron walkways linking the ward blocks on first and second floors were particularly oppressive; Fiona remembers a Polish man who was regularly sent out there for making too much noise. Nursing was custodial, and very behind the times, with a token economy system used for discipline. Following refurbishment, the nurse education centre was the only modern building in the hospital. The entrance was kept locked, but a long-stay female patient sneaked in on several occasions, and urinated on the plush armchairs in the staff room. Perhaps this was a statement against luxuries afforded to others.

Transferred to the Staff Development Department at the Nightingale School of Nursing, Lemmer initiated a management of change project at Tooting Bec in 1985. The ineffectual training for nursing assistants was scrapped, as the project focused on the whole team on five psychogeriatric wards. Nurses did not plan or review individualised care, but simply maintained a ward routine. Applying Donabedian's[30] quality evaluation framework of structure, process and outcome, Lemmer observed that the ward sisters' main concern was the structural input: the organisation of human and physical resources, and documentation. Sisters had little autonomy as senior nurses were unwilling to relinquish their inherited power. However, Lemmer saw that change depended on leadership; merely training nursing assistants would not make any real difference. To redirect the nursing effort to a person-centred, outcome-orientated approach, Lemmer facilitated a collective effort, with group work as the vehicle of change. Staff support meetings and sisters' groups were held regularly; 'quality circles' were facilitated by senior nurse Kathleen McClafferty as a forum for staff to discuss and solve problems. Sisters moved from the conventional shift pattern to a 9 a.m. to 5 p.m. day, thereby enhancing supervision and support for staff. Group meetings tended to focus on concrete matters rather than abstract issues such as role conflict, and the project did not produce dramatic results. However, new norms evolved, as nurses began to take more professional responsibility, and nursing assistants relinquished archaic institutional practices. Quality improvement was achieved not by top-down decree but as a bottom-up, participatory endeavour.

In 1986 'Project 2000'[31] was announced as a reorientation of nurse training from an apprenticeship to studying at institutes of higher education, with clinical experience as supernumerary learners free from rostered service. As previously recommended by Briggs,[32] a common foundation programme was introduced, whereby all nursing students would study together for the first half of their training, with placements in medical, surgical, geriatric and psychiatric wards. The second half of the training would be branch-specific in teaching and clinical experience. For the first time, recruits would begin their careers as students not only in name, but in an academic environment that would encourage self-directed learning and critical enquiry. Nurse training, indeed, became nurse education.

Project 2000 wiped out hundreds of small hospital-based schools of nursing, and in psychiatric hospitals this was a visible sign of the changing times. Most nurse tutors were relocated to the premises of a polytechnic college or university, alongside counterparts from other branches of nursing and midwifery. For professional and social reasons, nursing fitted neither in a medical school, nor in a social science or humanities department. In most institutes, a department of nursing was created. Relabelled as lecturers, experienced tutors such as co-author PN found themselves reporting to superiors with limited understanding of psychiatric nurse training or practice. Typical of the newly created directors of nurse education was Margaret Howard at Bath School of Nursing. Sceptical towards the theoretical input to psychiatric nurse training, Howard believed that tutors were offering little more than a hodgepodge of left-wing ideas and sociological speculation, of limited value in caring for patients and promoting their recovery. She saw general nursing as a practical occupation, based on logical premises with demonstrable effectiveness, in contrast to what she perceived as the subjectivity and fragile epistemological foundation of psychiatric nursing. Howard's way was to bring the latter into line with the general nursing curriculum. Project 2000 reduced the amount of time devoted to psychiatric nursing, as students were immersed in anatomy and physiology, pathology and aseptic procedures; some mental health recruits became disillusioned and left in the first year. Annie Altschul criticised the homogenisation of nursing as an administrative convenience that neglected the special skills needed for mental health practice.[33]

Academic trailblazers

Far removed from the insular world of the mental institution, a few ambitious nurses took advantage of the new opportunities arising in the higher education environment. An early bird was Bryn Davis, who was the recipient of DHSS funding for nursing scholarship in the 1970s, culminating in a doctorate. Bryn's distinguished career had begun in 1956, when he declared himself as a conscientious objector to National Service. Summoned to York Assizes for refusing the 'Queen's shilling', he was sentenced to two years of community service. His mother had qualified as a mental nurse at Storthes Hall in the 1930s, before leaving to get married and raise a family. Living in York after the war, she had worked at The Retreat for a few years. For his required period of service, Bryn decided to follow in her footsteps. As a Quaker institution, The Retreat had many other conscientious objectors among its staff.

> I was expected to do two years as an orderly. However, I was approached by the nurse tutors there soon after arriving and they discussed the possibility of my doing three years and qualifying as a mental nurse. I really had no definite idea what I was to do after the two years anyway. At home we had lots of my mother's books from her training which I had read and so the idea of training and getting involved in the subjects was attractive. So I agreed and started training in February 1957.[34]

After a delay of nine months due to a motorcycle accident, Bryn eventually passed the final examination in February 1961, but there were no vacancies at The Retreat. Instead of applying to one of the former county asylums in the area, he was advised by senior officers to try either The Maudsley or Holloway Sanatorium.[35] In May 1961 he found a job at the latter hospital. Initially Bryn lived in the male nurses' home, but after getting married in 1962 he secured one of the hospital-owned terraced cottages just outside the grounds. Bryn worked on all the male wards on a rotating relief for charge nurses on leave or sick. In 1963 he was seconded to SRN training at a general hospital in Windsor, and on his return in 1965 he became a charge nurse. Having heard from students that Bryn was a good teacher, in 1966 the nursing school interviewed him for tutor training.

> I was seconded to Battersea Polytechnic for the Sister Tutors course as it was called then. This was for two years. This I enjoyed immensely and fell in love with the academic world and further education and research. On my return to Holloway I entered the School of Nursing, quite a small one with principal tutor and three tutors. After a year, in 1969 I decided to approach Birkbeck College, London, to do psychology, inspired by the then principal tutor who had done just the same the year I joined. This was part-time evenings for three years after which, if successful, one was eligible for a full-time grant for the last, fourth year. My successful BSc then made me eligible for a DHSS Nursing Research Fellowship to do my PhD. These developments for nursing further education were the springboard for several of us to gain academic qualifications that led eventually to the development of nursing departments in universities.[36]

After his study at the London School of Economics, Bryn was appointed as deputy director of the highly reputed Nursing Research Unit at Edinburgh University. In the 1980s he moved to Brighton Polytechnic where he instituted a fellowship scheme for nurses. He observed that many psychiatric nurses had the aptitude for academic work, but lacked opportunities and encouragement for such endeavour.[37] The first fellowship was awarded to a nurse from Hellingly Hospital who had left school with no qualifications. Nurses were enabled to conduct research on contemporary issues such as the impact of hospital closure on patients, and the medical versus psychosocial model of mental illness. On becoming professor of nurse education at University of Cardiff, Bryn prepared a research strategy for the school, leading to the university funding doctoral research studentships. A slow trickle of PhD students, supervised by Bryn, contributed to a critical mass of nursing academe.

As chairs of nursing departments were created, mental health nursing gained greater credibility and influence in relation to other branches of nursing, and in the wider multidisciplinary sphere. Among the most notable figures was Julia Brooking. Having begun her nursing career at Cane Hill, Julia became senior lecturer in psychiatric nursing at The Maudsley and in 1989 she was appointed as professor of mental health nursing at University of Birmingham, where she played a major role in the academic development of her discipline.[38] However, while Brooking's textbook emphasised research as the basis for professional practice,[39] the infrastructure for nurses was a shanty town built on the perimeter of the medical metropolis. On his appointment at University of Birmingham, co-author PN found much difficulty in competing against medical schools for research funding. The lack of substantial grant income was reflected in the preponderance of small-scale, qualitative studies reported in journals in the 1980s and 1990s.[40]

In 1994 the *Journal of Psychiatric and Mental Health Nursing* was launched, edited by Bill Lemmer, opening with a commentary on the past, present and future of the discipline by Hildegard Peplau.[41] Its title reflected another important development. The label 'psychiatric nurse', although it continued to be widely used, was officially changed to 'mental health nurse'. The rationale for this change was twofold. First, mental health was cast as a positive approach, in contrast to the erstwhile stigmatised concept of mental illness. The second reason, which was not so explicitly stated, was that nurses would no longer be aides to a branch of medicine, but autonomous practitioners answerable to their own profession.

Last rites

Psychiatric nurses make good managers: pragmatic leaders who have worked up from the wards, experienced in dealing with the idiosyncrasies of patients and staff, and guided by professional ethics. Few make names for themselves, but an exception was Ray Rowden, a controversial character who deserves a place at the top table in the history of mental health nursing. Ray began his career at St Augustine's Hospital as a nursing auxiliary, qualifying as a nurse in 1973. He challenged bad practices in the hospital, and was an advocate for nursing students. After training as a general nurse, he returned to the mental health field in 1986. As one of the youngest chief executive officers in the NHS, at West Lambeth Community Mental Health Trust he took on the difficult mission of closing Tooting Bec Hospital.

Rowden had married a nurse from St Augustine's and fathered two children, but by the 1980s he was openly gay. His flamboyance was remarkable at a time of blatant prejudice against homosexuality. He spent lavishly on dandy clothes, and a pink shirt was his plumage. An enthusiast of ballet, he regularly took groups of patients to sit among the elite at Covent Garden. According to informants for this book, he was also a boorish drinker who was sexually promiscuous at conferences. Rowden was mocked behind his back but rarely challenged in person; he made allies of influential nursing officers and charge nurses. Although a left-wing maverick, he charmed Health Secretary Virginia Bottomley and Tory peer Baroness Julia Cumberlege, persuading them to place mental health higher on the agenda.[42] Co-author PN recalled that a favourite saying of Rowden's was his version of the carrot-and-stick approach: 'carrot up the arse, and hit them with the stick'. During his upheavals, some older nurses went off sick, suffering from stress and related physical health problems. Fiona Couper[43] recalls a stark contrast between his thuggish manner and the prim and proper tutors at the Nightingale School; the head of the school could not relate to the asylum culture, and Rowden saw her ideas for training Tooting Bec nurses as naive. In his view, nurses were not there primarily for the patients, but to earn money from a steady job with a salary boosted by unsocial hours and overtime. As a union man, he knew how to deal with staff and often held court in the social club, which Fiona described as 'a den of inequity'. Taking the reins of the macho management at Tooting Bec, Rowden shook the old culture and infused the insular hospital dynamics with his irrepressible energy.

One of Fiona's tasks at Tooting Bec was to invigilate at examinations for enrolled nurses, following a UKCC ruling on competence for drug administration. This caused consternation: on most wards at night SENs held the ward keys, and failure would result in loss of night shifts and overtime. Nurses blatantly cheated, but the blind were leading the blind. Officially three attempts were allowed, but some nurses were allowed several more chances. A few simply could not get through, and were eventually demoted in the national regrading of nurses.

Implemented in 1988, the UKCC grading structure was a logical division of responsibility and remuneration, but it caused resentment and some bitter disputes. Until then, a newly qualified staff nurse was essentially paid the same as one of twenty years' service (although the latter benefited from annual increments). Staff nurse posts were divided into D and E grades, with a deputy charge nurse at F and charge nurse at G. This reform faced much opposition across the nursing profession, and particularly in the more militant branch of psychiatric nursing. The COHSE campaign of literally working to grade and threatened strike action were condemned by a RCN spokesman, who argued that 'if the issue of working to grade went to court nurses would be leaving themselves wide open to the charge that they had breached their contracts.' He accused NUPE and COHSE of 'sailing very close to the wind' by advising nurses not to drug ward rounds or go into locked wards:

> Nurses could end up before their statutory body because they didn't go to the aid of patients when they were qualified to do so.[44]

In the early 1990s most of the mental hospitals remained in use, although the number of workers now exceeded that of the residents. Lessons were learned from elsewhere, but closure was a protracted and stressful process. Management faced powerful professional interests and a heavily unionised workforce,[45] seemingly incapable of adapting to a changing environment. Without the nurses, the patients could not survive; without the patients, there would be no jobs – this was the unwritten contract as perceived by many nurses. In 1995 co-author NM attended a multidisciplinary meeting at a rehabilitation ward at Netherne to consider the transfer of a young schizophrenic woman to a group home, which had a vacancy. The ward manager tried to delay the move, arguing: 'She will need rehabilitation.' Yet she had been on this ward for three years. It seemed that he was jealously guarding his flock.

According to Peter Senge,[46] bureaucratic organisations are handicapped by 'learning difficulties', whereby workers are concerned with their own narrow positions rather than the collective product, externalising of blame, reactive rather than proactive management, seeing immediate events but not longer-term patterns, and a misconception that learning is derived from experience thus giving trial and error ascendancy over rational planning. As Kurt Lewin[47] explained, the homeostatic tendency in organisations can only be overcome if sufficient energy is applied to produce change. In the mental hospitals, managers needed to understand the driving and resisting forces. Lewin's model entailed a three-stage process: unfreezing the existing state by showing the need for change, moving to the planned position, then refreezing by reinforcing new group behaviour. Schein (1987) elaborated Lewin's process with psychological mechanisms at each stage. In unfreezing, change is encouraged by withdrawal of support for old behaviours. In moving to a new position, workers learn that change is possible and desirable. In refreezing, new behaviours are internalised, and significant relationships are formed in the new environment.

However, attitudes were not the only barrier to progress. In the Epsom Cluster, a stumbling block was the multitude of 'out of area' patients. The first task in planning resettlement was to identify patients by their responsible health authority. Earmarked as the first of the Epsom hospitals to close, Long Grove was managed by Kingston and Esher District Health Authority, but as well as accommodating many patients from the catchment area of Richmond, Twickenham and Roehampton Health Authority, hundreds of long-stay residents originated in the east end of London. These old Cockneys, born in earshot of the Bow Bells, were in danger of becoming 'stateless'. The system, it seemed, was waiting for them to die.

In July 1985 the Epsom Cluster Steering Group announced that Long Grove would close within five years, enabled by Kingston and Esher Health Authority building a new mental health unit at Tolworth Hospital, opening of community facilities in Roehampton, and transfer of remaining patients to neighbouring Horton and West Park. Below a banner headline 'Hospital axed' in the *Epsom Herald*, Maurice Smith of the TGWU argued that the 600 staff 'will be fighting this closure all the way. They don't want to be part of the government's asset-stripping of the health service'.[48] In fact, Long Grove was far from empty by 1990. Insufficient bridging finance from the regional health authority to the district authorities was compounded by a sudden slump in the property market. This was not the best time to be relying on sale of hospital land. Four hundred patients remained at Long Grove, and serious concerns arose on the conditions for those left behind, and a demoralised workforce. The Mental Health Act Commission visited the hospital four times from 1988 to 1990, finding lack of therapeutic activity, deterioration in standards of care, and wards devoid of personal effects and comforts. As half-empty wards merged, patients were moved around like a game of musical chairs.

To keep staff on board in the closure process, and to allay rumour, monthly meetings were held, including sessions for night staff. After lengthy negotiations, the health authorities and trade unions agreed that there would be no compulsory redundancies at the Epsom Cluster, as had been agreed by Riverside Health Authority when Banstead moved into Horton. Although there was a surplus of staff, many nurses were approaching the early retirement age of fifty. A personnel team interviewed 528 Long Grove workers on their job opportunities. The Epsom Cluster Agreement required health authorities to give Long Grove staff first chance to apply for any vacancies. By the end of 1991 almost all of the nurses had accepted jobs in the new services in the community, or transfer to Horton or West Park (the latter run by Mid-Surrey Health Authority). A few members of staff refused to apply for redeployment, but in doing so forfeited their rights; the health authorities held firm, and exemplary dismissals were made. Ultimately, just six nurses were made redundant.

In June 1991 the regional health authority proposed to close the hospital sooner rather than later. By then there were 157 patients from Kingston and Esher, seventy-five from Richmond, Twickenham and Roehampton, and 113 from distant parts of London. In October, while the foundations were being laid at Tolworth, final closure of Long Grove was set for March 1992. The regional authority had decided that it would not wait until community facilities were in place. In the last months, some of the remaining patients moved into hostels and homes in the community, but the majority were transferred to neighbouring hospitals. Five wards containing 117 patients, mostly from the old catchment areas of east and south London, went to West Park. A total of 195 patients moved to Horton, while awaiting the opening of Tolworth and of community services by Richmond, Twickenham and Roehampton Health Authority. Another ward of Richmond patients went to West Park. Horton took five psychogeriatric wards, two admission wards and Addison Ward, the ward for disturbed patients. Nurses followed their patients, and were recontracted to Riverside or Mid-Surrey. On the day before closure, Roy Galley, chairman of Kingston and Esher Health Authority, thanked the staff:

> As you are fully aware, Long Grove Hospital is now virtually closed and the patients housed in new accommodation. This whole exercise has been a daunting task and, I believe, the right step to take as the first move in creating new mental health services which will be soundly based for the future. Although there have been problems, I believe that the whole operation of closure and of opening new facilities has been very successful for the vast majority of patients, relatives, staff and other carers. You have made your own personal contribution to this success and I thank you very much for all your hard work and dedication.[49]

On 1 April 1992, when Guildford Ward was decanted to West Park, one Polish man refused to budge. The ward having been emptied of furniture and closed, he wandered along the deserted corridors. There was no bed, no nurses and no kitchen, but the patient could not be persuaded to go to his new home. It seemed that the only course of action would be to 'section' him, but eventually a combined force of senior managers and West Park nurses coaxed him into the mini-bus. The incident demonstrated the human impact of a hospital closure programme, and the need to put people first, as a government committee emphasised:

> Any fool can close a long-stay hospital: it takes more time and trouble to do it properly and compassionately.[50]

With the influx from Long Grove, staff at Horton Hospital felt that their jobs were safe. The budget had increased with the migrations from Banstead and Long Grove. Long-stay patients were gradually being discharged, but many were accommodated in group homes built in the hospital grounds. Peter Walsh,[51] having recently been appointed as community and assessment services manager for Riverside, was given one of the transferred wards from Long Grove in his broad remit, and was dismayed to find members of staff who he had previously sacked returning to Horton.

In 1993 Peter was appointed service director, but this was a poisoned chalice: he became responsible for closing Horton. As he recalled: 'I went from poacher to gamekeeper.' Holding fortnightly meetings with forty-two charge nurses, he faced much hostility to the closure programme. Peter persuaded nurses that while they could not reverse the decision to close Horton, with their active involvement they could have influence on the process. Some older charge nurses accepted the inevitable and tried to make the move into the community go as smoothly as possible for their patients. Others were extremely resistant and constantly undermined the positive messages conveyed by management, perpetuating anxiety among patients and colleagues.

Many nurses believed that as Horton had been refilled by patients from other hospitals, perhaps it would get another reprieve. Yet the resident population was falling irreversibly, and as half-empty wards merged with other half-empty wards, large parts of the Victorian structure were abandoned. Horton had a very unhappy atmosphere, according to Peter, plagued by management power struggles, union militancy, and rampant overspending. The hospital had lacked the strong leadership necessary for managing change, and negativity festered. The unions fought every decision, and managers were subjected to *ad hominem* insults in meetings. Sometimes managers used patients as pawns: if a charge nurse was being awkward, a batch of the most challenging patients might be sent to his ward. Peter tried to make management more transparent and supportive, but it did not take long before a serious confrontation: the COHSE steward threatened to shut the kitchen after a trifling comment Peter had made. He was not always supported by his own superiors, and his job was always at risk.

> I was under immense pressure. I stopped drinking. I couldn't have a hangover, as I needed to be on top form the next morning.[52]

Peter was losing sleep, and his wife could not understand why he stayed. His light at the end of the tunnel was the definite closure date. However, it was a rocky road, and he knew that he was detested. On one occasion a nurse of Sicilian origin threatened him with a visit by the Mafia. Every day, when managers left their offices to go home, they staggered their departure for safety. Peter would get to his car, lock the doors and not drive off until the next manager had done the same. Some senior colleagues could not cope with death threats, but Peter had a good working relationship with many of the charge nurses, and persevered. Several nurses refused to accept redeployment. They wanted redundancy, but this was costly and unnecessary, as there were numerous jobs in the community. In Peter's view, members of staff were poorly advised by the union leader, who used them to fight his own issues with management. Peter attended forty-three employment tribunals, where claims of constructive dismissal were rejected, and nurses lost their jobs. Twenty years on, the relief was palpable in Peter's voice:

Horton closed on 30th June 1996 – the date is etched in my memory.[53]

Community care and its casualties

Some nurses were enriched by hospital closure. Care homes for the mentally ill proliferated in the 1990s, as it was realised that the remaining patients in hospital needed 24-hour support in the community. Homes providing intensive nursing care were run by voluntary organisations or housing associations, but many residential care homes were privately owned. Opening a home for people leaving a psychiatric hospital was a potentially lucrative venture, as copious health authority funds followed each patient. Among the keenest entrepreneurs were Mauritian nurses, who had striven and saved for so many years. As observed by informants for this book, some unremarkable nurses became proprietors in the new care market, driving limousines and buying racehorses at Epsom.

In many cases the patients and nursing staff from the last remaining wards moved to a group home together. This minimised the trauma of the move, but the danger of such familiarity was the tendency for recreating a hospital atmosphere in the community. In a carehome for people discharged from Netherne, run by Hexagon Housing Association, co-author NM found some truth in the adage that 'you can take the nurse out of the institution, but you cannot take the institution out of the nurse'. A sharp contrast was apparent between the attitudes and practices of the ex-Netherne staff and those who had never worked in a mental hospital: the experience of the former had taught them to avoid taking any risks; they administered cigarette supplies and generally treated residents as irresponsible. While residents appeared to enjoy their new status, having their own rooms in a relatively normal domestic setting , institutional language persisted as care staff named the lounge as the 'day-room' and bedside cabinets as 'lockers'. Although they no longer looked out to expansive hospital grounds, residents of this Edwardian villa enjoyed a spacious 100-foot garden, surrounded by the tall trees of surrounding properties. They sat outside smoking in variable states of dress, away from prying eyes. Sadly, the adjacent house was demolished and a massive four-storey apartment block was built along the entire plot. Their garden now overlooked by countless windows, the residents stayed indoors. Perhaps this was symbolic of care in the community.

A study by John Barnes and Graham Thornicroft in Southend showed considerable variation in living conditions for discharged patients.[54] Mentally ill residents of bed-and-breakfast houses appeared to have the least contact with community mental health services, and a higher rate of readmission. However, their accommodation was normally close to the town centre and amenities, and they had more liberty than afforded to residents of care homes. The problem of 'transinstitutionalisation' was compounded by increasing reliance on unqualified workers, many of whom had poor English and limited knowledge of mental health.

Unless the home manager actively promoted a liberal, person-centred approach, inevitably staff resorted to a controlling regime. Barnes and Thornicroft found that homes employing psychiatric nurses were the least restrictive, but this was inhibited not only by cost, but also by ideological eschewal of a nursing culture in a social care setting.

Another group home for Netherne patients with severe mental disorder at Horley in Surrey, where co-author NM was deputy manager, was on a tree-lined avenue of large houses now in their third chapter of use. Originally owned by affluent families, these residences had later become staging posts for nearby Gatwick Airport. One by one they had been converted to care homes for people with mental disorder or intellectual disabilities, conveniently close to the local high street. On Monday to Friday the residents were conveyed to The Vale, the workshop that had moved from Netherne to an industrial estate in Redhill. To an outsider the work of untangling and repackaging bundles of headphones for British Airways may have seemed tedious, but daily occupation fitted the normalising philosophy of care, and spared residents from existential void. In an enlightening article in the *Independent* newspaper in December 1993, reporter Melanie McFadyean[55] interviewed several people who had been discharged from Tooting Bec to a patchwork of care homes in the Clapham district. Mostly their comments were positive: common themes were dignity and choice. However, little therapeutic activity was provided: as on the wards, residents spent their days smoking, drinking weak tea and staring vacantly at the television; their main incentive for going out was to collect 'dog-ends' from the park.

Promisingly, a study of patients discharged from Tooting Bec found that people living on the same street as group homes were accepting of their new neighbours[56]. Prejudice, it seemed, was reduced by contact. Yet all the good work in nurturing a tolerant and caring community was being undone. The problem was not with people in staffed homes but those who had apparently been dumped on the streets. On 17 December 1992 Jonathan Zito was chatting to his brother while awaiting an underground train at Finsbury Park. A stout and dishevelled black man was acting bizarrely on the platform, ignored by other passengers. Suddenly, without provocation, this man lurched towards Zito, stabbing him three times in the face. Christopher Clunis had paranoid schizophrenia, and in his sqaulid bedsit police found a large supply of antipsychotic medication, as well as letters from social workers and the hospital. Clunis was convicted of manslaughter and sent to Rampton Hospital under Sections 37/41 of the Mental Health Act. An enquiry found a catalogue of errors by the services involved in Clunis' care, and warned that such a tragedy was likely to recur if people with severe mental disorder were not adequately monitored and treated.[57]

Fears about homicidal maniacs let loose were heightened by sensational reporting in the tabloid press. Newspaper articles often used psychiatric jargon without explanation, and shocking incidents contributed to an exaggerated association of mental illness with dangerousness.[58] Despite evidence that violence was not disproportionately common in schizophrenia or any other mental illness, care in the community was becoming harder to sell to a society that suspected the policy as either reckless ideology or uncaring expedience. Fears were justifiable: no death of an innocent member of the public could be tolerated as a collateral footnote to an otherwise positive venture. Furthermore, reports of enquiries suggested that serious incidents were preventable.

In its simplistic belief that discharged psychiatric patients had been abandoned, a sceptical society was ignorant of the crucial work of doctors and nurses in the community. By the mid-1990s community mental health teams (CMHT) had become the standard model for mental health provision. Each covering a locality of the catchment area of a NHS trust, CMHTs comprised a multidisciplinary team of consultant psychiatrists and other medical ranks, CPNs, a psychologist and an occupational therapist; social workers were either integrated or based at local authority offices. Much overlap became apparent in the work of nurses and social workers, although some distinctions were drawn: CPNs monitored medication and physical health, while the latter were adept in navigating the housing and welfare benefit systems. Duplication was not so much of a problem as the gaps left by specialisation, as Elaine Murphy argued:

> There are too many highly-qualified, expensive professionals employed in mental health services who work within traditional professional roles, and too few 'generic' mental health workers willing to turn their hands to a variety of practical and emotional support work.[59]

Community psychiatric nursing was becoming a victim of its own success. Skilled nurses had freed themselves from the control of psychiatrists, working instead with general practitioners who gladly accepted their input. Many CPNs gained certificates in counselling, but their psychotherapeutic forays led them away from chronic cases to people with depression or social phobia. This reorientation was demonstrated by a study of the community nursing service in Salford: CPNs spent an average of 25 minutes with neurotic patients but only 9 minutes with the psychotic.[60] In 1994 the Audit Commission report *Finding a Place* found that in CMHTs where the majority of patients on caseloads had mild mental disorder, the professional group with the smallest proportion of severely mentally ill people was nursing. The report recommended that common mental health problems should be managed in primary care, leaving psychiatric services to deal with patients with enduring illness and complex needs; the latter were more prone to self-neglect and crises, often culminating in admission to hospital under the Mental Health Act. Nurses were summoned to return from the 'worried well' to the type of patients who would once have been institutionalised for life.

Nurses had more autonomy in community mental health services, but working alone with a caseload was relatively stressful. CPNs were vulnerable to investigation and disciplinary consequences should a suicide or killing be attributable to their omission. Meanwhile tension arose within CMHTs, due to blurring of role boundaries, lack of staff support and weak management.[61] The Care Programme Approach, introduced in response to scandals, increased nurses' responsibilities and documentary burden, but many psychiatrists refused to engage in this process, in distrust of an encroaching managerialism and a plethora of standardised procedures and targets.[62] Although the CMHT was meant to be comprehensive, failings in assessment and management of risk had repeatedly been found by enquiries, leading to new types of service. As many of the highly publicised homicides had been committed by patients with paranoid delusions who had stopped taking medication and avoided contact with mental health workers, assertive outreach teams were introduced to closely monitor patients of high risk and low compliance. Crisis teams, operating beyond normal working hours, offered help to patients in urgent need.

Tragedies involving discharged psychiatric patients caused schism between mental health campaigners. Mind was generally supportive of patients' right to live in the community, and at its annual conference in 1986 an offshoot Survivors Speak Out was founded. This radical anti-establishment group, politically left wing, denounced the psychiatric system for its perceived cruelty by means of medication, ECT and detention. In their definition, all patients discharged from mental hospitals were victims. By contrast, groups for carers of people with psychiatric illness were critical of care in the community. The National Schizophrenia Fellowship, run by relatives of schizophrenic patients, was surpassed in this respect by a new organisation. In 1987, after Marjorie Wallace wrote a series of articles on community care in *The Times*, a television documentary exposed the unhappy lot of discharged patients in boarding houses. In response to an outpouring from concerned relatives, Wallace founded Schizophrenia – a National Emergency (SANE). Counteracting the liberal stance of Mind, SANE opposed hospital closure. It was never representative of the broad population of mental health service-users, but its argument chimed with public opinion, and Wallace was often first to comment in the media on the latest serious incident. Wallace was unable to halt policy, but as most of the large mental hospitals in the London area had closed at the turn of the millennium,[63] the insufficiency of acute psychiatric beds was becoming a serious problem. In many acute units, bed occupancy constantly exceeded 100 per cent, and a rapid turnover was the only means of freeing space for admissions.

In the 1970s the hospitals were scandalised; in the 1990s, it was care in the community. Just as the latter had been proposed as a solution to the problems of institutional neglect, in the 1990s the solution to neglect in the community was to bring back asylum. Just as all psychiatric nurses had been unfairly tainted by abuses in hospitals, now they were associated with a callous system of neglect. Frank Dobson, Secretary for Health in the new Labour government elected on a landslide in 1997, played to the gallery when he declared in the House of Commons:[64]

Care in the community has failed.

Dobson wanted to show that the government had heard people's concerns, and would act to prevent more calamities. Proponents were dismayed by this sweeping dismissal, but he did not really intend a major reversal of policy. Dobson was making a subtle distinction between 'community care' and 'care in the community'. At best, the former implied a naïve ideal of collective compassion instead of professional care, but the latter was mostly invisible to opinionated critics. The public needed to be aware of the range of community mental health services, and the best way to do this was to make mental health a priority in a major programme of investment in the NHS.

We shall remember them

For the final curtain, mental hospitals had ceremonies of great poignancy, with eulogies and hymns, and a last supper. Ex-staff and ex-patients came to pay their last respects, and many tears were shed. Psychiatrists Piezchniak and Murphy[65] described the event at Cane Hill in 1992, attended by 500 people, many dressed as for a funeral:

> The day of the ceremony was sunny. The mourners walked through the beautiful but now overgrown grounds to the splendid turreted façade. Outside were parked several large black limousines…The dignitaries were ushered into the boardroom for a glass of sherry while others were offered tea and biscuits in the main hall.

Cane Hill buildings were then boarded up by the regional health authority. Visiting the site in 1999, co-author NM[66] persuaded a security guard to do an escorted tour. Starting at the administrative offices with oak-panelled boardroom and medical library, they then ventured along the former male corridor. This side of the hospital had closed last, and although it had been uninhabited for seven years, an institutional odour lingered. However, the overpowering smell was of dampness, with fungi growing on the walls and puddles from leaks in the dilapidated structure. Entering one of the vast wards upstairs, an apparent green carpet was actually a complete covering of moss. Linen cupboards had items bearing the old London County Council stamp. At the bend of the main corridor they passed the 'Top to Toe' boutique and looked towards the female side. It was an apocalyptic scene. The corridor had become a canal, and falling debris frequently splashed in the deep trench of dark water. Ash and birch trees rose towards gaps in the roof, their foliage festooned with shards of glass. This afterworld was out of bounds.

Some mental hospitals continued into the twenty-first century. Hospitals with a forensic or medium-secure unit had a stay of execution, although eventually other buildings on the site were closed. Kevin Halpin,[67] manager of the Trevor Gibbens Unit at Oakwood, observed the dismantling of the former Kent County Asylum as a reverse chronological sequence. Prefabricated offices from the 1970s and the industrial workshop were first to go, followed by Northdowns House, the red-brick admission unit described in Chapter 3. In 1992 a female corpse was discovered in the disused Martin Ward on the top floor at Hermitage House. An escaped patient from the secure unit was found guilty of her murder; he had also apparently been secreting stolen goods in the underground tunnels. With liability risk, health authorities had no choice but to provide 24-hour security on their empty buildings, but such large sites were difficult to protect. A late nineteenth-century addition, Hermitage House was knocked down in 1997 after a spate of arson attacks, leaving St Andrews House (the original block), Queen's House and the medical superintendent's villa and gate lodges. These forlorn yet forbidding structures were eventually converted to luxury apartments. In 2001, co-author NM visited the marketing office in the former Ash Ward, and asked the young saleswoman whether she knew the former use of the buildings. Tentatively, she responded: 'It was a hospital'. A psychiatric hospital, he suggested. 'Maybe, but only the doctors could afford to live here now', she reassured.

There were three phases in the disposal of mental hospitals. The earliest closures were swiftly followed by complete demolition, as developers ensured that all evidence of the asylum were obliterated, in the belief that buyers would be deterred by a stigmatised and allegedly haunted site. Demand was low: the hospitals were typically far from a town centre and its employment and entertainment opportunities, and before the tide of mass immigration, the British population was stable and falling in some areas. By the mid-1990s local conservationists and national bodies such as English Heritage were applying pressure to preserve the more ornate features of these defunct institutions. The reception block with its fine stonework, the chapel, gate lodges and medical superintendent's residence were fenced off for refurbishment. To their surprise, developers found that an apartment in the renovated Victorian administrative block could sell for more than a newly built house in the grounds. Not only did the grandeur appeal, but also the quirk of living in a former asylum.

In the third phase most of the nineteenth-century buildings were retained, although this may have seemed an unlikely outcome at the time of closure. A lucky survivor was Denbigh Hospital, where vigorous marketing of the 120-acre site and listed hospital buildings drew little interest after the last patients departed in 1995. A year later a potential buyer emerged, but the planning application was rejected. A similar fate was suffered by other developers, partly due to concerns that the site would become a ghost town of second homes, and that outsiders would dilute the Welsh language culture. Meanwhile the North Wales Health Authority was fighting a costly losing battle against vandals and thieves. Doors, lead flashing and the old hospital clock were plundered. Fortunately, Denbigh was saved for the benefit of its new residents, and for local heritage.

Abandoned to the ravages of nature, thieves and arsonists, great legacies of Victorian philanthropy were being lost forever. Woodilee, the first of the Scottish parochial asylums, had fallen into disrepair after evacuation of most of the original block on 13 March 1987 ('Black Friday' to the staff), on discovery of serious structural deficits. Within a few years the chapel, main hall and iconic twin towers were demolished, although the hospital remained in use until 2001. The new housing estate built on the site bears little sign of its past as the largest psychiatric hospital in Scotland. By contrast, some hospitals were fully converted. At Netherne a family can enjoy a panoramic view over the North Downs from a living-room atop the water-tower, while residents in the old ward blocks have barbecues in gardens where patients once mingled on airing-courts. Architectural masterpieces have been brought back to their former glory: Friern, Warley, and the stunning neo-Gothic Holloway Sanatorium. Many have gate security – now to keep people out.

Where we are now

The bed manager scanned the whiteboard in the busy office of an acute psychiatric ward. 'What about this man, RD,' she asked. 'He's been in for two weeks – can he go on weekend leave?' The nurse-in-charge was sceptical, but an urgent admission was imminent, and there was no room. So RD was informed that he was ready for a trial period at home, and his bed was swiftly changed for the new arrival. Such is life in the modern psychiatric ward.

Two decades after the closure of the large mental institutions, care in the community is no longer a major public controversy. After the scandals of the 1990s, more robust structures and processes were established, with a revised legal framework, and today the majority of mental health care is provided outside hospital. Yet community is no panacea for mental disorder, and concern is growing over the reduction in hospital beds – down to 20,000 in England. As observed by leading psychiatrist Peter Tyrer,[68] whereas in the past patients were excluded from society, now they are excluded from hospital. The threshold for admission is higher than ever, while the throughput of patients has accelerated. Patients who would until recently have been admitted to hospital are now served by home treatment teams. With the intensive support of three or four visits per day, patients are helped from crisis to recovery, but a heavy burden of risk and responsibility is carried on the shoulders of practitioners. Arguably, we are approaching the point of 'peak community care', whereby the proportion of care and treatment reaches the maximum level attainable in the community. As stress in the system rises, the pot may soon boil over.

Instead of being considered as components of a whole system, hospital and community have become a false dichotomy, as criticised by Thornicroft and Tansella:[69]

> There is no compelling argument and no scientific evidence favouring the use of hospital services alone. On the other hand, there is also no evidence that community services alone can provide satisfactory and comprehensive care. Both the evidence available so far, and accumulated clinical experience, therefore support a balanced approach, incorporating elements of both hospital and community care.

Debate has tended to focus on the number of beds, rather than the type. Currently, patients spend a short time in hospital before returning to the same social adversities that contributed to their admission. For better continuity of care, the pace of treatment should be slowed to allow a smoother transition between hospital and community. For some patients, a longer period of inpatient care may be necessary, providing social as well as medical treatment. With active therapeutic endeavour and discharge planning from the outset, such facilities should not revert to the hopeless 'back wards' of old.

History is not merely an indulgent or eccentric interest, but a deep well of experience, from which lessons should be learned. The meaning of the mental hospital is contested, as discussed by Hector Parr and colleagues following the closure of Craig Dunain Hospital in the north of Scotland. As the site of the old institution, halfway between Inverness and Loch Ness on the A82 road, was being sold off, local people expressed ambivalence towards its legacy. Some ex-patients perceived the hospital as oppressive, but others regretted the loss of a therapeutic landscape, where they had enjoyed the extensive grounds, featuring a wood and a pond where they fed ducks. One patient, Angus McPhee, who resided at Craig Dunain from 1946 to the mid-1990s, was renowned as 'the weaver of grass':

> From the moment of his admission from the island of South Uist, McPhee was off outside gathering lengths of couch grass, leaves of various kinds and other items like sheep's wool, using these materials to weave the most remarkable objects that he stored beneath bushes of holly or rhododendron. Hats, bonnets, jackets, vests, trousers, waders, boots, harnesses, pouches and ropes: all of these were among his creations.[70]

The tranquil, natural environment of Craig Dunain was a polar opposite to New Craigs, a smaller mental health unit built nearby. Patients felt like they had moved from a country manor estate to an office block. This sterile building with its entry buzzer and car park lacks the green spaces, the café, corridors and the sense of community of the former asylum. Yet Craig Dunain also evoked sad or troubling memories. Many patients had whiled away the years scouring the bleak Nightingale wards in search of cigarette butts. Others remembered the trauma of being held down by nurses for an injection, or kept for days on close observation. Perhaps the asylum was like the Chestnut Tree Café in George Orwell's dystopian *1984*, where Winston sat sipping tea, freed of all responsibilities but also of any purpose in life.[71] Patients at hospitals like Craig Dunain were neutralised by the system, and to see them as happy campers would ignore the limits of their situation. Yet the concept of asylum, despite its faults in practice, remains persuasive.

Mental health nursing is at a crossroads. As we have shown, it has a history of constancy and change. Undoubtedly it has progressed, from the controlled and controlling regime of asylum attendants, to the empowered and empowering practice of modern nurses in the community. However, it would be a misleading to portray a singular discipline. In the past, the role and environment of nursing was relatively static; while there were differences between types of ward, there was a collective spirit, reinforced by sport, the social club and the trade union. Today, mental health nursing has an ambiguous function, and practitioners in multidisciplinary community teams have an ambivalent identity. Jobs are advertised for a 'mental health practitioner', who could be a social worker or occupational therapist, and in practice these disciplines are interchangeable.

Meanwhile there has been a steady process of deprofessionalisation in residential care, where the majority of staff comprises unqualified workers. People with enduring psychotic illness demonstrate the limits of the medical model, and the need for social care, yet mental health nurses are no longer performing this role. Another development is a renewed focus on physical health. With evidence that people with schizophrenia lose an average of fifteen years of life expectancy, policy-makers and the nursing profession have emphasised the need for better knowledge and skills in diseases such as diabetes mellitus, which tend to be neglected by both psychiatric patients and their carers. A revised nursing curriculum will reduce the mental health input to the final year, but there is a growing movement to replace specialised nurse training with a generic course.[72]

Our story shows recurring themes in the development of mental health nursing. Direction has mostly come from the heights of officialdom or 'experts' with vested interests, instead of from within the discipline. Therapeutic approaches have come and gone, partly because they have not convinced staff of their viability or value. Too many patients have been damaged by an impersonal, centrally controlled system, which has lacked accountability. State interference has inhibited systemic alliances between patient, family and mental health practitioner. Generally, nurses have not been assertive in challenging management or policy-makers, or in suggesting new ways of organising and delivering care. Mental health nursing has had episodes of darkness and light, but its *raison d'être* is unchanged. Whether patients are seen at home or on a ward, the essence of nursing is in a therapeutic relationship: the form changes, but the content remains. As the mental health system continues to evolve, nurses should be at the forefront of policy as well as practice. Libertarian and institutional modes of care are not necessarily in opposition, and nurses should advocate for patients who need more than occasional monitoring in the community. The wheel does not need reinventing, but it will surely revolve.

Notes

1 Hassall C, Rose S (1989).
2 Hassall C, Rose S (1989).
3 Personal communication (NM, 2014).
4 Personal communication (NM, 2013).
5 Personal communication (NM, 2013). Not all of the patients knew what was happening. Another informant stated that Banstead patients were taken straight from their breakfast to hospital transport, without explanation.
6 The nurses' homes were retained for prison use, and some of the farm buildings survive.
7 Personal communication (NM, 2015).
8 When the industrial workshop was transferred from Banstead, it occupied a basement previously used for colonic lavage (washout of the bowels).
9 Knowles DJ (1986): Closure of Banstead Hospital (letter). *Lancet.*
10 King D (1991): *Moving on from Mental Hospital to Community Care.*

11 King D (1991). 57.
12 COHSE (1984): *The Future of Psychiatric Services (The Mallinson Report)*. London: COHSE. As an example of him putting patients first, in 1974 Mallinson dissuaded nurses from going on strike at Highcroft Hospital (www.macearchive.org/archive).
13 Personal communication (NM, 2015).
14 Handy C (1993): *Understanding Organizations* (4th edition)
15 Graham C (1994): Sir Roy Griffiths (obituary). *Independent.*
16 Mocon A (1994): *Collaboration in Community Care in the 1990s.*
17 Murphy E (1990): *After the Asylums: Community Care for People with Mental Illness.*
18 Thatcher M (1993): *The Downing Street Years.* 608.
19 Brent & Harrow Health Authority (1993): *Mental Health Reprovision: a Strategic Framework.* 7.
20 Leff J (1997): The outcome for long-stay non-demented patients. In *Care in the Community: Illusion or Reality?* (ed. J Leff).
21 Nolan P (1993). 148.
22 Roper N, Logan WW, Tierney A (1981): *Learning to Use the Process of Nursing.*
23 Ward MF (1985): *The Nursing Process in Psychiatry.*
24 Lyttle JR (1986): *Mental Disorder: its Care and Treatment*
25 McCrae N (1992): Who needs care plans? Nursing Times.
26 McCrae N (2011): Whither nursing models? The value of nursing theory in the context of evidence-based practice and multidisciplinary health care. Journal of Advanced Nursing.
27 Lemmer B, Smits M (1989): *Facilitating Change in Mental Health.*
28 Lemmer B, Smits M (1989). 40.
29 Personal communication (NM, 2014). The nurse education centre at Tooting Bec was a satellite of the Nightingale School of Nursing, which was based at Gassiot House at St Thomas' Hospital. The course was ENB811 Community Psychiatric Nursing.
30 Donabedian A (1969): Some issues in evaluating the quality of care. *American Journal of Public Health.*
31 UKCC (1986): *Project 2000: A New Preparation for Practice.*
32 Davies C, Beach A (2000): *Interpreting Professional Self-Regulation: a History of the United Kingdom Central Council for Nursing, Midwifery and Health Visiting.*
33 Altschul A (1997): A personal view of psychiatric nursing, In *The Mental Health Nurse: Views of Practice and Education* (ed. S Tilley).
34 Personal communication (PN, 2015).
35 Thomas Holloway, an industrialist who made his money selling pills and ointments for common maladies, founded the sanatorium and nearby eponymous college as a way of buying into high society. Officially opened by the Prince of Wales in 1885, Holloway Sanatorium was intended as a temporary refuge for ladies and gentlemen of the middle classes, and was of suitably grand design inside and out.
36 Personal communication (PN, 2015).
37 Davis B (1990): Research and psychiatric nursing. In *Psychiatric and Mental Health Nursing* (eds W Reynolds, D Cormack).
38 Co-author PN worked with Julia Brooking at University of Birmingham, where he too became a professor of nursing.
39 Brooking JI, Ritter S, Thomas B (eds 1992): *A Textbook of Psychiatric and Mental Health Nursing.*
40 Yonge O, Austin W, Qiuping Z, Wacko M, Wilson S, Zaleski J (1997): A systematic review of the psychiatric/mental health nursing research literature 1982-1992. *Journal of Psychiatric and Mental Health Nursing.*
41 Peplau HE (1994): Psychiatric mental health nursing: challenge and change. *Journal of Psychiatric and Mental Health Nursing.*
42 Snell J (2014): Ray Rowden (obituary). *Nursing Standard.*
43 Personal communication (NM, 2014).

44 *Daily Mail* (21 November 1988): Pay row nurses 'risking court action'.
45 As well as long-term decline in membership, the unions were weakened by restrictive legislation by the Thatcher administration. To boost collective bargaining, on 1 July 1993 COHSE, NUPE and the National and Local Government Officers (NALGO) joined forces to form Unison, which became the largest trade union in Britain.
46 Senge PN (1990): *The Fifth Discipline: the Art and Practice of the Learning Organization*.
47 Lewin K (1952).
48 Quoted in Day T (1993). 56.
49 Quoted in Day T (1993). 113.
50 Social Services Committee (1985): *Community Care with Special Reference to Adult Mentally Ill and Mentally Handicapped People*.
51 Personal communication (NM, 2015). Peter's managerial portfolio included wards and community teams dispersed over a wide area: Level 9 at Charing Cross Hospital, one ward at Gordon Hospital, the psychiatric unit at a small hospital in Ealing, two CMHTs, and also two wards at Horton).
52 Personal communication (NM, 2015).
53 Personal communication (NM, 2015). Actually, Horton did not completely shut down. The forty-bed Henry Rollin Unit, which had opened in September 1992 for male and female forensic patients, remained in the old block before it was transferred out by West London Mental Health Trust in 1998. In 1995 the Wolvercote Clinic, specialising in intensive treatment of convicted pædophiles, opened in the grounds; despite its international reputation, in 2002 the unit was moved due to local opposition. Although the old asylum buildings were demolished, Horton Haven, a rehabilitation unit for sixty-seven patients, survives to this day. Peter remained a director of mental health services in the area, retiring from Central and North West London NHS Trust in 2015.
54 Barnes J, Thornicroft G (1993): The last resort? Bed and breakfast accommodation for mentally ill people in a seaside town. *Health Trends*.
55 McFadyean M (1993): Breaking out of the asylums. *Independent* (19 December).
56 Wolff G (1997): Attitudes of the media and the public. In *Care in the Community: Illusion or Reality?* (ed. J Leff).
57 Quoted in Cold JW (1994): The Christopher Clunis enquiry. *Psychiatric Bulletin*,.
58 Scott J (1994): What the papers say. *Psychiatric Bulletin*.
59 Murphy E (1991). 174.
60 Wooff K, Rose S, Street J (1989).
61 Patmore C, Weaver T (1991): *Community Mental Health Teams: Lessons for Planners and Managers*.
62 Lelliott P (1997): Should psychiatrists support CPA, guidelines and routine outcome measurement? *Psychiatric Bulletin*.
63 With a few exceptions, such as Springfield, where some services continue today.
64 Dobson F (1998): Frank Dobson outlines third way for mental health (press release). Department of Health.
65 Piezchniak P, Murphy D (1992): Death of a hospital. *Psychiatric Bulletin*.
66 NM visited closed or closing mental hospitals across Britain in the late 1990s, including almost all of the institutions southern England, Gartloch and Hartwood near Glasgow, the 'Saints' in Northumberland, and the large Lancashire asylums. He walked along the tunnels underneath Bexley, climbed the water tower at Horton, and had close encounters with salivating Alsatian guard-dogs. Fellow explorers were psychology trainee Angela and social worker Charles.
67 Personal communication (NM, 1998).
68 Tyrer P (2013): A solution to the ossification of community psychiatry. *Psychiatrist*.
69 Thornicroft G, Tansella M (2004): Components of a modern mental health service: a pragmatic balance of community and hospital care: overview of systematic evidence. *British Journal of Psychiatry*.

70 Parr H, Philo C, Burns N (2008): 'That awful place was home': reflections on the contested meanings of Craig Dunain Asylum. *Scottish Geographical Journal.*
71 Orwell G (1949): *Nineteen Eighty-Four.*
72 Britain is one of merely four countries in the world with registration as a mental health nurse. Everywhere else, nurses working in mental health do post-registration training in this specialty.

Appendix

Mental hospitals in Great Britain

This table shows the county / borough / district mental institutions later operated by the NHS. The royal chartered asylums in Scotland are also included (most became district asylums). Originally, asylums were officially titled by the county or other local authority but were also known by their location – for example, Kent County Asylum / Barming Heath. Many mental hospital names were changed on the NHS takeover in 1948. Bed capacity is shown for 1971.[1]

Hospital	Original name	Year opened	Original authority	Number of beds (1971)	Notes
London & South-East England					
St Bernards'	Hanwell	1831	Middlesex	2191	
Friern	Colney Hatch	1851	Middlesex	2131	
Banstead		1877	Middlesex	1602	
Cane Hill		1883	Middlesex	1769	
Napsbury		1905	Middlesex	1702	
Shenley		1934	Middlesex	1881	
Stone House	Dartford	1866	City of London	459	
Tooting Bec		1903	MAB	1715	
Claybury		1893	London	1713	
Bexley	Bexley Heath	1898	London	1879	
Horton		1902	London	1587	
Long Grove		1907	London	1635	
The Maudsley		1923	London	c150	Used as war hospital on completion in 1915
West Park		1924	London	1673	

Hospital	Original name	Year opened	Original authority	Number of beds (1971)	Notes
Springfield	Wandsworth	1841	Surrey	1546	
Brookwood		1867	Surrey	1593	
Netherne		1909	Surrey	1494	
Warlingham Park		1896	Croydon	847	
Warley	Brentwood	1853	Essex	2022	
Severalls		1913	Essex	1630	
Goodmayes	Ilford	1901	West Ham	1270	
Runwell		1937	Southend	1050	
Oakwood	Barming Heath	1833	Kent	1563	
St Augustine's	Chartham	1875	Kent	1339	
St Francis'	Haywards Heath	1859	Sussex	1010	
Hellingly		1903	East Sussex	1010	
Graylingwell		1897	West Sussex	916	
St John's	Stone	1853	Buckingham-shire	800	
Fairmile	Moulsford	1870	Berkshire, Reading & Newbury	800	
Littlemore		1846	Oxford & Oxfordshire	c500	
Fairfield	Arlesey	1860	Bedfordshire, Hertfordshire & Hunting-donshire	1268	Replaced original Bedford Asylum
Hill End		1899	Hertfordshire	793	
Broadmoor		1863	State criminal lunatic asylum	920	

South-West England

St Lawrence's	Bodmin	1820	Cornwall	1256	
Exminster		1845	Devon	1860	Beds include Wonford House (originally private asylum) and Digby

Hospital	Original name	Year opened	Original authority	Number of beds (1971)	Notes
Digby		1886	Exeter		
Moorhaven	Blackadon	1891	Plymouth	737	
Mendip	Wells	1848	Somerset & Bath	855	
Tone Vale	Cotford	1896	Somerset	727	
Glenside	Fishponds	1861	Bristol	950	
Barrow		1939	Bristol	405	
Horton Road	Gloucester	1823	Gloucester-shire	573	
Coney Hill		1885	Gloucester-shire	633	
Herrison	Dorchester	1863	Dorset	1057	Replaced original asylum (1832)
Roundway	Devizes	1851	Wiltshire	1012	
Knowle	Fareham	1852	Hampshire	1209	
Park Prewett		1921	Hampshire	1331	
St James'	Milton	1879	Portsmouth	917	
Whitecroft		1896	Isle of Wight	410	
West Midlands					
All Saints	Winson Green	1851	Birmingham	778	
Rubery Hill		1882	Birmingham	873	
Hollymoor		1905	Birmingham	642	
Central	Hatton	1852	Warwickshire	1133	
Powick		1852	Worcester & Worcester-shire	949	
Barnsley Hall		1907	Worcester-shire	650	
St George's	Stafford	1818	Staffordshire	1170	Beds include Coton Hill (originally private asylum)
St Matthew's	Burntwood	1865	Staffordshire	1119	
St Edward's	Cheddleton	1899	Staffordshire	1175	

Hospital	Original name	Year opened	Original authority	Number of beds (1971)	Notes
Shelton	Bicton Heath	1845	Salop & Wenlock	1062	
St Mary's	Burghill	1871	Hereford & Herefordshire	540	

East Midlands & East Anglia

Hospital	Original name	Year opened	Original authority	Number of beds (1971)	Notes
Saxondale	Radcliffe	1902	Nottingham-shire	728	Replaced original county asylum (1810)
Mapperley		1880	Nottingham	534	
The Pastures	Mickleover	1853	Derbyshire	895	
Kingsway	Derby	1888	Derby	688	
The Towers	Humberstone	1869	Leicester	769	
Carlton Hayes	Narborough	1904	Leicestershire & Rutland	786	Replaced original asylum (1833)
St John's	Bracebridge Heath	1852	Lincolnshire	1062	
Rauceby	Kesteven	1902	Lincolnshire	589	
The Lawn	Lincoln	1820	Lincolnshire	129	Original county asylum, built for private patients
St Andrew's	Thorpe	1814	Norfolk	963	
Hellesdon	Norwich	1828	Norwich	682	
St Audry's	Melton	1829	Suffolk	1065	
St Clement's	Ipswich	1870	Ipswich	419	
Fulbourn		1858	Cambridgesh-ire	793	
St Crispin	Berrywood	1876	Northamp-tonshire	870	
Rampton		1912	State criminal mental hospital	1177	Built as overflow for Broadmoor; in NHS mostly used for mental handicap

Hospital	Original name	Year opened	Original authority	Number of beds (1971)	Notes
North-West England					
Lancaster Moor	Lancaster	1816	Lancashire	1836	Beds include 172 at Ridge Lea
Rainhill		1851	Lancashire	2256	
Prestwich		1851	Lancashire	1915	
Whittingham		1869	Lancashire	2233	
Winwick		1897	Lancashire	2117	
Garlands		1862	Cumberland & Westmoreland	934	
West Cheshire	Upton	1829	Cheshire	1601	Beds include Moston
Parkside	Macclesfield	1871	Cheshire	1453	
North-East England					
Stanley Royd	Wakefield	1818	West Riding, Yorkshire	1775	
Middewood	Wadsley Park	1872	West Riding, Yorkshire	1583	
High Royds	Menston	1888	West Riding, Yorkshire	1622	
Scalebor Park		1895	West Riding, Yorkshire	457	Built for private patients
Storthes Hall		1904	West Riding, Yorkshire	1698	
Clifton		1849	York & East Riding	773	
Broadgate	Walkington	1871	East Riding, Yorkshire	600	
Naburn		1906	York	439	
De la Pole	Willerby	1883	Kingston upon Hull	910	
St Luke's	Middlesbrough	1898	Cleveland	516	
Winterton	Sedgefield	1859	Durham	1504	
St George's	Morpeth	1859	Northumberland	1148	

Hospital	Original name	Year opened	Original authority	Number of beds (1971)	Notes
St Mary's	Stannington	1914	Gateshead	790	
St Nicholas'	Gosforth	1869	Newcastle	1117	
Cherry Knowle	Ryhope	1895	Sunderland	908	
Wales					
Denbigh		1848	North Welsh counties	916	
Pen-y-Fal	Abergavenny	1851	Monmouth-shire, Her-efordshire, Brecon & Radnor	1044	
St David's	Carmarthen	1865	Carmarthen, Pembroke & Cardigan	1000	
Mid Wales	Talgarth	1906	Brecon & Radnor	461	
Morgannwg	Bridgend	1864	Glamorgan	1752	
Whitchurch		1908	Cardiff	729	
Cefn Coed		1932	Swansea	666	
St Cadoc's	Caerleon	1865	Newport	516	
Scotland					
Gartnavel Royal		1814	Chartered asylum	730	
Woodilee		1875	Barony	1258	
Gartloch		1896	Glasgow City	963	
Leverndale	Hawkhead	1895	Govan	1100	
Hartwood		1895	Lanark	1810	
Dykebar		1909	Renfrew	451	
Argyll & Bute	Argyll	1863	Argyll	560	
Ailsa	Glengall	1878	Ayr	650	
Crichton Royal		1839	Chartered asylum	1086	Became Dum-fries District Asylum
Dingleton	Melrose	1872	Roxburgh, Berwick & Selkirk	418	

Hospital	Original name	Year opened	Original authority	Number of beds (1971)	Notes
Herdmanflat	Haddington	1866	East Lothian	202	
Royal Edinburgh	Morningside	1813	Chartered asylum	924	Initially for private patients only; West House opened 1842 for paupers
Bangour Village	Bangour	1906	Edinburgh	1132	
Rosslynlee		1874	Midlothian & Peebles	370	
Bellsdyke	Larbert	1869	Stirling	1072	
Stratheden	Cupar	1866	Fife & Kinross	990	
Murthly	Perth	1864	Perthshire	425	
Murray Royal	James Murray's	1829	Chartered asylum	304	
Royal Dundee Liff	Royal Dundee	1882	Chartered asylum	626	Replaced original asylum (opened 1820); became Dundee District Asylum 1903
Royal Cornhill	Royal Aberdeen	1800	Chartered asylum	855	
Kingseat		1904	Aberdeen	752	
Sunnyside Royal	Montrose Royal	1781	Chartered asylum		
Bilbohall	Elgin	1835	Unincorporated public asylum	188	Became Elgin District Asylum 1859
Ladysbridge	Banff	1865	Banff	522	Converted to mental subnormality hospital 1960
Craig Dunain	Inverness	1864	Northern counties	977	

Hospital	Original name	Year opened	Original authority	Number of beds (1971)	Notes
Carstairs		1957	State criminal mental hospital	412	Used as war hospital on completion in 1939; opened in 1948 as state institution for mental defectives; became state mental hospital 1957

Other large institutions used as psychiatric hospitals in NHS era

Hospital	Location	Original name / function	Number of beds (1971)	Notes
Bethlem Royal	Beckenham (previously Lambeth 1815–1930)	Bethlehem Hospital for the Care of the Insane (monastery 1247; became hospital for insane 16th century)	503	Merged with The Maudsley Hospital as NHS teaching hospital, 1948 (total beds for both hospitals shown)
Belmont	Sutton, Surrey	Orphanage (1853); poorhouse; wartime base of Maudsley Hospital (1939)	500	Transferred to NHS, 1948 (beds include 100 at adjacent Henderson Hospital)
Mabledon	Dartford	NHS neurosis unit for Polish soldiers (moved from Tunbridge Wells 1955)	211	Reclassified as psychiatric hospital, 1959
Holloway Sanatorium	Virginia Water, Surrey	Private asylum (1884)	515	Transferred to NHS, 1948
St Andrew's	Northampton	Northampton General Lunatic Asylum (charitable institution, 1838)	500	Some beds used by NHS (50 in 1971); remains in use as charitable psychiatric hospital
Highcroft	Birmingham	Aston Union Poorhouse (1836)	1206	Transferred to NHS, 1948
Warneford	Radcliffe	Charitable asylum for private patients (1826)	174	Transferred to NHS, 1948

Hospital	Location	Original name / function	Number of beds (1971)	Notes
St Nicholas'	Great Yarmouth	Naval hospital (1811)	241	Transferred to NHS, 1958
Old Manor	Salisbury	Fisherton House Asylum (c1820); renamed 1925	620	Transferred to NHS, 1955
Bootham Park	York	York Asylum (1777)	186	Transferred to NHS, 1948
The Retreat	York	Voluntary hospital (1791)	275	Remains in use as private hospital
Springfield	Manchester	Crumpsall Poorhouse (1857)	642	Transferred to NHS, 1948
Moston	Cheshire	Moston Hall Military Hospital (1940s)	376	Became NHS psychiatric hospital, 1960
Cheadle Royal	Cheadle	Manchester Royal Lunatic Hospital (charitable institution, 1849; replaced lunatic hospital of 1763)	400	Remains in use as private hospital
Ely	Cardiff	School for orphans (1862); poorhouse	610	Transferred to NHS, 1948; also used for mental handicap (included in bed number)
Ravenscraig	Greenock, Renfrewshire	Smithston Poorhouse (1879)	481	Transferred to NHS, 1948

Note

1 Institute of Health Service Administrators (1971): *The Hospitals Year Book 1972*. London: Institute of Health Service Administrators. The year chosen was within the time worked by many of the informants for this book. Although long before definite closure plans, the population of mental hospitals had dropped by around a third since the peak in the 1950s.

References

Abel-Smith B (1960): *A History of the Nursing Profession*. London: Heinemann.

Ackner B (ed. 1964): *Handbook for Psychiatric Nurses* (8th edition). London: Baillière, Tindall & Cassell.

Ackner B, Harris A, Oldham AJ (1957): Insulin treatment of schizophrenia. *Lancet*, i: 607–611.

Adams JS (2009): *Challenge and Change in a Cinderella Service: a History of Fulbourn Hospital, Cambridgeshire, 1953–1995*. PhD thesis (Open University).

Altschul A (1957): *Aids to Psychiatric Nursing*. London: Baillière Tindall.

Altschul A (1972): *Patient–Nurse Interaction: a Study of Interaction Patterns in Acute Psychiatric Wards*. Edinburgh: Churchill Livingstone. 191.

Altschul A (1997): A personal view of psychiatric nursing. In *The Mental Health Nurse: Views of Practice and Education* (ed. S Tilley). Oxford: Blackwell Science.

Andrews J (1997): A failure to flourish? David Yellowlees and the Glasgow School of Psychiatry, part I. *History of Psychiatry*, 8: 177–212.

Andrews J, Scull A (2001): *Undertaker of the Mind: John Monro and Mad-Doctoring in Eighteenth-Century England*. Oakland CA: California University Press.

Ankers WB (1976): A good report, but … *Nursing Times*, 1 July: 997–999.

Anton-Stephens D (1954): Preliminary observations of the psychiatric uses of chlorpromazine (Largactil). *Journal of Mental Science*, 100: 543–557.

Ardern P (2001): John Greene (obituary). *Guardian*. 23 May.

Arton M (1998): *The Professionalisation of Mental Nursing in Great Britain, 1850–1950*. PhD thesis (University College London).

Associate member (1909): *Asylum News*, 15 December: 121–122.

Asylum Journal (1854): Suicide of Dr Grahamsley, Medical Superintendent of the Worcester County and City Pauper Lunatic Asylum. 7: 105–106.

Asylum News (October 1913): Unrest in the West Riding Asylums. 105.

Asylum News (15 January 1901): Notes and news. 2.

Asylum News (15 February 1901): Notes and news. 12.

Asylum News (15 May, 1901): Notes and news. 37.

Asylum News (15 June 1902): Correspondence. 72.

Asylum News (15 October 1902): Notes and news. 89.

Asylum News (15 February 1903): The fire at Colney Hatch Asylum. 15.

Asylum News (15 March 1903): Correspondence. 36.

Asylum News (15 March 1904): Correspondence. 28.

Asylum News (15 July 1904): Front cover.

Asylum News (15 January 1907): Correspondence. 8.

Asylum News (15 January 1910): Banquet in commemoration of the passing of the Asylum Officers' Superannuation Act. 3–4.

Azu-Okeke O (1992): Experiments with Nigerian village communities in the dual roles of Western psychiatric treatment centres and homes for indigenous Nigerian inhabitants. *Therapeutic Communities*, 13: 221–228.

Bailey MD (2003): *Battling Demons: Witchcraft, Heresy, and Reform in the Late Middle Ages.* University Park, PA: Pennsylvania State University Press.

Bain AJ (1940): The influence of Cardiazol on chronic schizophrenia. *Journal of Mental Science*, 86: 502–513.

Ball P (2006): *The Devil's Doctor.* London: William Heinemann.

Barham P (2007): *Forgotten Lunatics of the Great War.* New Haven CT: Yale University Press.

Barnes J, Thornicroft G (1993): The last resort? Bed and breakfast accommodation for mentally ill people in a seaside town. *Health Trends*, 25: 87–90.

Barraclough B (1986): David Clark in conversation with Brian Barraclough. *Bulletin of the Royal College of Psychiatrists*, 10: 42–49.

Bartlett P (1998): The asylum, the workhouse, and the voice of the insane poor in 19th-century England. *International Journal of Law and Psychiatry*, 21: 421–432.

Barton R (1959): *Institutional Neurosis.* Bristol: John Wright & Sons.

Barton R (1976): *Institutional Neurosis* (3rd edition). Bristol: John Wright & Sons.

BBC (1957): *The Hurt Mind: an Enquiry into Some of the Effects of Five Television Broadcasts about Mental Illness and its Treatment: Audience Research Report.* London: BBC.

BBC Radio 3 (December 1999): *Taking Over the Asylum.* London: BBC

Bean C (2014): *Investigation into the Contact that Jimmy Savile had with the Bethlem Royal and Maudsley Hospitals: a Report for the Board of Directors of the South London and The Maudsley NHS Foundation Trust.* www.slam.nhs.uk/media.

Beech I (2013): *Butter, Bands, Bandages and Bolshevism: Care, Conditions and Culture in Cardiff City Mental Hospital before WWI.* International Network for Psychiatric Nursing Research conference. University of Warwick. 5 September.

Bell BA (1996): Wylie McKissock – reminiscences of a commanding figure in British neurosurgery. *British Journal of Neurosurgery*, 10: 9–18.

Beresford A (1965): Integrating nursing service and mixing the sexes in a psychiatric hospital. *Nursing Times*, 3 December: 1666.

Berkshire Asylum (1903): *General Rules for the Government of the Asylum.* Moulsford: Berkshire Asylum.

Berrios GE (1995): Research into the history of psychiatry. In *Research Methods in Psychiatry: a Beginner's Guide* (eds C Freeman, P Tyrer). London: Gaskell. 296–303.

Berrios G, Porter R (1995, eds): *A History of Clinical Psychiatry: The Origins of Psychiatric Disorders.* London: Athlone.

Berthier M (1863): Qualifications of attendants upon the insane. *Journal of Mental Science*, 9: 56–62.

Best G (1979): *Mid-Victorian Britain 1851–75.* London: Fontana.

Bevan-Lewis W (1907): On the formation of character: an address to the nursing staff at the Retreat, York, delivered November 1st, 1906. *Journal of Mental Science*, 53: 121–137.

Bickford JAR (1955): The forgotten patient. *Lancet*, ii: 969–971.

Bickford JAR (1958): Shadow and substance: some changes in the mental hospital. *Lancet*, i: 423–424.

Bickford JAR, Miller HJB (1959): Exchange of patients by mental hospitals. *Lancet*, ii: 96–97.

Bingham S (1979): *Ministering Angels.* Oradell, NJ: Medical Economics Company.

Blacker CP (1946): *Neurosis and the Mental Health Services*. London: Oxford University Press.

Blugrass R (1978): Regional secure units and interim security for psychiatric patients. *British Medical Journal*, i: 489–493.

Board of Control for England and Wales (1925): *Report of the Board of Control's (England and Wales) Committee on Nursing in County and Borough Mental Hospitals*. London: HMSO.

Board of Control for England and Wales (1931): *The Seventeenth Annual Report of the Board of Control 1930*. London: HMSO.

Board of Control for England and Wales (1937): *The Twenty-Third Annual Report of the Board of Control 1936*. London: HMSO.

Board of Control for England and Wales (1939): *The Twenty-Fifth Annual Report of the Board of Control 1938*. London: HMSO.

Board of Control for England and Wales (1947): *Report on Prefrontal Leucotomy in 1,000 Cases*. London: HMSO.

Boschma G (2012): Community mental health nursing in Alberta, Canada: an oral history. *Nursing History Review*, 20: 103–135.

Bourn H (1953): The insulin myth. *Lancet*, ii: 964–968.

Bowen WAL (1965): Need for inspection (or survey) of psychiatric hospital services. In *Psychiatric Hospital Care: a Symposium* (ed. H Freeman). London: Bailliere, Tindall & Cassell. 151–164.

Braslow J (1997): *Mental Ills and Bodily Cures: Psychiatric Treatment in the First Half of the Twentieth Century*. Berkeley, CA: University of California Press.

Bray RE, Bird TE (1964): *The Practice of Psychiatric Nursing*. Edinburgh: E & S Livingstone.

Brent & Harrow Health Authority (1993): *Mental Health Reprovision: a Strategic Framework* (draft by T Walsh, 15th July).

Bristol Mental Hospital Visiting Committee (1939): *Opening of Barrow Hospital by Sir Laurence Brock, CB (Chairman of the Board of Control), May 3rd 1939*. Bristol: City and County of Bristol.

Broedel HP (2004): *The Malleus Maleficarum and the Construction of Witchcraft: Theology and Popular Belief*. Manchester: Manchester University Press.

Brooking JI, Ritter S, Thomas B (eds 1992): *A Textbook of Psychiatric and Mental Health Nursing*. London: Churchill Livingstone.

Brothwood J (1973): The development of national policy: some further aspects of mental health policy. In *Policy for Action: a Symposium on the Planning of a Comprehensive Psychiatric Service*. London: Oxford University Press. 13–31.

Browne I (2013): *The Writings of Ivor Browne: Steps Along the Road – The Evolution of a Slow Learner*. Cork: Atrium.

Browne WAF (1837): *What Asylums Were, Are, and Ought to Be: Being the Substance of Five Lectures Delivered Before the Managers of the Montrose Royal Lunatic Asylum*. Edinburgh: Adam & Charles Black.

Buchanan RD (2010): *Playing with Fire: the Controversial Career of Hans J Eysenck*. Oxford: Oxford University Press.

Buckinghamshire County Pauper Lunatic Asylum (1866): *Twelfth Annual Report on the Buckinghamshire County Pauper Lunatic Asylum*.

Builder (15 July 1865): Lunatic asylums. 495–496.

Busfield J (1986): *Managing Madness: Changing Ideas and Practice*. London: Hutchinson.

Cameron JL, Laing RD, McGhie A (1955): Patient and nurse: effects of environmental changes in the care of chronic schizophrenics. *Lancet*, ii: 1384–1386.

Campbell Clark A (1897): *Clinical Manual of Mental Disorders for Practitioners and Students*. London: Bailliere Tindall & Cox.

Callaway BJ (2000): *Hildegard Peplau: Psychiatric Nurse of the Century*. New York: Springer.

Cannadine D (2013): *The Undivided Past: History Beyond our Differences*. London: Allen Lane.

Carpenter M (1985): *They Still Go Marching On: a Celebration of COHSE's First 75 Years*. London: Confederation of Health Service Employees.

Carpenter M (1988): *Working for Health: the History of COHSE*. London: Lawrence & Wishart.

Carr EH (1990): *What is History?* London: Penguin.

Carrier J, Kendall I (1998): *Health and the National Health Service*. London: Athlone.

Casey N (1994): Trevor Clay (obituary). *Independent*, 26 April.

Chatterton C (2004): Caught in the middle? Mental nurse training in England 1919–1951. *Journal of Psychiatric and Mental Health Nursing*, 11: 30–35.

Chatterton CS (2007): '*The Weakest Link in the Chain of Nursing'? Recruitment and Retention in Mental Health Nursing, 1948-1968*. PhD thesis (University of Salford.

Cherry S, Munting R (2005): 'Exercise is the thing'? Sport and the asylum c1850–1950. *International Journal of the History of Sport*, 22: 42–58.

Chichester Observer (5 August 1939).

Chung MC, Nolan P (1994): The influence of positivistic thought on nineteenth century nursing. *Journal of Advanced Nursing*, 19: 226–232.

Clare A (1976): *Psychiatry in Dissent: Controversial Issues in Thought and Practice*. London: Tavistock.

Clark DH (1958): Administrative therapy: its clinical importance in the mental hospital. *Lancet*, i: 805–888.

Clark DH (1965): Ward therapeutic community and effects on hospital. In *Psychiatric Hospital Care: a Symposium* (ed. H Freeman). London: Baillière, Tindall & Cassell. 75–84.

Clark D (1974): *Social Therapy in Psychiatry*. Harmondsworth: Penguin.

Clark D (1981): The long term psychiatric patient and the future. In *The Future of the Mental Hospitals: a Report of MIND's 1980 Conference*. London: MIND. 37–41.

Clarke GW (1985): Having a keen desire to take up mental nursing. *History of Nursing*, 7: 25–28.

Clarke J (2014): Low life. *Spectator*, 23 August.

Clarke L (1993): The opening of doors in British mental hospitals in the 1930s. *History of Psychiatry*, 4: 527–551.

Clarke L (1997): Joshua Bierer: striving for power. *History of Psychiatry*, 8: 319–332.

Cochrane DA (1985): *The Colonisation of Epsom: the Building of the Epsom Cluster by the London County Council in its Historical Context*. London: South West Thames Regional Health Authority.

Cohen GL (1964): *What's Wrong with Hospitals*. Harmondsworth: Penguin.

COHSE (1984): *The Future of Psychiatric Services (the Mallinson Report)*. London: COHSE.

Cold JW (1994): The Christopher Clunis enquiry. *Psychiatric Bulletin*, 18: 449–452.

Commissioners in Lunacy (1859): *Twelfth Annual Report of the Commissioners in Lunacy for England and Wales*. London: HMSO.

Commissioners in Lunacy (1906): *Sixty-First Report of the Commissioners in Lunacy*. London: HMSO.

Commission of Lunacy for Scotland (1859): *Report of the Commission of Lunacy for Scotland 1857*. Edinburgh: HMSO.

Committee on Higher Education (1963): *Higher Education: Report of the Committee*. London: HMSO.

Conolly J (1847): *On the Construction and Government of Lunatic Asylums and Hospitals for the Insane*. London: John Churchill.

Cook LC (1958): The place of physical treatments in psychiatry. *Journal of Mental Science*, 104: 933–942.

Cook LC, Dax EC, Maclay WS (1952): The geriatric problem in mental hospitals. *Lancet*, i: 377–382.

Cooke EM (1895): A review of the last twenty years at the Worcester County and City Lunatic Asylum, with some conclusions derived therefrom. *Journal of Mental Science*, 46: 387–402.

Cookson C (1971): *Colour Blind*. London: Corgi.

Cooper D (1970): *Psychiatry and Anti-Psychiatry*. Frogmore: Paladin.

Cooper R, Bird J (1989): *The Burden: Fifty Years of Clinical and Experimental Neuroscience at the Burden Neurological Institute*. Bristol: White Tree.

County Council of Surrey (1929): *Rules for the Guidance of the Nurses, Attendants, and Servants in the Service of the Surrey County Mental Hospitals at Brookwood and Netherne*. Brookwood: County Council of Surrey.

Cormack D (1983): *Psychiatric Nursing Observed*. Edinburgh: Churchill Livingstone.

Cowper-Smith F (1977): Banstead Hospital. *Nursing Times*, 22/29 December: 41–44.

Crammer J (1990): *Asylum History: Buckinghamshire County Pauper Lunatic Asylum – St John's*. London: Gaskell.

Crawford P, Nolan P, Brown B (1998): Ministering to madness: the narratives of people who have left religious orders to work in the caring professions, *Journal of Advanced Nursing*, 28: 212–220.

Crichton Browne J (1898): Presidential address. *Asylum News*, 15 April: 32–35.

Crofts F (1998): *History of Hollymoor Hospital*. Studley: Brewin.

Crossley FH (1949): *The English Abbey* (3rd edition). London: BT Batsford.

Crossman RHS (1977): *The Diaries of a Cabinet Minister* (volume III). London: Hamish Hamilton & Jonathan Cape.

Crowther A, Ragusa A (2011): Realities of mental health nursing practice in rural Australia. *Issues in Mental Health Nursing*, 32: 512–518.

Croydon Area Health Authority (1976): *Report of the Committee of Inquiry: Warlingham Park Hospital*. Croydon: Croydon Area Health Authority.

Cubbin JK (2006): *The Waiting Room to Hell*. Universal Publishing Solutions Online.

Cunningham DE (1947): *Modern Mental Treatment: a Handbook for Nurses*. London: Faber.

Daily Mail (21 November 1988): Pay row nurses 'risking court action'. 9

Daily Telegraph (27 March 2012): Rowan Williams: fixation with gay rights, race and feminism threatens society. 14

Davies C, Beach A (2000): *Interpreting Professional Self-Regulation: a History of the United Kingdom Central Council for Nursing, Midwifery and Health Visiting*. Abingdon: Routledge.

Davis B (1990): Research and psychiatric nursing. In *Psychiatric and Mental Health Nursing* (eds W Reynolds, D Cormack). London: Chapman Hall.

Day T (1993): *More like Home: the Story of Long Grove Hospital and How it was Closed to Improve Mental Health Services*. Hove: Pavilion.

Department of Health and Social Security (1969): *The Facilities and Services of Psychiatric Hospitals in England and Wales 1966*. London: HMSO.

Department of Health and Social Security (1971): *Hospital Services for the Mentally Ill*. London: HMSO.

Department of Health and Social Security (1971): *The State Enrolled Nurse: a Report by the Sub-Committee of the Standing Nursing Advisory Committee*. London: HMSO.

Department of Health and Social Security (1972): *The Briggs Report: Report of the Committee on Nursing*. London: HMSO.

Department of Health and Social Security (1972): *Progress on Salmon*. London: HMSO.

Department of Health and Social Security (1977): *The Facilities and Services of Mental Illness and Mental Handicap Hospitals in England 1975*. London: HMSO.

Department of Health and Social Security (1979): *Report of the Committee of Enquiry into Mental Handicap Nursing.* London: HMSO.

Denham J (1965): Community care – basic needs and geographical factors: what local authorities should be providing *now*. In *Psychiatric Hospital Care: a Symposium* (ed. H Freeman). London: Bailliere, Tindall & Cassell. 144–152.

Dick D (1981): The place of the mental hospital in services which should begin at home. In *The Future of the Mental Hospitals: a Report of MIND's 1980 Conference.* London: MIND. 24–28.

Digby A (1985): Moral treatment at the Retreat, 1796–1946. In *The Anatomy of Madness: Essays in the History of Psychiatry; Volume II: Institutions and Society* (eds WF Bynum, R Porter, M Shepherd). London: Tavistock. 52–73.

Digby A (1996): Contexts and perspectives. In *From Idiocy to Mental Deficiency: Historical Perspectives on People with Learning Difficulties* (eds D Wright, A Digby). London: Routledge. 1–21.

Donabedian A (1969): Some issues in evaluating the quality of care. *American Journal of Public Health*, 59: 1833–1836.

Duckworth Williams SW (1864): *On the Efficacy of the Bromide of Potassium in Epilepsy and Certain Psychical Affections.* London: John Churchill & Sons.

Dumas S, Vedel-Petersen KO (1923): *Losses of Life Caused by War.* Oxford: Clarendon.

Eager R (1945): *The Treatment of Mental Disorders (Ancient and Modern).* Exeter: WV Cole & Sons.

Early DF (2003): *'The Lunatic Pauper Palace': Glenside Hospital Bristol 1861–1974.* Bristol: Friends of Glenside Hospital Museum.

Edinburgh District Lunacy Board (1897): *Report of Deputation from the Edinburgh District Lunacy Board Appointed to Visit Certain Asylums in France, Germany, and England, Recommended by the General Board on Lunacy.* Edinburgh: James Turner & Co.

Elgar E (2014): *Music for Powick Asylum* (performed by Innovation Chamber Ensemble). Thames Ditton: Somm Recordings.

Elkes J, Elkes C (1954): Effect of chlorpromazine on the behaviour of chronically overactive psychotic patients. *British Medical Journal*, ii: 560–565.

Ellis WC (1838): *A Treatise on the Nature, Symptoms, Causes and Treatment of Insanity, with Practical Observations on Lunatic Asylums.* London: Samuel Holdsworth.

Engels F (1845/2009): *The Condition of the Working Class in England.* Oxford: Oxford University Press.

Entwhistle C (1968): Overcrowding in mental hospitals (letter). *Lancet*, i: 116.

Etchell M (1863): *Ten Years in a Lunatic Asylum.* London: Simpkin, Marshall & Co.

Farman C (1974): *May 1926: the General Strike: Britain's Aborted Revolution?* Frogmore: Panther.

Farndale WAJ (1961): *The Day Hospital Movement in Great Britain.* Oxford: Pergamon.

Faulk M, Taylor JC (1986): Psychiatric interim regional secure unit: seven years' experience. *Medicine, Science and the Law*, 26: 17–22.

Firman C, Crump D (1985): Tooting Bec Hospital. *Nursing Mirror*, 160: 48.

Fisher RA, Lee JA (1930): Artificial light treatment in mental disease. *Nursing Mirror and Midwives' Journal*, 11 October: 52.

Fleming GWTH (1931): Some notes on mental disorder: epilepsy. *Nursing Mirror and Midwives' Journal*, 11 October: 439.

Fleming GWTH, Golla FL, Grey Walter W (1939): Electric-convulsion therapy of schizophrenia. *Lancet*, ii: 1353–1355.

Folkard MS (1957): *A Sociological Contribution to the Understanding of Aggression and its Treatment.* PhD thesis (University of London).

Foucault M (1967): *Madness and Civilization: a History of Insanity in the Age of Reason* (trans R Howard). London: Tavistock.

Freeman H (1965): Day hospitals. In *Psychiatric Hospital Care: a Symposium* (ed. H Freeman). London: Bailliere, Tindall & Cassell. 203–213.

Freeman H (1984): Mental health services in an English county borough before 1974. *Medical History*, 28: 111–128.

Freeman H (2010): Psychiatry in Britain, c1900. *History of Psychiatry*, 21: 312–324.

Freeman W, Watts J (1942): *Psychosurgery: Intelligence, Emotion and Social Behavior following Prefrontal Leucotomy for Mental Disorders.* Springfield, IL: Charles C Thomas.

Freeman T, Cameron JL, McGhie A (1958): *Chronic Schizophrenia.* London: Tavistock.

Fry A (2008): *Never Mind the Mind: Maudsley Hospital 1968–72 – a Narrative* (lecture notes). Institute of Psychiatry, King's College London. June.

Gallaher EB, Levinson DJ, Erlich I (eds 1957): *The Patient and the Mental Hospital.* Glencoe: Free Press.

Gardner J (1999): *Sweet Bells Jangled Out of Tune: a History of the Sussex Lunatic Asylum, Haywards Heath.* Brighton: James Gardner.

Gillespie JEON (1939): Cardiazol convulsions: the subjective aspect. *Lancet*, i: 391–392.

Gittins D (1998): *Madness in its Place: Narratives of Severalls Hospital, 1913–1997.* London: Routledge.

Glenister DA (2008): *Matrons, Mental Nurses and Madness: a Sociological Historiography of Mental Nursing from the Nurses Act 1943 to the Nurses Act 1969, Critically Adopting Some Sensitising Aspects of Giddens' Structuration Theory.* PhD thesis (London School of Economics).

Godin P (1996): The development of community psychiatric nursing: a professional project? *Journal of Advanced Nursing*, 23: 925–934.

Good R (1940): Some observations on the psychological aspects of Cardiazol therapy. *Journal of Mental Science*, 86: 491–501.

Gostin LO (1986): *Institutions Observed: Towards a New Concept of Secure Provision in Mental Health.* London: King Edward's Hospital Fund for London.

Graham C (1994): Sir Roy Griffiths (obituary). *Independent*, 29 March.

Granville JM (1877): *The Care and Cure of the Insane: Being the Reports of the Lancet Commission on Lunatic Asylums 1875-6-7, for Middlesex, the City of London, and Surrey, and a Review of the Work of Each Asylum.* London: Hardwicke & Bogue.

Greene B (1975): The rise and fall of the Asylum Workers Association. *Nursing Mirror*, 25 December: 53–55.

Guest T (2004): *A Life in Orange.* London: Granta.

Hall P (1991): The history of Powick Hospital. In *The Closure of Mental Hospitals* (eds P Hall, IF Brockington). London: Gaskell. 43–50.

Hamlett J, Hoskins L (2013): Comfort in small things? Control and agency in county lunatic asylums in nineteenth- and early twentieth-century England. *Journal of Victorian Culture*, 18: 93–114.

Hammond JL, Hammond B (1939): *Lord Shaftesbury.* Harmondsworth: Penguin.

Handy C (1993): *Understanding Organizations* (4th edition). Harmondsworth: Penguin.

Hare EH (1985): Old familiar faces: some aspects of the asylum era in Britain (part 1). *Psychiatric Developments*, 3: 245–255.

Harris EE (1957): Collingwood's theory of history. *Philosophical Quarterly*, 7: 35–49.

Hartley C (2003): *A Historical Dictionary of British Women* (2nd edition). Old Woking: Unwin.

Haslam J (1809): *Observations on Madness and Melancholy* (2nd edition). London: Longman.

Hassall C, Rose S (1989): Powick Hospital, 1978–86: a case register study. In *Health Service Planning and Research: Contributions from Psychiatric Case Registers* (ed. JK Wing). London: Royal College of Psychiatrists. 58–69.

Hawkins H (1870): *Work in the Wards*. London: Society for Promoting Christian Knowledge.

Healy D (2001): The dilemmas posed by new and fashionable treatments. *Archives of Psychiatric Treatment*, 7: 322–327.

Hemphill RE, Walter WG (1941): The treatment of mental disorders by electrically induced convulsions. *Journal of Mental Science*, 87: 256–275.

Henderson D, Gillespie RD (1936): *A Textbook of Psychiatry for Students and Practitioners* (4th edition). London: Oxford University Press.

Hereford County and City Asylum (1893): *Twenty-First Annual Report of the Committee of Visitors of the Hereford County and City Asylum 1893*. Hereford: Times.

Hereford County and City Asylum (1896): *Twenty-Fourth Annual Report of the Committee of Visitors of the Hereford County and City Asylum 1896*. Hereford: Times.

Hereford County and City Asylum (1912): *Fortieth Annual Report of the Committee of Visitors of the Hereford County and City Asylum 1912*. Hereford: Times.

Hereford County and City Asylum (1918): *Forty Sixth Annual Report of the Committee of Visitors of the Hereford County and City Asylum 1918*. Hereford: Times.

Hereford County and City Mental Hospitals (1934): *Sixty-Second Annual Report of the Committee of Visitors of the Hereford County and City Mental Hospitals, 1934*. Hereford: Times.

Hewitt H (1923): *From Harrow to Herrison House Asylum*. London: CW Daniel.

Higgins J (1981): Four years' experience of an interim secure unit. *British Medical Journal*, i: 889–893.

Hilton, C. (2005): The origins of old age psychiatry in Britain in the 1940s. *History of Psychiatry*, 16, 267–289.

Hitchcock T, Sharpe P (eds 1997): *Chronicling Poverty: The Voices and Strategies of the English Poor 1640–1840*. Basingstoke: Macmillan.

Holmes C (2006): The slow death of psychiatric nursing: what next? *Journal of Psychiatric and Mental Health Nursing*, 13: 401–415.

Hopper B (2011): *Better Court than Coroners: Memoirs of a Duty of Care* (volume I). Littlehampton: PerseVerance.

Hopper B (2012): *Lest we Forget: Memoirs of a Duty of Care* (volume II). Littlehampton: PerseVerance.

Hopton J (1999): Prestwich hospital in the twentieth century: a case study of slow and uneven progress in the development of psychiatric care. *History of Psychiatry*, 10: 349–369.

Houbert J (1981): Mauritius: independence and dependence. *Journal of Modern African Studies*, 19: 75–105.

Hughes PJ (1981): Saturday morning in the Whittingham Hospital café. In *The Future of the Mental Hospitals: a Report of MIND's 1980 Conference*. London: MIND.

Hunter R, Macalpine I (1974): *Psychiatry for the Poor: 1851 Colney Hatch Asylum – Friern Hospital 1973: a Medical and Social History*. London: Dawsons.

Hutton EL, Fleming GWTH, Fox FE (1941): Early results of prefrontal leucotomy. *Lancet*, i: 3–7.

Ingram ME (1939): *Principles of Psychiatric Nursing* (2nd edition). Philadelphia PA: WB Saunders.

Institute of Health Service Administrators (1971): *The Hospitals Year Book 1972*. London: Institute of Health Service Administrators.

Jayawardena C (1968): Migration and social change: a survey of Indian communities overseas. *Geographical Review*, 58: 426–449.

Jenkin P (1981): Mental health and mental illness services in the 80s. In *The Future of the Mental Hospitals: a Report of MIND's 1980 Conference*. London: Mind. 4–11.

John A (1961): *A Study of the Psychiatric Nurse*. Edinburgh: E & S Livingstone.

Johnson BCT (1969): *West Park: the First Sixty Years*. Epsom: West Park Hospital Management Committee.

Joint Committee of the Manchester Regional Hospital Board and the University of Manchester (1955): *The Work of the Mental Nurse*. Manchester: Manchester University Press.

Jones DAN (1968): Mental hospitals: a suitable cause for concern. *Sunday Times Magazine*: 29 September.

Jones K (1972): *A History of the Mental Health Services*. London: Routledge & Kegan Paul.

Jones K (1981): Re-inventing the wheel. In *The Future of the Mental Hospitals: a Report of MIND's 1980 Conference*. London: Mind. 17–23.

Jones K (1993): *Asylums and After: a Revised History of the Mental Health Services: From the Early 18th Century to the 1990s*. London: Athlone.

Jones K, Sidebotham R (1962): *Mental Hospitals at Work*. London: Routledge & Kegan Paul.

Jones M (1968): *Social Psychiatry in Practice: the Idea of the Therapeutic Community*. Harmondsworth: Penguin.

Journal of Mental Science (1881): Asylum reports for 1879. 27: 254.

Journal of Mental Science (1904): The management of the London County Council Asylums and the Horton Asylum scandal. 50: 751–754.

Kent County Mental Hospital (1927): A retrospect 1828–1927. In *A History of Oakwood Hospital 1828–1982*. Maidstone: Kent County Library.

Kessel N (1973): The district general hospital is where the action is. In *Policy for Action: a Symposium on the Planning of a Comprehensive Psychiatric Service* (eds R Crawley, G McLachlan). London: Oxford University Press. 53–64.

King D (1991): *Moving on from Mental Hospitals to Community Care: a Case Study of Change in Exeter*. London: Nuffield Provincial Hospitals Trust.

Kirkpatrick A, Feldman P (1983): Is anyone out there listening? Official enquiries into psychiatric hospitals. *Hospital and Health Services Review*, January: 17–20.

Knowles D (1969): *Christian Monasticism*. New York: McGraw–Hill.

Knowles DJ (1986): Closure of Banstead Hospital (letter). *Lancet*, ii: 1160–1161.

Kynaston D (2007): *Austerity Britain 1946–51*. London: Bloomsbury.

Kynaston D (2009): *Family Britain 1951–57*. London: Bloomsbury.

Laing J, McQuarrie D (1992): *50 Years in the System*. London: Corgi.

Lancet (1934): Shenley Mental Hospital, i: 1198–1200.

Larkin E (1937): Insulin shock treatment of schizophrenia. *Nursing Times*, 24 July, 723–724.

Le Fanu J (2011): *The Rise and Fall of Modern Medicine* (2nd edition). London: Abacus.

Leff J (1997): The outcome for long-stay non-demented patients. In *Care in the Community: Illusion or Reality?* (ed. J Leff). Chichester: Wiley. 69–91.

Leishman J (2004): Back to the future: making a case for including history of mental nursing in nurse education programmes. *International Journal of Psychiatric Nursing Research*, 10: 1157–1164.

Lelliott P (1997): Should psychiatrists support CPA, guidelines and routine outcome measurement? *Psychiatric Bulletin*, 21: 1–2.

Lemmer B, Smits M (1989): *Facilitating Change in Mental Health*. London: Chapman & Hall.

Lewin K (1952): *Field Theory in Social Science: Selected Theoretical Papers*. London: Tavistock.

Lewis A (1946): Ageing and senility: a major problem of psychiatry. *Journal of Mental Science*, 92: 150–170.

Lifton RJ (1988): *The Nazi Doctors: Medical Killing and the Psychology of Genocide.* New York: Basic.

Lockley D (2011): *The House of Cure: Life within the Leicestershire Lunatic Asylum.* Anchorprint.

Lodge Patch I (undated, c1985): *Springfield: a Short History.* London: Friends of Springfield Hospital.

Lyttle JR (1986): *Mental Disorder: its Care and Treatment.* Edinburgh: Baillière Tindall.

MacCammond I (1963): *The Argyll and Bute Hospital 1863–1963.* Lochgilphead: Argyll & Bute Hospital.

Main TF (1946): The hospital as a therapeutic institution. *Bulletin of the Menninger Clinic,* 10: 66–70.

Malster R (1994): *St Lawrence's: the Story of a Hospital 1870–1994.* Caterham: Lifecare NHS Trust.

Marsh H (2014): *First Do No Harm: Stories of Life, Death and Brain Surgery.* London: Phoenix.

Marsh J (2012): *The Liberal Delusion: the Roots of our Current Moral Crisis.* Bury St Edmunds: Arena.

Martin DV (1968): *Adventure in Psychiatry.* Oxford: Bruno Cassirer.

Martin JP (1984): *Hospitals in Trouble.* Oxford: Basil Blackwell.

Marx OM (1970): What is the history of psychiatry? *American Journal of Orthopsychiatry,* 4: 593–605.

Matthew. The Gospel according to Matthew. Holy Bible (New Testament), vii: 12.

Maudsley H (1870): *Body and Mind: an Inquiry into their Connection and Mutual Influence, Specially in Reference to Mental Disorders.* London: Macmillan & Co.

Maudsley H (1874): *Responsibility in Mental Disease.* London: Henry S King & Co.

May AR (1965): Observations on training the psychiatric nurse. In *Psychiatric Hospital Care: a Symposium* (ed. H Freeman). London: Baillière, Tindall & Cassell. 264–270.

McCrae N (1992): Who needs care plans? *Nursing Times,* 89: 48.

McCrae N (2006): 'A violent thunderstorm': Cardiazol therapy in British mental hospitals. *History of Psychiatry,* 17: 67–90.

McCrae N (2009): Beer in mental institutions: a historical perspective. In *Beer in Health and Disease Prevention* (ed. VR Preedy). Burlington: Academic Press. 60–72.

McCrae N (2009): Nonelectrical convulsive therapies. In *Electroconvulsive and Neuromodulation Therapies* (ed. CM Swartz). New York: Cambridge University Press. 17–44.

McCrae N (2011): Whither nursing models? The value of nursing theory in the context of evidence-based practice and multidisciplinary health care. *Journal of Advanced Nursing,* 68: 222–229.

McCrae N (2011): *The Moon and Madness.* Exeter: Imprint Academic.

McCrae N, Murray J, Huxley P, Evans S (2004): Prospects for mental health social work: a qualitative study of attitudes of service managers and academic staff. *Journal of Mental Health,* 13: 305–317.

McCusker J (1981): Mental hospitals – a view from the inside. In *The Future of the Mental Hospitals: a Report of MIND's 1980 Conference.* London: MIND. 70–71.

McFadyean M (1993): Breaking out of the asylums. *Independent* (19 December).

Menzies IEP (1960): A case study in the functioning of social systems as a defence against anxiety: a report on a study of the nursing service of a general hospital. *Human Relations,* 13: 95–121.

Metropolitan Asylum District (1872): *The Second Annual Report of the Committee of Management of the Metropolitan Imbecile Asylum, Caterham, Surrey 1871–72.* London: Harrison & Sons.

Michael P (2003): *Care and Treatment of the Mentally Ill in North Wales 1800–2000.* Cardiff: University of Wales Press.

Midgley G (2000): *Systemic Intervention: Philosophy, Methodology and Practice*. New York: Kluwer Academic / Plenum.

Milligan S (1976): *The New Barons: Union Power in the 1970s*. London: Temple Smith.

Mills E (1962): *Living with Mental Illness: a Study in East London*. London: Routledge & Kegan Paul.

Ministry of Health (1947): *Report on the Recruitment and Training of Nurses* (Wood Report). London: HMSO.

Ministry of Health (1962): *A Hospital Plan for England and Wales*. London: HMSO.

Ministry of Health and Ministry of Labour: Nursing Services Interdepartmental Committee (1945): *Report of the Subcommittee on Mental Nursing and the Nursing of the Mentally Handicapped*. London: HMSO.

Minski L (1936): Lectures on mental nursing XI: treatment and nursing. *Nursing Mirror and Midwives' Journal*, 26 October: 60–61.

Mocon A (1994): *Collaboration in Community Care in the 1990s*. Sunderland: Business Education Publishers.

Morrice JKW (1964): The ward as a therapeutic group. *British Journal of Medical Psychology*, 37: 157–165.

Morris P (1978): The scandal of the Prestwich secure unit. *Nursing Times*, 12 October: 8–9.

Morris R (1998): *Shelton: Past and Present*. Shrewsbury: Shropshire's Community and Mental Health Services NHS Trust.

Morten H (1897): Asylum attendants. *Nursing Notes*, 1 November: 141–143.

Moss MC, Hunter P (1963): Community methods of treatment. *British Journal of Medical Psychology*, 36: 85–91.

Murphy E (1990): *After the Asylums: Community Care for People with Mental Illness*. London: Faber & Faber.

Murray Royal Asylum (1869): *Special Regulation anent Dancing*. Perth: Murray Royal Asylum.

National Health Service (1968): *Findings and Recommendations Following Enquiries into Allegations Concerning the Care of Elderly Patients in Certain Hospitals*. London: HMSO.

National Health Service (1969): *Report of the Committee of Inquiry into Allegations of Ill-Treatment of Patients and Other Irregularities at the Ely Hospital, Cardiff*. London: HMSO.

National Health Service (1972): *Report of the Committee of Inquiry into Whittingham Hospital*. London: HMSO.

Nicoll J (1907): Mental nursing. *Asylum News*, 15 March: 18–19.

Nightingale GS (1990): *Warley Hospital Brentwood: the First Hundred Years 1853–1953* incorporating *Into the Second Century*. Brentwood: Warley Hospital Printing Department.

Nolan P (1987): Jack's Story. *History of Nursing Group at the Royal College of Nursing*, 2. London: RCN.

Nolan P (1993): *A History of Mental Health Nursing*. London: Chapman & Hall.

Nolan P (1999): Annie Altschul's legacy to 20th century British mental nursing. *Journal of Psychiatric and Mental Health Nursing*, 6: 267–272.

Nolan P, Hopper B (2000): Revisiting mental health nursing in the 1960s. *Journal of Mental Health*, 9: 563–573.

Nolan P (2005): The history of community mental health nursing. In *Handbook of Community Mental Health Nursing* (eds B Hannigan, M Coffey). London: Routledge. 7–18.

Nottingham Asylum (1875): *Nineteenth Annual Report of the State of the United Lunatic Asylum for the County and Borough of Nottingham, 1874*. Southwell: John Whittingham.

Nursing Mirror and Midwives' Journal (25 January 1930): Severalls Mental Hospital. 342–343.

Nursing Mirror and Midwives' Journal (15 March 1930): Occupational therapy in a mental hospital. 520.

Nursing Mirror and Midwives' Journal (4 July 1931): Springfield Mental Hospital: Princess Mary opens the nurses' home. 253.

Nursing Mirror and Midwives' Journal (19 November 1932): Advertisement. 27

Nursing Mirror and Midwives' Journal (15 September 1934): Devon Mental Hospital, Exminster: the wonderful year. 449–450.

Nursing Mirror and Midwives' Journal (25 January 1936): Cheshire County Mental Hospital: occupation and recreation at Macclesfield. 325.

Nursing Mirror and Midwives' Journal (13 February 1937): Friern Hospital for Nervous and Mental Disorders: a new home for the nurses. 393.

Nursing Mirror and Midwives' Journal (27 March 1937): Mental nursing in Holland. 531.

Nursing Mirror and Midwives' Journal (9 July 1938): The charge nurse describes her day in a mental hospital. 338.

Nursing Times (4 September 1937): Report. 546.

Nursing Times (4 September 1937): Long Grove Hospital, Epsom: the work of the male nurse. 538–540.

Nursing Times (30 October 1937): Trade unions as we understand them. 1069–1070.

Nursing Times (17 June 1939): The mental nurses' register. 741–742.

Nursing Times (28 November 1953): Friends of Menston Hospital. 1215–1216.

Nursing Times (13 November 1975): Seeking a better deal for overseas students. 1802–1803.

O'Doherty P (1912): A plea for cohesion among asylum workers. *Asylum News*, July: 63–64.

Ogdon JAH (1947): *Kingdom of the Lost*. London: Bodley Head.

Orwell G (1949): *Nineteen Eighty-Four*. London: Secker & Warburg.

Palmer E (1854): Description of the Lincolnshire County Asylum. *Asylum Journal*. 5: 72–75.

Parr H, Philo C, Burns N (2008): 'That awful place was home': reflections on the contested meanings of Craig Dunain Asylum. *Scottish Geographical Journal*, 119: 341–360.

Partridge M (1950): *Pre-frontal Leucotomy*. Oxford: Blackwell.

Patmore C, Weaver T (1991): *Community Mental Health Teams: Lessons for Planners and Managers*. London: Good Practices in Mental Health.

Pearce D (2011): Evacuation and deprivation: the wartime experience of the Devon and Exeter City Mental Hospitals. *History of Psychiatry*, 22: 332–343.

Peplau HE (1952): *Interpersonal Relations in Nursing*. New York: Putnam & Sons.

Peplau HE (1994): Psychiatric mental health nursing: challenge and change. *Journal of Psychiatric and Mental Health Nursing*, 1: 3–7.

Perinpanayagam MS (1973): Overseas postgraduate psychiatric doctors. *News and Notes* (supplement to the *British Journal of Psychiatry*), March: 11–12.

Peters UH (1985): *Anna Freud: a Life Dedicated to Children*. London: Weidenfeld & Nicholson.

Peters UH (1996): The emigration of German psychiatrists to Britain. In *150 Years of British Psychiatry* (volume 2): *The Aftermath* (eds H Freeman, G Berrios). London: Athlone.

Phillips UB (1968): *The Slave Economy of the Old South*. Baton Rouge LA: Louisiana State University Press.

Piezchniak P, Murphy D (1992): Death of a hospital. *Psychiatric Bulletin*, 16: 482–483.

Pilkington F (1958): *Moorhaven Hospital, Ivybridge, South Devon: Historical Review 1891–1958* (2nd edition). Plymouth.

Popper K (1976): *Unended Quest: an Intellectual Autobiography*. London: Fontana.

Porter R (1992, ed.): *Myths of the English*. London: Polity Press.

Powell E (1961): Opening speech. *Annual Conference of the National Association for Mental Health*. London: MIND.

Pratt D (1948): *Public Mental Hospitals in England: a Survey*. Philadelphia, PA: National Mental Health Foundation.

Procter G (1982): Oakwood Hospital 1928–1982. In *A History of Oakwood Hospital 1828– 1982*. Maidstone: Kent County Library.

Quarterly Review (1857): Lunatic asylums. 101: 358–393.

Ramon S (1985): *Psychiatry in Britain: Meaning and Policy*. London: Croom Helm.

Rapoport RN (1960): *Community as Doctor: New Perspectives on a Therapeutic Community*. London: Tavistock.

Reade C (1899): *Hard Cash: a Matter of Fact Romance*. London: Chatto & Windus.

Rees JR (1945): *The Shaping of Psychiatry by War*. New York: Norton & Co.

Rees L (1965): Drug therapy in perspective (discussion). In *The Scientific Basis of Drug Therapy in Psychiatry* (eds J Marks, CMB Pare). Oxford: Pergamon. 205–206.

Rees TP (1957): Back to moral treatment and community care. *Journal of Mental Science*, 103: 303–313.

Robb B (ed. 1967): *Sans Everything: a Case to Answer*. Edinburgh: Thomas Nelson.

Robertson CL (1860): A descriptive notice of the Sussex Lunatic Asylum. *Journal of Mental Science*, 33: 254.

Robertson CL (1861): Some results of night staffing at the Sussex Lunatic Asylum. *Journal of Mental Science*, 7: 391–398.

Robey T (2015): Art-house cinema. *Telegraph Magazine*, 10 January.

Robinson ADT (1989): Dorothea Dix: when will we see your likes again in Scotland? *Psychiatric Bulletin*, 13: 305–307.

Rollin HR (1990): *Festina Lente: a Psychiatric Odyssey*. London: Memoir Club.

Roper N, Logan WW, Tierney A (1981): *Learning to Use the Process of Nursing*. Edinburgh: Churchill Livingstone.

Rosenhan DL (1982) On being sane in insane places. In *Social Research Ethics* (ed. M Bulmer). New York: Holmes & Meier. 15–37.

Rowbotham S (1992): *Women in Movement: Feminism and Social Action*. London: Routledge.

Rowden R (1976): St Augustine's aftermath. *Nursing Times*, 1 July: 996–997.

Royal College of Nursing (1964): *A Reform of Nursing Education: First Report of a Special Committee on Nurse Education*. London: RCN.

Royal College of Psychiatrists (1980): Community psychiatric nursing: a discussion document by a working party of the Social & Community Services Section. *Bulletin of the Royal College of Psychiatrists*, August: 114–118.

Royal Commission on Lunacy and Mental Disorder (1926): *Report of the Royal Commission on Lunacy and Mental Disorder*. London: HMSO.

Royal Commission on the Law Relating to Mental Illness and Mental Deficiency (1957): *Report of the Royal Commission on the Law Relating to Mental Illness and Mental Deficiency*. London: HMSO.

Royal Medico-Psychological Association (1938): Discussion at annual meeting. *Journal of Mental Science*, 84: 685–692.

Royal Medico-Psychological Association (1954): *Handbook for Mental Nurses* (8th edition). London: Bailliere, Tindall & Cox.

Rubery Hill and Hollymoor Hospitals (1954): *Visit of the French Delegation – Monday 5th July 1954*. Birmingham: Rubery Hill and Hollymoor Hospital Management Committee.

Russell D (1997): *Scenes from Bedlam: a History of Caring for the Mentally Disordered at Bethlem Royal Hospital and the Maudsley*. London: Bailliere Tindall.

Russell D (1997): An oral history project in mental health nursing. *Journal of Advanced Nursing*, 26: 489–495.

Russell JI (1938): *The Occupational Treatment of Mental Illness*. London: Baillière, Tindall & Cox.

Russell R (1988): The lunacy profession and its staff in the second half of the nineteenth century, with special reference to the West Riding Lunatic Asylum. In *The Anatomy of Madness: Essays in the History of Psychiatry; Volume III: The Asylum and its Psychiatry* (eds WF Bynum, R Porter, M Shepherd). London: Routledge. 297–315.

Sainsbury P (1973): A comparative evaluation of a comprehensive community psychiatric service. In *Policy for Action: a Symposium on the Planning of a Comprehensive Psychiatric Service* (eds R Cawley, P McLachlan). London: Oxford University Press. 129–143.

Salvage J (1985): *The Politics of Nursing.* London: Heinemann.

Sandbrook D (2006): *Never Had it So Good: a History of Britain from Suez to The Beatles.* London: Abacus.

Sargant W (1967): *The Unquiet Mind.* London: Heinemann.

Sargant W, Slater E (1944): *Introduction to Physical Methods of Treatment in Psychiatry.* Edinburgh: E & S Livingstone.

Schama S (2009): *A History of Britain (volume 1): At the Edge of the World.* London: Bodley Head.

Schulz M (2012): Mental health services in Germany. In *Mental Health Services in Europe* (eds N Brimblecombe, P Nolan). London: Radcliffe.

Scott DH, Masterton JF, Hainsworth M, Mayne WS (1938): *Modern Mental Nursing.* London: Caxton.

Scott DJ, Philip AE (1985): Attitudes of psychiatric nurses to treatment and patients. *British Journal of Medical Psychology*, 58: 169–173.

Scott J (1994): What the papers say. *Psychiatric Bulletin*, 18: 489–491.

Scull A (1979): *Museums of Madness: the Social Organization of Insanity in 19th Century England.* London: Allen Lane.

Scull A (1995): Psychiatrists and historical 'facts', part one: the historiography of somatic treatments. *History of Psychiatry*, 6: 225–241.

Senge PN (1990): *The Fifth Discipline: the Art and Practice of the Learning Organization.* New York: Doubleday Business.

Sewart M (1930): The suicidal patient. *Nursing Mirror and Midwives' Journal*, 20 September: 450.

Shanley E (1980): Overseas nurses – effective therapeutic agents? *Journal of Advanced Nursing*, 5: 539–543.

Sharf A (1964): *The British Press and Jews under Nazi Rule.* London: Oxford University Press.

Shephard B (2003): *A War of Nerves: Soldiers and Psychiatrists in the Twentieth Century.* Cambridge MA: Harvard University Press.

Showalter E (1987): *The Female Malady: Women, Madness and English Culture, 1830–1980.* London: Little, Brown.

Sinton JA (1938): *Report on the Provision and Distribution of Malaria Therapy in England and Wales.* London: HMSO.

Skultans V (1979): *English Madness: Ideas on Insanity 1580–1890.* London: Routledge & Kegan Paul.

Smith JP (1976): The changing role of the large psychiatric hospital. *Nursing Mirror*, 4 November: 41.

Smith LD (1988): Behind closed doors; lunatic asylum keepers, 1800–60. *Social History of Medicine*, 1: 301–327.

Smith S (1973): Psychiatric units and relation to mental hospitals. In *Psychiatric Hospital Care: a Symposium* (ed. H Freeman). London: Bailliere, Tindall & Cassell. 214–222.

Snell J (2014): Ray Rowden (obituary). *Nursing Standard*, 29: 34.

Social Services Committee (1985): *Community Care with Special Reference to Adult Mentally Ill and Mentally Handicapped People.* London: HMSO.

Somerset County Asylum (1852): *Fourth Report of the Somerset County Asylum for Insane Paupers 1851*. Wells: Samuel Backhouse.

South East Thames Regional Health Authority (1976): *Report of Committee of Enquiry St Augustine's Hospital, Chartham, Canterbury*. Croydon: South East Thames Regional Health Authority.

Spratley VA, Stern ES (1952): *History of the Mental Hospital at Hatton in the County of Warwick 1852–1952* (2nd edition). Hatton: Hatton Hospital.

Stafford Clark D (1963): *Psychiatry Today* (2nd edition). Harmondsworth: Penguin.

Steppe H (1992): Nursing in Nazi Germany. *Western Journal of Nursing Research*, 14: 744–753.

Stern ES (1957): 'Operation Sesame'. *Lancet*, i: 577–578.

Stevenson J, Cook C (2009): *The Slump, Britain in the Great Depression*. London: Routledge.

Surrey Area Health Authority (1980): *The Provision of Services for the Mentally Ill*. Surrey Health Authority.

Taylor R (2001): Death of neurasthenia and its psychological reincarnation: a study of neurasthenia at the National Hospital for the Relief and Cure of the Paralysed and Epileptic, Queen Square, London, 1870–1932. *British Journal of Psychiatry*, 179: 550–557.

Thatcher M (1993): *The Downing Street Years*. London: HarperCollins.

Thomas RW, Wilson IGH (1938): *Report on Cardiazol Treatment and on the Present Application of Hypoglycaemic Shock Treatment in Schizophrenia*. London: HMSO.

Thompson EP (2002): *The Making of the English Working Class*. Harmondsworth: Penguin.

Thompson P (1978): *The Voice of the Past: Oral History*. Oxford: Oxford Oral History.

Thomson M (1992): Sterilisation, segregation and community care: ideology and solutions to the problem of mental deficiency in inter-war Britain. *History of Psychiatry*, 3: 473–498.

Thornicroft G, Tansella M (2004): Components of a modern mental health service: a pragmatic balance of community and hospital care: overview of systematic evidence. *British Journal of Psychiatry*, 185: 283–290.

Tooth GC, Brooke EM (1961): Trends in the mental hospital population and their effect on future planning. *Lancet*, i: 710–713.

Tooth GC, Newton MP (1961): *Leucotomy in England and Wales 1942–1954*. London: HMSO.

Towell D (1975): *Understanding Psychiatric Nursing: a Sociological Study of Modern Psychiatric Nursing Practice*. London: RCN.

Tredgold AF (1908): *Text-Book of Mental Deficiency*. London: Bailliere Tindall & Cox.

Trimingham A (2008): *Out of the Shadows: a History of Mental Health Care in Sussex*. Lewes: Pomegranate.

Tuke DH (1882): *Chapters in the History of the Insane in the British Isles*. York: Kegan Paul/ Trench.

Tuke DH (1885): On alcohol in asylums, chiefly as a beverage. *Journal of Mental Science*, 132: 535–550.

Tuke S (1813/1964): *A Description of The Retreat: an Institution near York for Insane Persons of the Society of Friends* (revised edition). London: Dawsons.

Tyrer P (2013): A solution to the ossification of community psychiatry. *Psychiatrist*, 37: 336–339.

UKCC (1986): *Project 2000: A New Preparation for Practice*. London: United Kingdom Central Council for Nursing, Midwifery and Health Visiting.

Valentine R (1996): *Asylum, Hospital, Haven: a History of Horton Hospital*. London: Riverside Mental Health Trust.

Vaughan GF, Leiberman DM, Cook LC (1955): Chlorpromazine in psychiatry. *Lancet*, i: 1083–1087.

'Veritas' (1906): How to improve the conditions of the asylum service. *Asylum News*, 15 December: 114–115.

Vincent J (1948): *Inside the Asylum*. London: George Allen & Unwin.

Vines G (1983): Sacked nurse takes ECT case to Europe. *New Scientist*, 17 March: 708.

Walk A (1961): The history of mental nursing. *Journal of Mental Science*, 107: 1–17.

Wall BA (1977): *A World of its Own: Chester's Psychiatric Hospitals 1829–1976*. Chester: Cheshire Area Health Authority.

Walton J (1981): The treatment of pauper lunatics in Victorian England: the case of Lancaster Asylum 1816–1870. In *Mad Doctors and Madmen: the Social History of Psychiatry in the Victorian Era* (ed. A Scull). London: Athlone. 166–197.

Wansbrough SN (1971): The future of industrial therapy. *Lancet*, i: 1009–1010.

Ward MF (1985): *The Nursing Process in Psychiatry*. Edinburgh: Churchill Livingstone.

Warelow P, Edward K (2007): Evidence-based mental health nursing in Australia: our history and our future. *International Journal of Mental Health Nursing*, 16: 57–61.

Warr P (1957): *Brother Lunatic*. London: Neville Spearman.

Weeks KF (1965): The Plymouth Nuffield Clinic: a community mental health centre. In *Psychiatric Hospital Care: a Symposium* (ed. H Freeman). London: Bailliere, Tindall & Cassell. 14–22.

Weil Pl (1950): 'Regressive' electroplexy in schizophrenia. *Journal of Mental Science*, 96: 514–520.

Welch JC, Frogley G (1993): *A Pictorial History of Netherne Hospital*. Redhill: East Surrey Health Authority.

Whitaker R (2002): *Mad in America: Bad Science, Bad Medicine, and the Enduring Mistreatment of the Mentally Ill*. New York: Basic.

White E (1993): Community psychiatric nursing 1980 to 1990: a review of organisation, education and practice. In *Community Psychiatric Nursing: a Research Perspective* (volume 2; eds C Brooker, E White). London: Chapman & Hall. 1–26.

White EW (1900): The remodelling of an old asylum. *Journal of Mental Science*, 46: 457–468.

Whitehead A (1970): *In the Service of Old Age: the Welfare of Psychogeriatric Patients*. Harmondsworth: Penguin.

Wilkinson D (1994): Douglas Bennett: In Conversation. *Psychiatric Bulletin*, 18: 622–626.

Willmuth LR (1979): Medical views of depression in the elderly: historical notes. *Journal of the American Geriatrics Society*, 27: 494–499.

Wilson IGH (1936): *A Study of Hypoglycaemic Shock Treatment in Schizophrenia*. London: HMSO.

Wiltshire County Asylum (1892): *Report of the Committee of Visitors for the Year 1891 and Forty-First Annual Report of the Medical Superintendent of the Asylum for the Insane Poor of the County of Wilts*. Devizes: George Simpson.

Wiltshire County Asylum (1900): *Forty-Ninth Annual Report of the Wilts County Asylum for the Year 1900 and Financial Statements for 1899–1900*. Devizes: George Simpson.

Wing JK, Brown GW (1961): Social treatment of chronic schizophrenia: a comparative survey of three mental hospitals. *Journal of Mental Science*, 107: 847–861.

Wing JK, Brown GW (1970): *Institutionalism and Schizophrenia: a Comparative Study of Three Mental Hospitals 1960–1968*. London: Cambridge University Press.

Wing JK, Monck E, Brown GW, Carstairs GM (1964): Morbidity in the community of schizophrenic patients discharged from London mental hospitals in 1959. *British Journal of Psychiatry*, 110: 10–21.

Winslow FB (1867): *Light: its Influence on Life and Health*. London: Longmans & Co.

Winter J (2006): *Remembering War*. New Haven CT: Yale University Press.

Winterton P (1938): *Mending Minds: the Truth about our Mental Hospitals*. London: Peter Davies.

Wolfensberger W (1972): *The Principle of Normalization in Human Services*. Toronto: National Institute on Mental Retardation.

Wolff G (1997): Attitudes of the media and the public. In *Care in the Community: Illusion or Reality?* (ed. J Leff). Chichester: Wiley. 145–163.

Wooff K, Rose S, Street J (1989): Community psychiatric nursing services in Salford, Southampton and Worcester. In *Health Service Planning and Research: Contributions from Psychiatric Case Registers* (ed. JK Wing). London: Royal College of Psychiatrists. 73–80.

Worth J (2009): *Shadows of the Workhouse: the Drama of Life in Post-War London*. London: Phoenix.

Wortis J (1959): The history of insulin shock treatment. In *Insulin Treatment in Psychiatry* (eds M Rinkel, HE Himwich). New York: Philosophical Library.

Yonge O, Austin W, Qiuping Z, Wacko M, Wilson S, Zaleski J (1997): A systematic review of the psychiatric/mental health nursing research literature 1982–1992. *Journal of Psychiatric and Mental Health Nursing*, 4: 171–177.

Index

Milton Keynes UK
Ingram Content Group UK Ltd.
UKHW031143141024
449569UK00024B/1112